GROWTH FACTORS AND THE CARDIOVASCULAR SYSTEM

DEVELOPMENTS IN CARDIOVASCULAR MEDICINE

121. S. Sideman, R. Beyar and A. G. Kleber (eds.): Cardiac Electrophysiology, Circulation, and Transport. Proceedings of the 7th Henry Goldberg Workshop (Berne, Switzerland, 1990). 1991. ISBN 0-7923-1145-0.

122. D. M. Bers: Excitation-Contraction Coupling and Cardiac Contractile Force. 1991. ISBN 0-7923-1186-8.

123. A.-M. Salmasi and A. N. Nicolaides (eds.): Occult Atherosclerotic Disease. Diagnosis, Assessment and Management. 1991. ISBN 0-7923-1188-4.

124. J. A. E. Spaan: Coronary Blood Flow. Mechanics, Distribution, and Control. 1991. ISBN 0-7923-1210-4.

125. R. W. Stout (ed.): Diabetes and Atherosclerosis. 1991. ISBN 0-7923-1310-0.

126. A. G. Herman (ed.): Antithrombotics. Pathophysiological Rationale for Pharmacological Interventions. 1991. ISBN 0-7923-1413-1.

127. N. H. J. Pijls: Maximal Myocardial Perfusion as a Measure of the Functional Significance of Coronary Arteriogram. From a Pathoanatomic to a Pathophysiologic Interpretation of the Coronary Arteriogram. 1991. ISBN 0-7923-1430-1.

128. J. H. C. Reiber and E. E. v. d. Wall (eds.): Cardiovascular Nuclear Medicine and MRI. Quantitation and Clinical Applications. 1992. ISBN 0-7923-1467-0.

129. E. Andries, P. Brugada and R. Stroobrandt (eds.): How to Face "the Faces" of Cardiac Pacing. 1992. ISBN 0-7923-1528-6.

130. M. Nagano, S. Mochizuki and N. S. Dhalla (eds.): Cardiovascular Disease in Diabetes. 1992. ISBN 0-7923-1554-5.

131. P. W. Serruys, B. H. Strauss and S. B. King III (eds.): Restenosis after Intervention with New Mechanical Devices. 1992. ISBN 0-7923-1555-3.

132. P. J. Winter (ed.): Quality of Life after Open Heart Surgery. 1992. ISBN 0-7923-1580-4.

133. E. E. van der Wall, H. Sochot, A. Righetti and M. G. Niemeyer (eds.): What is new in Cardiac Imaging? SPECT, PET and MRI. 1992. ISBN 0-7923-1615-0.

134. P. Hanrath, R. Uebis and W. Krebs (eds.); Cardiovascular Imaging by Ultrasound. 1992. ISBN 0-7923-1755-6.

135. F. H. Messerli (ed.): Cardiovascular Disease in the Elderly, 3rd ed. 1992. ISBN 0-7923-1859-5.

136. J. Hess and G. R. Sutherland (eds.); Congenital Heart Disease in Adolescents and Adults. 1992. ISBN 0-7923-1862-5.

137. J. H. C. Reiber and P. W. Serruys (eds.): Advances in Quantitative Coronary Arteriography. 1992. ISBN 0-7923-1863-3.

138. A.-M. Salmasi and A. S. Iskandrian (eds.): Cardiac Output and Regional Flow in Health and Disease. 1993. ISBN 0-7923-1911-7.

139. J. H. Kingma, N. M. van Hemel and K. I. Lie (eds.): Atrial Fibrillation, a Treatable Disease? 1992. ISBN 0-7923-2008-5.

140. B. Ostadal, N. S. Dhalla (eds.): Heart Function in Health and Disease. 1993. ISBN 0-7923-2052-2.

141. D. Noble and Y.E. Earm (eds.): *Ionic Channels and Effect of Taurine on the Heart.* Proceedings of an International Symposium (Seoul, Korea, 1992). 1993. ISBN 0-7923-2199-5.

142. H.M. Piper (ed.): *Ischemia-reperfusion in Cardiac Surgery.* 1993. ISBN 0-7923-2241-X.

GROWTH FACTORS AND THE CARDIOVASCULAR SYSTEM

edited by

Peter Cummins
Department of Physiology
University of Birmingham
School of Medicine
Birmingham, UK

KLUWER ACADEMIC PUBLISHERS
Boston / Dordrecht / London

Distributors for North America:
Kluwer Academic Publishers
101 Philip Drive
Assinippi Park
Norwell, Massachusetts 02061 USA

Distributors for all other countries:
Kluwer Academic Publishers Group
Distribution Centre
Post Office Box 322
3300 AH Dordrecht, THE NETHERLANDS

Library of Congress Cataloging-in-Publication Data

Growth factors and the cardiovascular system / edited by Peter
  Cummins.
        p. cm. -- (Developments in cardiovascular medicine; v. 147)
  Includes index.
  ISBN 0-7923-2401-3 (alk. paper)
  1. Heart--Physiology. 2. Heart--Pathophysiology. 3. Growth factors.
  I. Cummins, Peter, 1947-   . II. Series.
  [DNLM: 1. Cardiovascular System--growth & development. 2. Growth
  Substances--physiology. W1 DE997VME v. 147 1993 / WG 102 G884 1993]
  QP102.G76   1993
  612.1'7--dc20
  DNLM/DLC
  for Library of Congress   93-11507
                                                             CIP

Copyright © 1993 by Kluwer Academic Publishers

Printed on acid-free paper.

Printed in the United States of America

Contents

List of Contributors   ix

Foreword: Bernard Swynghedauw   xiii

Preface: Peter Cummins   xv

Introduction

1.   Growth Factors: In vivo function and mechanism of action   1
     Carl-Henrik Heldin, Lena Claesson-Welsh, Kohei
     Miyazono and Bengt Westermark

Section one: Growth factors in the heart

2.   Fibroblast and transforming growth factors in the heart: A role   17
     in cardiac growth ?
     Peter Cummins

3.   Growth factors and the cardiac extra-cellular matrix   31
     Lydie Rappaport and Jane Lise Samuel

Section two: Growth factors and the cardiac myocyte

4.   Transforming growth factor-ß : Localization and possible   45
     functional roles in cardiac myocytes.
     Anita B. Roberts and Michael B. Sporn

5.   Basic fibroblast growth factor in cardiac myocytes: expression   55
     and effects
     Elissavet Kardami, Raymond R. Padua, Kishore Babu S.
     Pasumarthi, Lei Liu, Bradley W. Doble, Sarah E. Davey and
     Peter A. Cattini.

6.   Growth factor signal transduction in the cardiac myocyte: 77
     Functions of the serum response element
     Michael D. Schneider, Thomas Brand, Robert J. Schwartz and
     W. Robb MacLellan

7.   Effects of growth factors on human cardiac myocytes   105
     Bruce I. Goldman and John Wurzel

Section three: Growth factors and angiogenesis

8.   Growth factors and development of coronary collaterals   119
     Hari S. Sharma and Rene Zimmerman

9.   The role of growth factors in angiogenesis   149
     Robert J. Schott and Linda A. Morrow

Section four: Growth factors and atherosclerosis

10. Atherosclerosis and platelet derived growth factors   169
     Gordon A. A. Ferns and Claire Rutherford

11. Effects of TGF-ß on vascular smooth muscle cell growth   189
     Peter L. Weissberg, D.J. Grainger and James C. Metcalfe

12.   Some aspects of growth signal transduction in vascular   207
      smooth muscle cells
      Andrew C. Newby and Nicholas P. J. Brindle

13.   Basic FGF's role in smooth muscle cell proliferation: A basis   227
      for molecular atherectomy
      Ward Casscells, Douglas A. Lappi and Andrew Baird

Section five: Growth factors and cardiovascular disease:
Clinical and therapeutic implications

14.   Role of transforming growth factor ß in cardioprotection of   249
      the ischemic-reperfused myocardium
      Allan M. Lefer

15.   Platelet-derived growth factor release after angioplasty   261
      P. Macke Consigny

16.   Platelet-derived growth factor (PDGF) receptor induced by   275
      vascular injury
      Glenda E. Bilder

17.   Growth factors and hypertension: Implications for a role in   287
      vascular remodelling
      Abdel-Ilah K. El Amrani and Francine El Amrani

18.   Transforming growth factor-ß induction in carcinoid heart   311
      disease
      Johannes Waltenberger

Section six: Growth factor effects on the myocardium

19.   Adrenergic stimulation and growth factor activity   321
      Carlin S. Long and Paul C. Simpson

viii

20. Effects of transforming growth factor-beta on cardiac   337
     fibroblasts
     Mahboubeh Eghbali

21. Transforming growth factor ßs and cardiac development   347
     Rosemary J. Akhurst, Marion Dickson and
     Fergus A. Millan

     Index   367

List of contributors

Rosemary J.Akhurst
Department of Medical Genetics
University of Glasgow
Yorkhill
GLASGOW G3 8SJ
UK

Co-authors: Marion Dickson and Fergus
A. Millan

Glenda E. Bilder,
Rhone-Poulenc Rorer Central Research
500 Arcola Road
PO Box 1200
Collegeville
PENNSYLVANIA 19426-0107,
USA

Ward Casscells
Cardiology Division
University of Texas Health Center and
Texas Heart Institute
PO Box 20708
Houston
TEXAS 77030
USA

Co-authors: Douglas A. Lappi, and
Andrew Baird

P. Macke Consigny
Department of Radiology
Division of Physiologic Research
11th and Walnut
Thomas Jefferson University
Philadelphia,
PENNSYLVANIA 19107
USA

Peter Cummins
British Heart Foundation Molecular
Cardiology Research Group
Department of Physiology
The Medical School
University of Birmingham
BIRMINGHAM B15 2TT
UK

Co-authors: Francine El Amrani, and
Abdel-Ilah K. El Amrani

Mahboubeh Eghbali
Department of Anesthesiology
Yale University School of Medicine
333 Cedar Street, PO Box 3333
New Haven
CONNECTICUT 06510
USA

Abdel-Ilah K. El Amrani
Molecular Cardiology Research Group
Department of Physiology
The Medical School
University of Birmingham
BIRMINGHAM B15 2TT
UK

Co-authors: Francine El Amrani and
Peter Cummins

Gordon A.A. Ferns
The William Harvey Research
Institute and Department of Chemical
Pathology
St Bartholomew's Hospital Medical
College, Charterhouse Square
LONDON EC1M 6BQ
UK

Co-author: Claire Rutherford

Bruce I. Goldman
Department of Pathology
School of Medicine
Temple University
Broad and Ontario Streets
Philadelphia
PENNSYLVANIA 19140
USA

Co-author: John Wurzel

Carl-Hendrik Heldin
Ludwig Institute for Cancern Research
Uppsala Branch
Box 595, Biomedical Centre
S-751 24 UPPSALA
Sweden

Co-authors: Lena Claesson-Welsh,
Kohei Miyazono and Bengt Westermark

Elissavet Kardami
Division of Cardiovascular Sciences,
St. Boniface General Hospital Research
Center and Department of Physiology
University of Manitoba
351 Tache Avenue
Winnipeg
MANITOBA R2H 2A6
Canada

Co-authors: Raymond R. Padua, Kishore
Babu S. Pasumarthi, Lei Liu, Bradley
W. Doble, Sarah E. Davey, and Peter A.
Cattini

Allan M. Lefer,
Department of Physiology
Jefferson Medical College
Thomas Jefferson University
1020 Locust Street
Philadelphia
PENNSYLVANIA 19107-6799
USA

Carlin S. Long
Cardiology Section and Research
Service
Division of Cardiology 111-C
Veterans Administration Medical
Center and Cardiovascular Research
Institute and Department of Medicine
4150 Clement Street
San Francisco
CALIFORNIA 94121
USA

Co-author: Paul C. Simpson

Andrew C. Newby
Department of Cardiology
University of Wales College of
Medicine
Heath Park
CARDIFF CF4 4XN
UK

Co-author: Nicholas P.J. Brindle

Lydie Rappaport
U127 INSERM
Hopital Lariboisiere
41 Bld Chapelle
75010 PARIS
France

Co-author: Jane Lise Samuel

Anita B. Roberts
Laboratory of Chemoprevention
Building 41
National Cancer Institute
Bethesda
MARYLAND 20892
USA

Co-author: Michael B. Sporn

Michael D. Schneider
Molecular Cardiology Unit
Section of Cardiology
Department of Medicine
One Baylor Plaza, Room 506C
Houston
TEXAS 77030
USA

Co-authors: Thomas Brand, Robert
J. Schwartz and W. Robb MacLellan

Robert J. Schott
Cardiac Unit
Massachusetts General Hospital
and Harvard Medical School
Boston,
MASSACHUSETTS 02115
USA.

Co-author: Linda A. Morrow

Hari S. Sharma
Max-Planck Institute
Department of Experimental
Cardiology and Kerckhoff Klinik
Benekestrasse 2
D-6350, BAD NAUHEIM
Federal Republic of Germany

Co-author: Rene Zimmermann,

Johannes Waltenberger
Ludwig Institute for Cancer Research
Uppsala Branch
Box 595, Biomedical Centre
S-751 24 UPPSALA
Sweden

Peter L. Weissberg
British Heart Foundation Vascular
Smooth Muscle Cell Group
Department of Biochemistry
University of Cambridge
Tennis Court Road
CAMBRIDGE CB8 1QW
UK

Co-authors: D.J. Grainger and
James C. Metcalfe

Foreword

Nature is totally amoral! There are at least 3-4 million people in France alone who suffer from arterial hypertension, and whose cardiovascular system is submitted day and night to both a haemodynamic and hormonal stress. In all cases, the vasculature hypertrophies as does the myocardium. This growth process is obviously mainly detrimental at the outset since it lowers compliance of the arteries and makes them stiffer. In contrast, myocardial hypertrophy is initially beneficial since the growth process multiplies the number of contractile units and by so doing improves external work. In addition, according to Starling's law, wall stress is lowered. Growth factors play a major role in this amoral process as a trigger for hypertrophy at the vascular level, and very likely at the level of the myocardium.

Another major point of interest is the role of growth factors as determinants of restenosis after angioplasty and also of atherogenesis. Several chapters in this book are directly or indirectly concerned with this problem which is far from being purely academic since several groups are currently trying to control these processes by gene transfer. Certainly, one of the major clinical questions arising from such studies is why restenosis is not more frequent in clinical practice. After de-endotheliazation, the biologist would predict on the basis of recent studies on growth factors, and in contrast with current clinical opinion, that hypertrophy would occur in all cases with more or less complete restenosis. However, the most pessimistic clinical studies in fact find no more than 30 to 50% of restenosis.

This book is a superb summary of the work emerging from the major teams involved in studies on Growth Factors in cardiovascular research and, both as a clinician and as an experimental investigator, I have to thank one of the leaders in this field, Peter Cummins, for performing such a fine job and for contributing such a significant piece of scientific work.

Bernard Swynghedauw MD PhD
Directeur de Recherches à l'INSERM
Directeur de l'Unité 127 de l'INSERM
a l'Hopital Lariboisiére à Paris

Preface

During the past ten years there has been a remarkable expansion in the literature devoted to the role of polypeptide growth factors in the cardiovascular system. This has however to be seen against a background of an even larger body of research on growth factors in general and in other organ systems in particular. In large part this has been a real benefit to cardiovascular researchers who have been able to investigate a relatively untouched area while having the benefits of major advances from workers in other systems. It also means that readers of this volume should be able to relate the findings described to the wider area of inter- and intra-cellular signalling.

It is for this reason that the Introduction to this volume examines the *in vivo* function and mechanism of action of growth factors in the broadest context. Growth factors have been classified in terms of their receptors and signal transduction mechanisms and the possible intracellular mechanisms of action discussed. Here, in addition to growth factors that are well known to be implicated in cardiovascular function, there is mention of growth factor families whose immediate relevance to the cardiovascular system is not immediately apparent. Past experience should make us all cautious of dismissing these as irrelevant. Is there a single growth factor that has not made itself apparent somewhere in the cardiovascular system when the appropriate search has been conducted ?

In preparing this volume I have tried to follow certain objectives in the organisation of the different Sections. The first aim has been to examine the overall evidence for the role of specific growth factor expression in the different cellular compartments of the whole heart. Given that growth factors are well known to act by both autocrine and paracrine mechanisms we must not lose sight of the fact that some of the major cellular mechanisms of action almost certainly originate in adjacent cellular or extra-cellular compartments. For this reason it is imperative that there is a balance in future research between studies *in vivo* and *in vitro*.

Notwithstanding these considerations there can be little doubt that one of the major areas of activity in the past five years has been the possible role of growth factors in the proliferation (or lack of proliferation !) and enlargement of cardiac myocytes. This is dealt with both in Section One and at length in Section Two where studies on isolated cardiac myocytes are incorporated.

The following two Sections examine the role of growth factors in perhaps less controversial areas, namely angiogenesis and atherosclerosis. These are intentionally placed together given the considerable degree of overlap attached to the role of smooth muscle cell growth in these activities. Nonetheless an attempt has been made to distinguish between normal and abnormal growth factor functions.

The possible clinical and therapeutic involvement of growth factors in cardiovascular disease is the subject of Section Five. A brief examination of the diverse topics addressed in this section, namely ischemic protection, hypertension, vascular injury and angioplasty, and carcinoid heart disease should provide ample evidence of the pivotal role of growth factors. There are likely to be few conditions where we can conclusively exclude a role for these ubiqitous molecules. This naturally leads us back to the more fundamental and wide ranging actions of growth factors in the heart in Section Six.

This is the first volume devoted entirely to the role of growth factors in the cardiovascular system and as such I hope it fills an important niche. It should be of interest to both to the basic researcher and the clinician. In addition researchers from other areas will also hopefully find much to interest them here. Perhaps there are even areas in this rapidly expanding field where the cardiovascular system has led the way !

I have been fortunate in being able to persuade all the leading researchers in the field from around to world to contribute to this volume. They have had a free hand and in consequence the reader should find many stimulating and provocative ideas.

The genesis of this book arose out of a small Symposium on the 'Role of growth factors in the heart' held at the XIIIth Congress of the European Society of Cardiology in Amsterdam in August 1991. The Symposium organised by the Working Group on 'Pathophysiology of the Cardiac Myocyte' was the first to deal exclusively with growth factors in this context at the European Society and met with much enthusiasm. This was shared by Kluwer Academic, in particular Melissa Welch, the Editor of the Medical Division, to whom I must give thanks for making this volume possible.

Peter Cummins
Department of Physiology
The Medical School
University of Birmingham
Birmingham, UK

1. Growth factors: In vivo function and mechanism of action

CARL-HENRIK HELDIN, LENA CLAESSON-WELSH,
KOHEI MIYAZONO and BENGT WESTERMARK

Introduction

The control of mammalian cell growth is in part regulated by peptide factors that stimulate or inhibit cell proliferation. The number of identified growth regulatory peptides have increased considerably during the last years, as a result of the purification and characterization of new factors or isolation of cDNAs for structurally related factors. For a description of the structural and functional properties of the more well characterized factors, see [1]. The known factors can be assigned to different families according to their structural and functional properties (Table I). Most of the factors of Table I stimulate cell proliferation, whereas *e.g.* TGF-ß's, TNF's and IFN's generally inhibit cell growth. However, a single factor can act both as a growth stimulator and a growth inhibitor depending on cell type and culture condition [reviewed in ref. 2]. Moreover, growth regulatory factors have also other effects on cells, *e.g.* to stimulate or inhibit cell locomotion and chemotaxis; several factors also affect cell differentiation. Most growth regulatory factors act locally, through autocrine or paracrine mechanisms, a fact which is important to keep in mind when their *in vivo* function is discussed.

The purpose of the present review is to discuss in general the mechanism of action of growth regulatory factors and their possible *in vivo* function. This review will focus on general concepts; for deeper discussions of specific topics the reader is referred to the cited review articles and to other chapters of this volume.

Table I. Families of growth regulatory factors

Family	Examples of factors	Receptors	Receptor type
Platelet-derived GF (PDGF)	PDGF-AA PDGF-AB PDGF-BB	PDGF-R-α PDGF-R-β	PTK PTK
	Vascular endothelial GF Placenta GF	Flt-1 ?	PTK
Epidermal GF (EGF)	EGF TGF-α	EGF-R (ErbB)	PTK
	Amphiregulin Neu differentiation factor Heparin binding EGF	? Neu (ErbB2) ?	PTK
Fibroblast GF (FGF)	FGF-1 (aFGF) FGF-2 (bFGF) FGF-3 (Hst) FGF-4 (Int-2) FGF-5 FGF-6 FGF-7 (KGF)	FGF-R-1 FGF-R-2 FGF-R-3 FGF-R-4	PTK PTK PTK PTK
Hepatocyte GF (HGF)	HGF HGF receptor antagonist	HGF-R (Met)	PTK
Insulin-like GF (IGF)	Insulin IGF-I IGF-II	Insulin-R IGF-I-R IGF-II-R/Man-6-P rec	PTK PTK
Neurotrophins	Nerve GF Brain-derived Neurotrophic factor Neurotrophin-3 Neurotrophin-4	Trk[1] TrkB[1] TrkC[1]	PTK PTK PTK
Neuropeptides	Gastrin-releasing peptide Vasopressin Endothelin	GRP-R Vasopressin-R ET-R	7TMR 7TMR 7TMR
Interleukin (IL)	IL-1α IL-1β IL-1 receptor antagonist IL-2	IL-1-R IL-2-R-α IL-2-R-β	ILR
	IL-3 IL-4 IL-5 IL-6 IL-7 IL-8[4]	IL-3-R-α[2] IL-4-R IL-5-R-α[2] IL-6-R[3] IL-7-R IL-8-R-A IL-8-R-B	ILR ILR ILR ILR ILR 7TMR 7TMR
	IL-9	IL-9-R	ILR
Colony stimulatory factor (CSF)	G-CSF M-CSF GM-CSF Stem cell factor Erythropoietin	G-CSF-R CSF-1-R (Fms) GM-CSF-R-α[2] SCF-R (Kit) EPO-R	ILR PTK ILR PTK ILR

Family	Examples of factors	Receptors	Receptor type
Melanocyte growth stimulatory activity (MGSA)	MGSA[4]	IL-8-R-B	7TMR
Transforming GF-β (TGF-β)	TGF-β1 TGF-β2 TGF-β3	} TGF-β type II-R	PSK
	Activin	Activin-R	PSK
	Inhibin	?	
	BMP-2	?	
	BMP-3	?	
	BMP-4	?	
	BMP-5	?	
	BMP-6	?	
	BMP-7	?	
Interferon (IFN)	IFN-α IFN-β	} IFN-α/β-R	
	IFN-γ	IFN-γ-R	
Tumor necrosis factor (TNF)	TNF-α TNF-β	} { TNF-R1 TNF-R2	
Leukemia inhibitory factor (LIF)	LIF	LIF-R[3]	ILR
	Oncostatin M	Oncostatin-M-R[3]	ILR
	Ciliary neurotrophic factor	CNTF-R[3]	ILR

The table lists polypeptide factors which stimulate or inhibit cell growth or differentiation. Families of factors where there is some information about the corresponding receptors, have been included. Brackets indicate that a ligand binds to more than one receptor, or vice versa. Abbreviations: GF, growth factor; R, receptor; PTK, protein tyrosine kinase; PSK, protein serine/threonine kinase; ILR, interleukin receptor; 7TMR, G-protein coupled receptor that spans the cell membrane seven times. For references see the reviews cited in the text. Some recent entries in the table are not covered in these reviews; further information can be obtained from the authors.

Footnotes:

[1] Members of the neurotrophin family also bind with lower affinity to a receptor with structural similarity to the TNF receptors.

[2] The receptors for IL-3, IL-5 and GM-CSF share a common β_c subunit which is important for signal transduction.

[3] The receptors for IL-6, LIF, Oncostatin M and CNTF share a common signal transducer, gp130.

[4] IL-8 and MGSA are structurally related and cross-react for receptor binding.

Receptors for growth regulatory factors

Growth regulatory factors exert their effects on cells via binding to specific receptors on the cell surface. The main types of receptors for such factors are depicted schematically in Figure 1. Several of the receptors have an intrinsic protein tyrosine kinase activity. Studies of members of this receptor family have recently yielded some insight into the signal transduction pathways [reviewed in ref. 3] (see below).

Members of the interleukin receptor family (also called hematopoietin receptor family) have a characteristic motif in the extracellular part, a single transmembrane spanning domain and only a short cytoplasmic tail [reviewed in ref. 4]. These receptors therefore often depend on the interaction with another component, a signal transducer, to trigger the mitogenic pathway. Activation of several members of the interleukin receptor family leads to stimulation of protein tyrosine kinase activity. This could occur through the association of a cytoplasmic tyrosine kinase with the activated receptor complex, or activation of a tyrosine kinase further downstream in the signal transduction pathway.

Members of the TGF-ß family bind to many different types of receptors [reviewed in ref. 5]. The known receptors which have roles in signal transduction have intrinsic serine/threonine kinase activities. Thus, the down stream signalling most likely involves the phosphorylation of specific substrates on serine/threonine residues, but knowledge about the identity of such substrates is still lacking.

Finally, some compounds that have growth promoting effects on certain cell types, *e.g.* certain neuropeptides and thrombin, bind to receptors that transverse the cell membrane seven times [reviewed in ref. 6]. Signalling through these seven-transmembrane-segment receptors occurs via G-protein mediated pathways. Certain receptors in this family also bind ligands that are not proteins or peptides; some of these ligands stimulate cell growth, *e.g.* serotonin and lysophosphatidate. However, it is likely that the majority of receptors in this family do not have as their primary function to regulate cell growth.

Signal transduction via tyrosine kinase receptors

The principle structure of the protein tyrosine kinase receptors is depicted in Figure 1. These receptors have an extracellular ligand binding domain that is connected to the cytoplasmic kinase domain through a single transmembrane segment. Binding of the respective ligands to the receptor leads to activation of the receptor kinase and to

Receptors for Growth Regulatory Factors

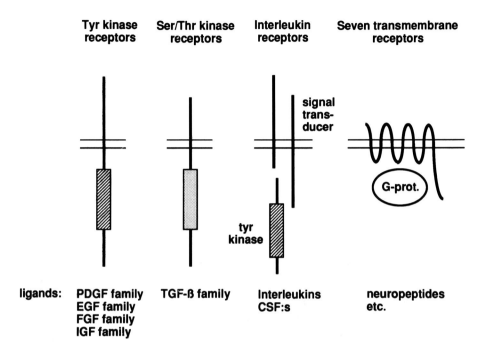

Figure 1. Schematic illustration of different families of receptors for growth regulatory factors.

autophosphorylation of the receptors on tyrosine residues, as well as to tyrosine phosphorylation of specific cytoplasmic substrates. The mechanism of activation of these receptors involves ligand-induced receptor dimerization; interposition of the receptors allows phosphorylation *in trans*. This "autophosphorylation" seems to have two consequences; it locks the kinase in an active configuration, and it provides attachment sites for down-stream components in the signal transduction pathway [reviewed in refs.1,7].

Several enzymes have been shown to associate with autophosphorylated tyrosine kinase receptors, and these are candidates for being involved in the transduction of the signal leading to cell growth and chemotaxis (Figure 2). One is phospholipase C-γ (PLC-γ), an enzyme that cleaves phosphatidylinositol 4,5 bisphosphate (PI-4,5-P_2) to diacylglycerol and inositol trisphosphate, components that activates protein kinase C (PKC) and mobilizes Ca^{2+} from intracellular stores, respectively. Receptor association leads to the phosphorylation of PLC-γ on tyrosine residues, which causes an increase in its enzymatic activity [reviewed in ref. 8]. Despite the potential importance of both Ca^{2+} and PKC in growth stimulation, activation of PLC-γ seems not to be obligatory for growth stimulation.

Another enzyme that utilizes PI-4,5-P_2 as a substrate also becomes associated with autophosphorylated tyrosine kinase receptors, *i.e.* phosphatidylinositol-3'-kinase (PI-3-K) [reviewed in ref. 9]. This enzyme consists of a regulatory subunit, p85, which binds to the receptors, and a catalytic subunit, p110 [10]. Its product PI-3,4,5-P_3 has a potentially important, albeit still unknown, role in the signal transduction pathway.

GTPase activating protein (GAP) is a molecule that interacts with Ras and thus potentially influences the signalling through Ras-dependent pathways. It has been found to bind to certain autophosphorylated tyrosine kinase receptors; the functional implication of this interaction in relation to Ras signalling or mitogenicity is, however, unknown [11].

Src is the prototype for a family of tyrosine kinases without transmembrane domains. Members of this family have been shown to associate with activated tyrosine kinase receptors [12].

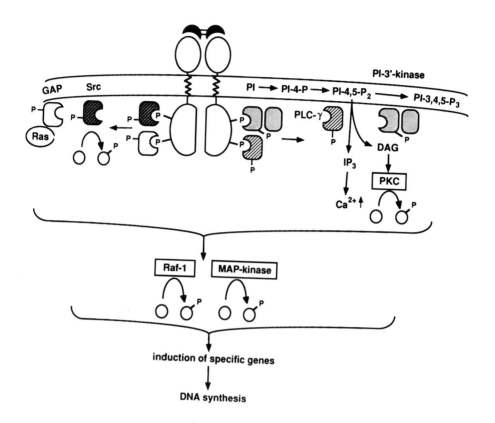

Figure 2. Schematic illustration of intracellular signalling pathways in PDGF-stimulated cells. For discussion, see the text.

All the above mentioned receptor associated molecules contain one or two copies of a conserved motif denoted SH2 domains (from Src homology region 2). It has been shown that these domains mediate the binding to autophosphorylated regions of receptors [reviewed in ref. 13]. There is some specificity in this interaction; not all tyrosine kinase receptors bind all SH2 domain-containing molecules, and each SH2 domain show a preference for certain of the autophosphorylation sites in a given receptor. As an example, the β-receptor for PDGF, which binds all four of the putative substrates discussed above, has been shown to have at least six autophosphorylation sites. Two of these, that are located in the carboxyterminal tail of the receptor, mediate the binding of PLC-γ [14]. The kinase domain of the PDGF receptor contains an insert sequence of about 100 amino acids without homology to kinases. This region contains three autophosphorylated tyrosine residues; two of these are involved in the binding of PI-3-K and the third binds GAP [15; 16]. The sites in different receptors that have been shown to bind PI-3-K are surrounded by a common motif of amino acids, *i.e.* -Tyr(P)-Met/Val-Xxx-Met-. Other motifs might determine the specificity of binding of other SH2 domain containing proteins, although this remains to be elucidated.

Certain of the SH2-domain-containing proteins have intrinsic catalytic properties, like PLC-γ, GAP and Src. In these cases the interaction with the receptor may lead to a change in the catalytic properties, via phosphorylation on tyrosine residues or via a conformational change induced upon interaction with the autophosphorylated receptor. However, there is also another class of SH2-domain-containing molecules, that does not have any intrinsic catalytic activity and whose function might be that of adapters. One example is p85, the regulatory subunit of PI-3-K [reviewed in ref. 9]. Another example is IRS-1, a 185 kDa major substrate for the insulin receptor which potentially can mediate interaction with multiple signal transduction molecules [17]. The function of the adapters might be to translocate molecules to the receptors at the cell membrane. These possible functions of the SH2-domain-mediated interactions, *i.e.* activation via tyrosine phosphorylation, activation via conformational changes or translocation of an enzymatic activity to the cell membrane, need not be mutually exclusive.

Downstream signalling

Growth stimulation of cells is characterized by activation of a cascade of phosphorylation events (Figure 2). This includes phosphorylation by the tyrosine kinase receptors, as described above, as well as phosphorylation further downstream, involving the activation of other tyrosine kinases, *e.g.* in the Src family. Moreover, serine/threonine kinases are activated. One example is PKC which is activated by PLC-γ-mediated diacylglycerol production [reviewed in ref. 18]. Other examples are the Raf-1 kinase [reviewed in ref. 19] and MAP kinases (also called extracellular signal regulated kinases, ERKs) [reviewed in ref. 20], which have been shown to become activated after growth stimulation via tyrosine kinase receptors, as well as via interleukin receptors. Both these serine/threonine kinases are activated by phosphorylation events, but the mechanism whereby the signals are transduced from the activated growth factor receptors to the kinases, remains to be elucidated. The substrates for these kinases and their exact role in the mitogenic pathway, also remain to be determined.

Given that TGF-β acts via receptors with serine/threonine kinase activity, phosphorylation on serine or threonine residues of specific proteins is likely to be part also of growth inhibitory pathways.

Ligand-induced receptor activation leads to the induction of a host of genes within 5 min to a couple of hours. A systematic investigation revealed that about 80 genes were induced after growth factor stimulation of 3T3 cells [21]. Amongst those were found *e.g.* matrix molecules and their receptors, cytoskeletal proteins, growth factors and growth inhibitors, as well as transcription factors. Whereas the former molecules may affect cell proliferation indirectly, the induction of certain transcription factors may be of direct importance for growth regulation, *e.g.* by regulating the components involved in the DNA synthesis machinery.

Possible *in vivo* function of growth regulatory factors

Several of the growth regulatory factors listed in Table I appear to have important functions during the embryonal development [reviewed in ref. 22]. The specific spatial and temporal expression of certain growth factors and their receptors during the embryonal development suggests that they control cell growth, migration and differentiation through paracrine mechanisms. Some of the factors involved are freely diffusible, but others are restricted in their diffusion through interaction with the extracellular matrix, yet others are anchored to the producer cell by a transmembrane domain.

An extensively studied example of embryonic induction is the induction of mesodermal tissues in the frog Xenopus. In this system, vegetal blastomeres secrete factors that induce adjacent animal ectoderm to differentiate into mesoderm, *e.g.* muscle and notochord. Members of the FGF family, the TGF-β family and the Wnt (Wingless/Int-1) family, have been shown to mimic different aspects of mesoderm induction. Members of these families have also been found to be expressed in the developing nervous system [reviewed in ref. 22].

In a few cases specific functions for certain growth factors during the latter part of the developmental process have been demonstrated. One example is the differentiation of glial cells in the rat optic nerve; PDGF and CNTF derived from type-1 astrocytes control the differentiation of O-2A progenitor cells into oligodendrocytes and type-2 astrocytes [reviewed in ref. 23].

Analysis of the molecular basis of naturally occurring mouse mutations have given further insight into the role of growth factors during the mammalian development. Two mouse mutants, *Steel (Sl)* and *Dominant White Spotting (W)*, which have analogous defects in the maturation of melanocytes, hematopoietic cells and germ cells, have arisen through mutations in the genes for SCF or its receptor, c-Kit [reviewed in ref. 24]. Another mouse mutant *Patch (Ph)*, which like *Sl* and *W* is characterized by a "spotted" fur coat, involves the deletion of the PDGF α-receptor. *Ph* mice with homozygous deletions of the PDGF α-receptor die in midgestation with abnormalities in the neural tube, fluid retention and craniofacial abnormalities. Additional information about the role of specific factors during the embryonal development is expected in the near future through the analysis of the phenotypes of mice with deletions introduced in specific genes.

In the adult organism, members of the interleukin family have as their function to regulate the immune response, and colony stimulating factors to regulate hematopoiesis. Furthermore, members of the PDGF, EGF, TGF-β, IGF, and FGF families may promote wound healing of soft tissues, whereas bone morphogenic proteins, that are members of the TGF-β family, have been shown to have a positive effect in healing of bone fractures [reviewed in ref. 25]. In wound healing as well as during the embryonal development, angiogenesis, *i.e.* the ability to stimulate ingrowth into a tissue of blood vessels, is important [reviewed in ref. 26]. The most potent stimulators of angiogenesis are members of the FGF family. Another important aspect of wound healing is the ability to stimulate the production of matrix molecules. TGF-βэs have been shown to have a particularly powerful effect on matrix production, and promotes wound healing despite the fact that they inhibit the growth of most cell types in the soft tissues. Another example of a growth factor with a function during tissue regeneration is HGF which increases markedly after liver injury and thus most likely has an important role during liver regeneration [reviewed in ref. 27].

Adverse effects *in vivo* of growth regulatory factors

Perturbation of the normal mitogenic pathway of growth factors may contribute to the loss of growth control that characterizes malignant cells. There are examples that transformed cells overproduce autocrine growth factors, express too large amounts of growth factor receptors, or express constitutively active, mutated forms of the components of the intracellular mitogenic pathway [reviewed in ref. 28]. It is also possible that loss of growth inhibitory pathways, through the lack of a specific growth inhibitor, or lack of the cognate receptor or other downstream elements, is important in certain forms of tumors. Studies of human tumors have given ample evidence that the constitutive activation of growth stimulatory pathways is important in certain forms of tumors. There is still less evidence that the suppression of growth inhibitory pathways may account for the loss of growth control in tumors, but such data is anticipated in the future.

An excess of cell growth is characteristic also of certain non-malignant disorders including atherosclerosis and fibrotic processes. Excess activity of PDGF may be involved in the atherosclerotic process; at sites of endothelial cell injury, PDGF released from platelets or macrophages may stimulate the migration and proliferation of smooth muscle cells in the intima layer of vessels, which is an early sign of atherosclerosis [reviewed in ref. 29]. In fact, the infusion of neutralizing PDGF antibodies was shown to prevent the development of atherosclerosis in rat carotid arteria after de-endothelialization [30].

PDGF, and other factors, may also be involved in the development of myelofibrosis and fibrotic lesions in chronic inflammatory conditions, *e.g.* in liver cirrhosis, scleroderma, and lung fibrosis. Firm evidence in support of this notion is still lacking, but

PDGF has been found to occur in excess amounts in certain fibrotic tissues [31]. Furthermore, TGF-β may be involved in the development of glomerulonephritis; inhibition of TGF-β activity was found to prevent the development of experimentally induced glomerulonephritis [32].

Abnormal IL-6 production has been suggested to be involved in a number of diseases, including glomerulonephritis, rheumatoid arthritis and other autoimmune diseases [reviewed in ref. 33]. Autoimmune diseases are likely to involve overactivity of many different factors. IL-2 was recently linked to the development of autoimmune diabetes [34]. Moreover, the synovial fluid of patients with rheumatoid arthritis contain high concentrations of different interleukins, IFN-γ, TNF-α, PDGF and TGF-β. These factors may mediate the excessive inflammatory response, the pronounced proliferative response of synovial cells and other cells, the fibrotic reactions seen in later stages, as well as the phases of remission through immunosuppression by TGF-β [reviewed in ref. 35].

Future perspectives

Research during recent years has provided an initial insight into the *in vivo* function of growth regulatory factors and their possible involvement in diseases. Moreover, an outline of the mechanisms of signal transduction of growth regulatory factors is emerging through the structural and functional characterization of receptors for such factors, and of intracellular components that are controlled by growth regulatory factors.

The now available technology to knock out genes will most likely give additional valuable information about the normal function of growth regulatory factors. The overexpression of such factors or their receptors in transgenic mice will furthermore be informative in relation to their role in disease. Such data will be complemented by investigations of normal and pathological tissues by immunohistochemistry and *in situ* techniques for mRNA detection.

Regarding signal transduction, the challenge for the future will be to understand how the signals generated at the cell membrane are transduced through the cytoplasm to the nucleus. Moreover, the interplay between components in different signal transduction pathways will be important to elucidate.

Finally, the availability of large quantities of growth regulatory factors, obtained through recombinant techniques, will now make it possible to explore their clinical utility. The fact that certain growth regulatory factors may be involved in adverse reactions, makes the development of specific inhibitors highly warranted. It is anticipated that both agonists and antagonists for growth regulatory factors will be important future therapeutic tools.

Acknowledgements

We thank Ingegärd Schiller for valuable help in the preparation of this review.

References

1. Sporn MB, Roberts AB. editors. In: Handbook of Experimental Pharmacology. Springer-Verlag, Heidelberg.1990; 95.
2. Sporn MB, Roberts AB. Peptide growth factors are multifunctional. Nature 1988; 332: 217-219.
3. Ullrich A, Schlessinger J. Signal transduction by receptors with tyrosine kinase activity. Cell 1990; 61: 203-212.
4. Miyajima A, Kitamura T, Harada N, Yokota T, Arai K-I. Cytokine receptors and signal transduction. Annu Rev Immunol 1992; 10: 295-331.
5. Massagué J. Receptors for the TGF-β family. Cell 1992; 69: 1067-1070.
6. Moolenaar WH. G-protein-coupled receptors, phosphoinositide hydrolysis, and cell proliferation. Cell Growth & Differ 1991; 2: 359-364.
7. Cantley LC, Auger KR, Carpenter C, Duckworth B, Graziani A, Kapeller R, Soltoff S. Oncogenes and signal transduction. Cell 1991; 64: 281-302.
8. Wahl M, Carpenter G. Selective phospholipase C activation. BioEssays 1991; 13: 107-113.
9. Downes CP, Carter AN. Phosphoinositide 3-kinase: A new effector in signal transduction? Cellular Signalling 1991; 3: 501-513.
10. Hiles ID, Otsu M, Volinia S, Fry MJ, Gout I, Dhand R, Panayotou G, Ruiz-Larrea F, Thompson A, Totty NF, Hsuan JJ, Courtneidge SA, Parker PJ, Waterfield MD. Phosphatidylinositol 3-kinase: Structure and expression of the 110 kd catalytic subunit. Cell 1992; 70: 419-429.

11. Molloy CJ, Bottaro DP, Fleming MS, Gibbs JB, Aaronson, SA. PDGF induction of tyrosine phosphorylation of the GTPase activating protein. Nature 1989; 342: 711-714.

12. Kypta RM, Goldberg Y, Ulug ET, Courtneidge SA. Association between the PDGF receptor and members of the src family of tyrosine kinases. Cell 1990; 62: 481-492.

13. Koch CA, Anderson D, Moran MF, Ellis C, Pawson T. SH2 and SH3 domains: Elements that control interactions of cytoplasmic signaling proteins. Science 1992; 252: 668-674.

14. Rönnstrand L, Mori S, Arvidsson A-K, Eriksson A, Wernstedt C, Hellman U, Claesson-Welsh L, Heldin C-H. Identification of two C-terminal autophosphorylation sites in the PDGF β-receptor: involvement in the interaction with phospholipase C-γ. EMBO J 1992; 11: 3911-3919.

15. Fantl WJ, Escobedo JA, Martin GA, Turck CW, del Rosario M, McCormick F, Williams LT. Distinct phosphotyrosines on a growth factor receptor bind to specific molecules that mediate different signaling pathways. Cell 1992; 69: 413-423.

16. Kashishian A, Kazlauskas A, Cooper JA. Phosphorylation sites in the PDGF receptor with different specificities for binding GAP and PI3 kinase in vivo. EMBO J 1992; 11: 1373-1382.

17. Sun XJ, Rothenberg P, Kahn CR, Backer JM, Araki E, Wilden PA, Cahill DA, Goldstein BJ, White MF. Structure of the insulin receptor substrate IRS-1 defines a unique signal transduction protein. Nature 1991; 352: 73-77.

18. Nishizuka Y. The molecular heterogeneity of protein kinase C and its implications for cellular regulation. Nature 1988; 334: 661-668.

19. Rapp UR. Role of Raf-1 serine/threonine protein kinase in growth factor signal transduction. Oncogene 1991; 6: 495-500.

20. Cobb MH, Boulton TG, Robbins DJ. Extracellular signal-regulated kinases: ERKs in progress. Cell Regul 1991; 2: 965-978.

21. Almendral JM, Sommer D, MacDonald-Bravo H, Bruckhardt J, Perera,J, Bravo R. Complexity of the early genetic response to growth factors in mouse fibroblasts. Mol Cell Biol 1988; 8: 2140-2148.

22. Jessell TM, Melton DA. Diffusible factors in vertebrate embryonic induction. Cell 1992; 68: 257-270.

23. Lillie LE, Raff MC. Differentiation signals in the CNS: type-2 astrocyte development in vitro as a model system. Neuron 1990; 5: 111-119.

24. Besmer P. The kit ligand encoded at the murine Steel locus: a pleiotropic growth and differentiation factor. Current Opinion in Cell Biology 1991; 3: 939-946.

25. Robinson CJ. Growth factors in wound healing. TIBTECH 1992; 10: 301-302.

26. Folkman J, Shing Y. Angiogenesis. J Biol Chem 1992; 267: 10931-10934.

27. Nakamura T. Structure and function of hepatocyte growth factor. Progress in Growth Factor Research 1991; 3: 67-85.

28. Aaronson SA. Growth factors and cancer. Science 1991; 254: 1146-1153.

29. Ross R. Medical Progress - The pathogenesis of atherosclerosis - an update. N Engl J Med 1986; 314: 488-500.

30. Ferns GAA, Raines EW, Sprugel KH, Motani AS, Reidy MA, Ross R. Inhibition of neointimal smooth muscle accumulation after angioplasty by an antibody to PDGF. Science 1991; 253: 1129-1132.

31. Martinet Y, Rom WN, Grotendorst GR, Martin GR, Crystal RG. Exaggerated spontaneous release of platelet-derived growth factor by alveolar macrophages from patients with idiopathic pulmonary fibrosis. N Engl J Med 1987; 317: 202-209.

32. Border WA, Okuda S, Languino LR, Sporn,MB, Ruoslahti E. Suppression of experimental glomerulonephritis by antiserum against transforming growth factor $\beta 1$. Nature 1990; 346: 371-374.

33. Hirano T, Akira S, Taga T, Kishimoto,T. Biological and clinical aspects of interleukin 6. Immunology Today 1990; 11: 443-449.

34. Heath WR, Allison J, Hoffmann MW, Schönrich G, Hämmerling G, Arnold B, Miller JFAP. Autoimmune diabetes as a consequence of locally produced interleukin-2. Nature 1992; 359: 547-549.

35. Klareskog L, Rönnelid J, Gudmundsson S, Karlsson-Parra A. Rheumatoid arthritis. Current Opinion in Immunology 1991; 3: 912-916.

2. Fibroblast and transforming growth factors in the heart: A role in cardiac growth ?

PETER CUMMINS, ABDEL-ILAH K. EL AMRANI and
FRANCINE EL AMRANI

Introduction

Growth of the heart either during normal development or as a result of abnormal hemodynamic stimuli is a poorly understood process at the molecular and cellular level. In many respects this lack of understanding is common to other organ systems and centres on the roles played by a variety of extra- and intracellular signalling molecules in the cell cycle and growth process. The number of cell types in the heart is diverse including myocytes, fibroblasts, endothelial and smooth muscle cells. While much is known about signalling mechanisms in some of these cells in the isolated state it is clear that a significant degree of cross talk must exist in vivo to coordinate growth of myocardium, blood vessels and extra-cellular matrix. Polypeptide growth factors almost certainly play a key role in the sequence of events leading to growth of all these cell masses. However, central to the problem of cardiac adaptive growth is the function, if any, of peptide growth factors in the cardiac myocyte. The following article will examine the involvement of two key growth factors in relation to the cardiac myocyte.

Growth of the cardiac myocyte

Cardiac myocytes are widely accepted as being terminally differentiated cells incapable of division in the adult. This has obvious major implications for the response of the heart to both hemodynamic stress and injury. Following cardiac overload the myocardium enlarges first in a truly adaptive and normal physiological response. In addition to a change in cell size accompanied by increased DNA synthesis there are also transitions in the forms of many of the protein types expressed. There are however natural limitations to these processes. Once myocytes enlarge beyond a certain size the diffusion distances to capillaries become too great. Protein switching can also only occur until there is a maximum expression of one particular, albeit better suited, isoform. It may be that these limiting stages are related to, or even coincide with, the change from normal adaptive growth to abnormal function and eventual heart failure.

Given the consequences of this inability of cardiac myocytes to divide it is suprising that there are circumstances in which cytokinetic division does occur. During the fetal period, the heart enlarges both by hyperplasia and hypertrophy of cardiac myocytes [1]. Mitotic division and cytokinesis then declines and soon after birth, myocytes cease hyperplasia and further muscle growth is by cellular hypertrophy. Injury to cardiac muscle results in hypertrophy or scar formation by non-muscle cells which can further compromise cardiac performance.

However the situation is possibly not as clear as the above suggests. Indeed it is possible that the inability of cardiac myocytes to undergo cytokinesis is a property that may be repressed and not irreversibly lost [2]. As outlined above myocytes proliferate in the developing heart although the rate of division declines rapidly during the late fetal and early postnatal stages [1]. Rumyantsev demonstrated that adult atrial myocytes underwent DNA synthesis, nuclear division and possibly limited cytokinesis by ventricular overload subsequent to experimental myocardial infarction [3]. Amphibian ventricular and atrial myocytes undergo mitosis 15-20 days following wounding of the myocardium, even to the extent of regeneration of the tip of the excised ventricle [4]. *In vivo*, SV40 T antigen has been coupled to the promoter for the gene for atrial natriuretic factor and injected into fertilised mouse eggs. Some of the transgenic mice developed tumours of the atrium due to uncontrolled division of myocytes which in most other respects appeared normal [5].These findings suggest it is necessary to look beyond the limitations posed by past thinking. Rather the focus should be on understanding the normal signalling processes by which the cardiac myocyte proliferates and then enlarges.

Candidate growth factors

Almost certainly a large number of growth regulatory molecules will be implicated in controlling the normal and abnormal growth of the cardiac myocyte. They would be required to act both intra- and extra-cellularly. Messages would need to be conveyed from one cell type to another and between adjacent cardiac myocytes. Actions in different intracellular compartments would need to be coordinated. The polypeptide growth factors are well suited to this role. They are well known to be multifunctional agents with a ubiquitous distribution. Moreover their actions are not always fixed but can change depending on location, concentration and co-existing peptides.Although several growth factors have been tentatively suggested as having a role in myocyte growth (eg. insulin-like growth factors, myotrophin, non-myocyte-derived growth factor), two classes of growth factors, namely the transforming and fibroblast growth factors, have been implicated in signalling processes involving the cardiac myocyte [6,7]. Attention has focussed in particular on transforming growth factor ß (TGF ß) and acidic (aFGF) and basic (bFGF) fibroblast growth factors.

The family of transforming growth factor ß peptides

The structural prototype of this gene superfamily family of proteins with diverse activities that regulate cell growth and division is TGFß. TGFß1, a major isoform, is a dimer of two identical peptides of 112 residues. Other members of the family include the activins, inhibins, Mullerian inhibiting substance in mammals and the decapentaplegic gene complex transcript which controls morphogenesis in *Drosophila*. The family includes embryogenic morphogens, regulators of endocrine function, and broad spectrum as well as specialised regulators of cell proliferation and differentiation [8]. TGF ß is a potent regulator of myogenesis in *in vitro* models [9,10]. It appears to act at an early stage of commitment to differentiation in mouse and rat myoblasts rather than inhibiting expression of differentiated functions *per se.* [9,10]. It has either no effect or possibly supresses cell proliferation of myoblasts [10].

The family of fibroblast growth factor peptides

The FGF's are multifunctional. They can induce cell proliferation, stimulate or suppress specific cellular protein synthesis, induce changes in differentiated function and in cell motility, and influence cell survival and the onset of senescence in a wide variety of target tissues. This family includes aFGF, bFGF, the hst/K-fgf gene product in Kaposi's sarcoma, the int-2 proto-oncogene, FGF-5 and FGF-6. It is now clear that they are present in a wide range of organs, solid tissues, tumours and cultured cells [11]. FGF's are characterised by their ability to bind heparin, an important functional property. aFGF and bFGF seem to differ only in their potency. Both aFGF and bFGF elicit proliferation of isolated skeletal muscle myoblasts and block myogenic differentiation, probably between the Go and G1 transition [7]. In contrast, TGF-ß supresses the induction of muscle specific proteins including myosin heavy chains and actin in the absence of proliferative growth [9,10]. Interestingly, the action of FGF's on skeletal muscle can be inhibited by TGF ß suggesting a possible model for regulation of myoblast proliferation in vivo [9].

When considering the possible candidates for growth factor action on the cardiac myocyte it must be remembered that a range of growth factors are present in non-myocyte cells in the heart. While some of these, such as the fibroblast growth factors are well known to act on capillary endothelial cells to induce angiogenesis [12] (see Section Three) it does not preclude their actions on other cells. Indeed the sequestration of a growth factor in one cell and release to act on another is a well established mechanism of action. As such there is growing evidence for the presence of transforming and fibroblast growth factors in myocyte and non-myocyte compartments and for their involvment in the regulation of cardiac growth and diffentiation.

Evidence for cardiac transforming growth factors

Immunohistochemical techniques have demonstrated that transforming growth factor ß1 is present in the hearts of adult and neonatal mice [13]. Antibody staining demonstrated localisation in both cardiac myocytes and in interstitial connective tissue. In part this depended on the nature of the different antibodies employed. Thompson et al. [13] used antibodies raised to the amino-terminal 30 residues of TGF ß1 which were distinguished on the basis of their relative intra- and extra-cellular immunoreactivities with results suggesting a possible differential TGF ß isoform distribution. Staining of myocyte cytoplasm and extra-cellular matrix was present with intensity of staining being similar in neonatal and adult hearts. Interestingly, given the possible different growth potentials of atrial compared with ventricular myocytes, there was stronger TGF ß1 staining in the former. Support for different isoforms comes from the finding that a 2.4 Kb mRNA transcript was detected in both adult and neonatal whole mouse heart extracts but additional 0.8 and 1.1 Kb transcripts were present in the adult [13]. Levels of TGFß mRNA do not correlate with the distribution of immunoreactive TGFß1 as a differential localisation is often observed [13,14,15,16]. It may be that certain cells synthesise and release TGFß into the extracellular matrix of adjacent cells which then respond accordingly. Other studies on the mouse heart using antibodies specific for the three major isoforms of TGFß have however failed to confirm a differential location [14]. In mouse embryos between 12.5 and 18.5 days, antibodies to TGFß1, 2 and 3 all appeared to stain cardiac myocytes. There was differential staining however of blood vessel endothelial cells with TGFß3 but not TGFß1 showing positive staining [14].

Using polyclonal antibodies to porcine TGF-ß1 and also a cDNA probe, Eghbali [17] has found that both the protein and mRNA are present in the myocardium. However, with freshly isolated cardiac myocytes and non-myocyte cells he was able to detect TGF-ß1 mRNA only in the non-myocyte fraction. Although the composition of non-myocyte cells is often poorly defined, in this study they were established to be 90-95% fibroblasts and 5-10% endothelial and smooth muscle cells presumably with minimal myocyte contamination. The antibodies employed were directed to the N-terminal 30 residues of TGFß [13]. Staining was shown to be intense around intramyocardial blood vessels and with no detectable staining in other parts of the heart. These findings therefore differ from those above in which staining of myocytes was observed [14]. While a role for TGF ß in the adult heart could be called into doubt by these findings the evidence for involvement during cardiogenesis is more firm. This aspect is dealt with in Section Six of this volume. Certainly TGF ß has been shown to mediate the transformation of epithelial to mesenchymal cells during cardiac embryogenesis in the developing endocardial cushion and valves of embryonic mice and chicks [13,18]. More recently, TGFß1 has been localised to mitochondria in cardiac myocytes [19] and TGFß1 mRNA to cardiac myocytes in the pig heart [20]. TGF ß1 gene expression has been determined in neonatal and maturing rat hearts [21]. mRNA increased after birth and remained elevated in the adult. Transcripts were localised to cardiomyocytes by in-situ hybridisation and immunoreactive TGF ß localised in the intracellular compartment at the light and electron microscope level. The variability in TGF ß localisation makes direct inferences about its role in relation to specific cell types difficult. This could be due to a variety of factors and in consequence several studies have focussed on isolated cardiac myocytes. Kardami [22, and see Section 2 in this volume] demonstrated that TGFß prevented proliferation of neonatal myocytes and inhibited DNA synthesis. This was in contrast to that of bFGF and indeed, TGFß cancelled the proliferative action of bFGF. Further evidence that myocytes are targets for TGFß and other growth factors has come from the studies of Parker and co-workers [23] who noted a re-expression of the 'fetal' contractile gene program which could be modified by the fibroblast growth factors. These transitions are similar to those following haemodynamic overload. This finding suggests that cardiac protein isoforms which have been shown to undergo well defined transitions during both development and haemodynamic overload [24,25] may be linked in some way to growth factor expression perhaps by sharing regulatory gene elements involved in cell proliferation and growth [7].

Evidence for cardiac fibroblast growth factors

The evidence that FGF's are expressed in the heart is better established [26], particularly with regard to their role in angiogenic processes [27]. Moreover, both aFGF and bFGF have been confirmed in isolated adult rat myocytes, [28]. Of particular interest is the finding that along with both aFGF and bFGF, TGFß is co-localised in the rat heart during embryonic and neonatal develpment [29]. This might suggest that as with the studies on isolated myocytes [22] there is a co-ordinated role for these growth factors which may act in an antithetical manner in the heart. The wide distribution of all three growth factors throughout the heart in the above study [29] contrasted with findings from the chick embryo in which immunostaining for bFGF protein was confined to the myocyte and decreased with development [30]. Co-localisation of aFGF peptide and fibroblast growth factor receptor (*flg*) transcripts to the developing fetal myocyte by immunocytochemistry, immunoelectron microscopy and in-situ hybridisation has been reported by Engelmann and co-workers [31]. Although localisation was observed in the neonatal / mature myocyte both *flg* mRNA and peptide were detected in non-muscle cell types. Of interest is the finding that bFGF has been localised to cardiac gap-junctions suggesting a possible role in cell-cell communication [32] .

As with TGF ß several studies to determine FGF localisation have been conducted on isolated cardiac myocytes. In general these have not provided conclusive evidence for a specific and unambiguous cell location. This may relate to the fact that FGF's are widely accepted to be located in the extra-cellular matrix. The fact that FGF's do not have classical N-terminal signalling sequences seen in secreted proteins that are extracellularly active [34] raises the question as to which cells they are synthesised in and how they might exert intracellular actions.

Whatever the cardiac location of the FGF's, studies in several laboratories, including the authors have quantitatively determined significant levels of FGF protein in the heart. Adult porcine, canine and bovine hearts were used to prepare between 100-500ug of purified aFGF / kg fresh heart which almost certainly underestimates the in vivo content [33,35]. Between 6-13 μg of purified bFGF /kg was isolated from bovine hearts in the same study [35]. Support for this underestimation in content comes from studies in the authors own laboratory which have indicated that bFGF content of the adult bovine myocardium is at least 300 μg /kg [36]. When fresh isolated myocytes have been examined, aFGF levels of 30-36ng / 10^6 cells and bFGF levels of 13ng / 10^6 cells have been reported [37].

Although in the case of TGFß it is possible to compare the cellular localisation of both the protein and mRNA by immunocytochemistry and in-situ hybridisation respectively, this is far more problematical in the case of both aFGF and bFGF. In common with the mRNA's for other members of the FGF superfamily they are very difficult to detect by conventional techniques, certainly in a quantitative fashion. This is mainly due to the very low number of mRNA copies present in vivo although whether this reflects the preparative situation or is due to rapid turnover and degradation is not clear. Confirmation of this anomaly comes from the studies of Speir and co-workers [37] who were able to clearly identify significant levels of bFGF protein in freshly isolated myocytes by mitogen assays with immunoneutralization, immunoblotting and radioimmmunoassay but were unable to detect bFGF mRNA by in-situ hybridisation. Unusually, after culturing of the myocytes bFGF mRNA was detectable. Whether this was due to release of some inhibitory molecule during culturing, the effects of medium or from co-existing non-myocyte cells is not clear. In cases where it has been possible to detect mRNA for the FGF's by conventional Northern hybridisation there appears to be agreement that the sizes are similar to those observed in other tissues at 3.8 Kb for aFGF and 7.1Kb for bFGF [38]. Using techniques which rely on hybridisation in solution, such as RNase protection analysis it has been possible to identify aFGF in the rat heart [39] although obviously with no indication as to size. bFGF mRNA was not detectable while in skeletal muscle the aFGF signal exceeded that of the detectable bFGF.

Evidence that both aFGF and bFGF are potent mitogens for isolated neonatal cardiac myocytes is well established although the degree of activity depends on a number of factors including serum conditions. Kardami [22] has demonstrated that bFGF in increasing concentrations enhances tritiated thymidine incorporation in both atrial and ventricular myocytes. This effect is inhibited in the presence of additional and comparable concentrations of TGFß while tri-iodothyronine has little or no effect. Similar results are observed when myocyte proliferation itself is examined as opposed to only DNA synthetic capacity [22]. Protein expression is also modified by FGF treatment of isolated myocytes. As with TGFß there are marked changes in the isoforms of some of the major contractile proteins. aFGF and bFGF both caused down-regulation of alpha myosin heavy chain mRNA and up-regulation of beta myosin heavy chain and alpha smooth muscle actin [23]. However, the two growth factors did not always exhibit identical effects. While aFGF down regulated alpha cardiac and skeletal actin mRNA's, bFGF had no effect on alpha cardiac actin and up regulated alpha skeletal actin mRNA. These changes are broadly similar to those seen in vivo in the adult following hemodynamic overload and mirror the effects of TGFß. The divergent response of alpha skeletal actin to aFGF and bFGF are dealt with at length in Section Two.

Expression of growth factor isoforms

One possible explanation for the inconsistencies in effects observed by the same growth factor in different systems could be due to the presence of different isoforms. It is well established as indicated previously that TGF ß exists as several different isoforms, certainly at least five. In many cases the precise distribution of these isoforms in the heart is not clear. Moreover, in studies on isolated cardiac myocytes, the effects of each of the different isoforms has not been clearly studied. TGFß also occurs in a high molecular weight latent complex in vivo. In the case of TGF ß1 in human platelets, this takes the form of a TGF ß1 molecule non-covalently associated with a disulphide-bonded complex of a dimer of the N-terminal propeptide of the TGF ß1 precursor and a third component denoted the TGF ß1 binding protein [8,40]. Certainly there is no doubt that the isoforms exhibit different biological activities [41].

aFGF and bFGF are also known to exist in a number of different isoforms. In the case of bFGF these are well established N-terminally extended forms which may display differential cell locations and developmental and physiological regulation [42,43,44,45].

Physiopathological role of TGFß and the FGF's

FGF's and TGFß are now known to be implicated in several areas of repair and regeneration after cardiac injury. The FGF's in particular are established as important mediators of angiogenesis. Exogenously added bFGF has been shown to enhance the recovery of blood flow after acute arterial occlusion in a rat model of severe hind limb ischemia [46]. The exact role of bFGF in the development of the collateral circulation in this model was not clear. However it was suggested that endothelial cell derived bFGF might influence platelet-derived growth factor mRNA which in turn was required for smooth muscle cell proliferation and media growth and thus collateral development. Alternatively, degradation following arterial occlusion in this model could have released extracellular matrix-bound bFGF [46]. Certainly bFGF is known to modify the proliferative and migratory capacity of endothelial cells and recent findings have demonstrated an ability of bFGF to upregulate the biosynthesis of specific integrins [47]. Moreover there was a differential regulation of other members of the integrin family by TGFß suggesting a coordinated role for these two growth factors in influencing interactions of microvascular endothelial cells with the extracellular matrix during neovascularization [47]. In contrast, after baloon catheter injury of the rat carotid artery [48], administration of neutralizing antibodies to bFGF failed to stop the chronic smooth muscle cell proliferation commonly seen after this damage suggesting that bFGF was not the major mitogen involved.

TGF ß has also been implicated in processes of repair following myocardial injury. TGF ß is up-regulated at both the protein and mRNA level in myocytes at the margin of experimentally infarcted areas in the rat between 24 and 48 hours after coronary artery ligation [49]. Normal ventricular myocytes stained strongly with TGFß1 antibody but this staining decreased in myocytes in the infarct zone within 1 hour of coronary artery ligation and had disappeared after 6 hours. Between 6 and 24 hours there was increased staining in viable myocytes which reached a maximum after 48 hours. This then persisted for up to 10 weeks after infarction. The normal 2.4 Kb TGFß1 mRNA transcript which was detected prior to infarction was present in addition to a 1.9 Kb transcript after infarction in the infarct zone only [48]. Similar staining of cardiac myocytes has been observed after coronary artery ligation in pigs [21]. However immunoblotting in this latter study showed a single band of 25 Kd both before and after ligation with no difference in the intensity of the signal. Two mRNA transcripts of 2.4 and 3.5 Kb were seen in control and infarcted hearts but the level of the larger transcript increased after infarction [21].

TGFß has also been demonstrated to prevent severe cardiac injury when injected i.v. immediately before or after experimental myocardial ischaemia [50]. In this respect it may be that the inhibition of superoxide radical formation by TGFß, which in turn preserves endothelial function may play a critical role in this protective effect [51]. While these findings might imply that the role of TGFß requires some form of cellular damage, perhaps via release of the growth factor from the extracellular matrix, it is clear from recent studies on stressed myocardium without injury that TGFß may play a more fundamental role in normal adaptive growth. Villareal and Dillman have found that mRNA levels of TGF-ß1 are increased 12 hours after experimental pressure-overload cardiac hypertrophy in the rat and that this preceedes increases for the extracellular matrix proteins fibronectin and collagen [52].

Conclusions

In the past few years there have been major advances in establishing a role for growth factor expression in the heart and the transforming and fibroblast growth factors have been key players in this field. Notwithstanding these advances far more questions have been raised than answered. There is still controversy as to their presence in, and association with the myocyte and in turn whether they play a role in normal or abnormal growth processes. Almost certainly they will be an integral part of the signalling process for this and other cells and for a variety of physiological functions. Future studies should establish their precise importance.

Acknowledgements

The authors work is supported by grants from the British Heart Foundation.

References

1.   Zak R, Kizu A, Bugaisky L. Cardiac hypertrophy: Its characteristics as a growth process. Amer J Cardiol 1979; 44: 941-946.

2.   Marino TA, Haldar S, Williamson EC, Beaverson K et al. Proliferating cell nuclear antigen in developing and adult rat cardiac muscle cells. Circ Res 1991; 69: 1353-1360.

3.   Rumyantsev P P. Interrelations of the proliferation and differentiation processes during cardiac myogenesis and regeneration. Int Rev Cytol 1977; 51: 187-273.

4.   Oberpriller J O. Nuclear characteristics of cardiac myocytes following the proliferative response to the mincing of the myocardium in the adult newt, Notophthalmus viridescens. Cell Tissue Res 1988; 253: 619-624.

5.   Field L J. Atrial natriuretic factor-SV 40 T antigen transgenes produce tumors and cardiac arrhythmias in mice. Science 1988; 239; 1029-1033.

6.   Schneider MD, Parker TG. Cardiac myocytes as targets for the action of peptide growth factors. Circulation 1990; 81: 1443-1456.

7.   Long CS, Kariya K, Karns L, Simpson PC. Trophic factors for cardiac myocytes. J Hypertension 1990; 8: Suppl. 7; S219-S224.

8.   Massague J. The transforming growth factor-ß family. Ann Rev Biochem 1990; 6: 597-641

9.   Florini J R, Magri K A. Effects of growth factors on myogenic differentiation. Am J Physiol 1989; 25: C701-C711.

10.   Florini J R. Hormonal control of muscle growth. Muscle and Nerve 1987; 10: 577-598.

11.   Baird A, Bohlen P. Fibroblast growth factors. 1990 In: Peptide growth factors and their receptors. Sporn MM, Roberts AB. eds Handbook of Exp Pharm 95; 369-418.

12.   Folkman J, Klagsbrun M. Angiogenic factors. Science 1987; 235: 442-447.

13.   Thompson NL, Flanders KC, Smith JM et al. Expression of transforming growth factor-beta 1 in specific cells and tissues of adult and neonatal mice. J Cell Biol 1989; 108: 661-669.

14.   Pelton RW, Saxena B, Jones M, Moses HL, Gold LI. Immunohistochemical localisation of transforming growth factor-ß1, 2 and 3 in the mouse embryo - expression patterns suggest multiple roles during embryonic development. J Cell Biol 1991; 115: 1091-1105.

15.   Schmid P, Cox D, Bilbe G, Maier R, Mcmaster GK. Differential expression of transforming growth factor ß1, 2 and 3 genes during mouse embryogenesis. Development 1991; 111: 117-130.

16.   Millan FA, Denhez F, Kondaiah P, Akhurst RJ. Embryonic gene expression patterns of transforming growth factor ß1, 2 and 3 suggest different developmental functions in-vivo. Development 1991; 111: 131-144.

17. Eghbali M. Cellular origin and diistribution of transforming growth factor-ß1 in the normal rat myocardium. Cell Tissue Res 1989; 256: 553-558.

18. Potts JD, Runyan RB. Epithelial-mesenchymal cell transformation in the heart can be mediated, in part, by transforming growth factor ß. Dev Biol 1989; 134: 392-401

19. Heine UI, Burmester JK, Flanders KC, Danielpour D, Munoz Ef, Roberts AB, Sporn MB. Localisation of transforming growth factor ß1 in mitochondria of murine heart and liver. Cell Regulation 1991; 2: 467-477.

20. Engelmann GL, Boehm KD, Birchenhall-Roberts MC, Ruscetti FW. Transforming growth factor-beta1 in heart development. Mechanisms of Development 1992; 38: 85-98.

21. Wunsch M, Sharma HS, Markert T, Bernotat-Danielowski S, Schott RJ, Kremer P, Bleese N, Schaper W. In-situ localisation of transforming growth factor-ß in porcine heart: enhanced expression after chronic coronary artery constriction. J Mol Cell Cardiol 1991; 23: 1051-1062.

22. Kardami E. Stimulation and inhibition of cardiac myocyte proliferation in vitro. Mol Cell Biochem 1990; 92: 129-135.

23. Parker TG, Schneider MD. Peptide growth factors can provoke 'fetal' contractile protein gene expression in rat cardiac myocytes. J Clin Invest 1990; 85: 507-514.

24. Cummins P. Transitions in human atrial and ventricular myosin light-chain isoenzymes in response to cardiac pressure overload-induced hypertrophy. Biochem J 1982; 205: 195-204.

25. Cummins P, Lambert J. Myosin transitions in the human and bovine heart: A developmental and anatomical study of heavy and light chain subunits in the atrium and ventricle. Circ Res 1986; 58: 846-858.

26. Parlow MH, Bolender DL, Kokan-Moore NP, Lough J. Localization of bFGF-like proteins as punctate inclusions in the preseptation myocardium of the chicken embryo. Dev Biol 1991; 146: 139-147

27. Banai S, Kaklitsch MT, Casscells W, Shou M, Shrivastav S, Correa R, Epstein SE, Unger EF. Effects of acidic fibroblast growth factor on normal and ischemic myocardium. Circ Res 1991; 69: 76-85.

28. Speir E, Yi-Fu Z, Lee M et al. Fibroblast growth factors are present in adult cardiac myocytes, in vivo. Biochem Biophys Res Commun 1988; 157: 1336-1340.

29. Spirito P, Fu Y-M, Yu Z-X, Epstein SE, Casscells W. Immunohistochemical localisation of basic and acidic fibroblast growth factors in the developing rat heart. Circulation 1991; 84: 322-332.

30.   Cosigli SA, Joseph-Silverstein J. Immunolocalisation of basic fibroblast growth factor during chicken cardiac development. J Cell Physiol 1991; 146: 379-385.

31.   Engelmann GL, Dionne CA, Jaye MC. Acidic fibroblast growth factor and heart development. Circ Res 1993; 72: 7-19.

32.   Kardami E, Stoski RM, Doble BW, Yamamoto T, Hertzberg EL, Nagy JI. Biochemical and ultrastructural evidence for the association of basic fibroblast growth factor with cardiac gap junctions. J Biol Chem 1991; 266: 19551-19557.

33.   Sasaki H, Hoshi H, Hong Y-M et al. Purification of acidic fibroblast growth factor from bovine heart and its localization in the cardiac myocytes. J Biol Chem 1989; 264: 17606-17612.

34.   Weiner HL, Swain JL. Acidic fibroblast growth factor mRNA is expressed by cardiac myocytes in culture and the protein is localized to the extracellular matrix. Proc Nat Acad Sci USA 1989; 86: 2683-2687.

35.   Quinkler W, Maasberg M, Bernotat-Danielowski S. Isolation of heparin-binding growth factors from bovine, porcine and canine hearts. Eur J Biochem 1989; 181: 67-73.

36.   Cummins P, Logan A, Cummins B. Basic fibroblast growth factor in the developing bovine heart. Biochem Soc Trans 1991; 19: 79S.

37.   Speir E, Tanner V, Gonzalez AM, Farris J, Baird A, Casscells W. Acidic and basic fibroblast growth factors in adult rat heart myocytes. Circ Res 1992; 71: 251-259.

38.   Cummins P, Beestone S, Chilton D. Fibroblast growth factor mRNA and protein expression in the developing heart. Eur Heart J 1991; 12: Suppl. 210

39.   Moore JW, Dionne C, Jaye M, Swain JL. The messenger RNA's encoding aFGF, bFGF and FGF receptor are coordinately downregulated during myogenic differentiation. Development 1991; 111: 741-748

40.   Kanzaki T, Olofsson A, Moren A, Wernstedt C et al. TGF-ß1 binding protein: A component of the large latent complex of TGF-ß1 with multiple repeat. Cell 1990; 61: 1051-1061.

41.   Danielpour D, Sporn MB. Differential inhibition of TGF-ß1 and TGF-ß2 activity by alpha-2 macroglobulin. J Cell Biochem 1989; 13B: 84-88.

42.   Giordano S, Sherman L, Lyman W, Morrison R. Multiple molecular weight forms of basic fibroblast growth factor are developmentally regulated in the central nervous system. Dev Biol 1992; 152: 293-303.

43.   Liu L, Kardami E. Hypothyroidism favors expression of high molecular weight basic FGF in the heart. J Cell Biochem 1991; Suppl. 15C: 171

44. Burgess WH, Maciag T. The heparin-binding fibroblast growth factor family of proteins. Ann Rev Biochem 1989; 58: 575-606

45. Cummins P, Chilton DC, Beestone S. Evidence for changes in acidic fibroblast growth factor peptides in the heart. J Cell Biochem 1993; 17D,219.

46. Chleboun JO, Martins RN, Mitchell CA, Chirila TV. bFGF enhances the development of the collateral circulation after acute arterial occlusion. Biochem Biophys Res Commun 1992; 185: 510-516.

47. Enenstein J, Waleh NS, Kramer RH. Basic FGF and TGF-ß differentially modulate integrin expression of human microvascular endothelial cells. Exp Cell Res 1992; 203: 499-503.

48. Olsen NE, Chao S, Lindner V, Reidy MA. Intimal smooth muscle cell proliferation after baloon catheter injury. Am J Path 1992; 140: 1017-1023.

49. Thompson NL, Bazoberry F, Speir EH et al. Transforming growth factor beta-1 in acute myocardial infarction in rats. Growth Factors 1988; 1: 91-99

50. Lefer AM, Tsao P, Aoki N et al. Mediation of cardioprotection by transforming growth factor beta. Science 1990; 249: 61-64

51. Lefer AM. Mechanism of the protective effects of transforming growth factor-ß in reperfusion injury. Biochem Pharmacol 1991; 42: 1323-1327

52. Villareal FJ, Dillmann WH. Cardiac hypertrophy-induced changes in mRNA levels for TGF-ß1, fibronectin and collagen. Am. J. Physiol. 1992; 262: H1861-H1866.

3. Growth factors and the cardiac extra-cellular matrix

LYDIE RAPPAPORT and JANE LISE SAMUEL

Introduction

The extracellular matrix (ECM) provides physical support to the tissue and plays an important role in the regulation of cellular function. It is a complex mesh of fibrillar collagens types I III, and V which associate directly with cells *via* membrane receptors or indirectly through basement membrane components such as fibronectin (FN), laminin, collagen type IV and proteoglycans [1]. Laminin, FN and collagen type IV contain specific sequences (RDG and YGSR sequences) which interact with integrins that are integral membrane proteins, thereby establishing a tight connection between the cells and ECM [2]. FN itself is present in both ECM and basal membrane, and either originates from the plasma (pFN) by exsudation at local sites or is synthetised locally by the tissular cells (cFN) [2]. Different isoforms of cFN originate from a single primary transcript by alternative splicing which is regulated during development [3,4,5] and pathological situations [4,6].

Several studies suggest that proteins of the ECM or trapped in the ECM (growth factors) can alter cellular growth and, either alone or in combination, be mitogenic. For instance some ECM components immobilize growth factors such as acidic and basic fibroblast growth factors (aFGF, bFGF), and transforming growth factors ß (TGFß 1,2, and 3) which are produced during ontogenic development [7,8] or pathological situations such as tissular regeneration and healing [9,10]. TGFßs stimulate specifically the transcription of FN gene in fibroblasts, but the cell growth is also stimulated by the fibronectin as well [11]. Some ECM components such as laminin contain growth factor peptide

32

sequence [12] which may be released by ECM-degrading enzymes; the genes coding for these enzymes are among the early genes activated by some of the growth factors such as bFGF (review in [8])

In this chapter the interactions between ECM components and growth factors (mainly TGFß) in the cardiovascular system during development and physiopathological situations will be considered and discuss in the light of what is known in other tissues and systems.

Extracellular matrix and growth factors in adult myocardium

The distribution and organization of the different ECM components in the heart are now well established (Figure 1) [1,13] but the function of

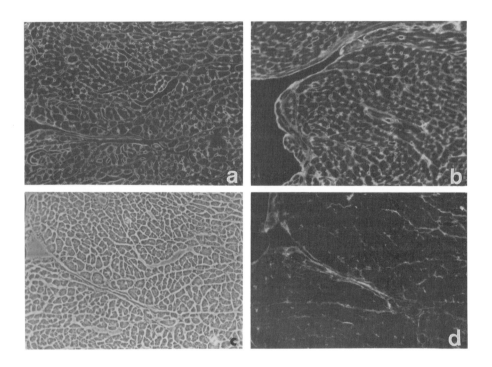

Figure 1. Distribution of laminin (a) FN (b), collagen I-III (d) in normal heart section. (c) is normal phase contrast image. (reprinted from [13] with permission)

each component is not yet completely understood. The fibrillar collagen network serves to maintain the architecture and the alignment of myocytes during the contraction cycle and to facilitate the transmission of myocyte-generated force to the ventricular chambers (review in [14]). Of equal importance, are the extracellular fluid, intercellular substances and ions essential for cell viability which constitute the interstitium. Fibronectin is distributed in a reticular pattern demonstrating a pericellular, pericapillary and interstitial location (Fig 1). Laminin and collagen IV surround the capillaries and the myocytes as well as the smooth muscle cells. Cardiac fibroblasts and smooth muscle cells (SMC) are mainly responsible for the synthesis collagen I and III and fibronectin while laminin and collagen type IV are synthetised by cardiomyocytes [1,15]. TGFß (Review in [7]), bFGF (16) aFGF., [17] are expressed by cardiac myocytes and others cells and stored in high amounts into the surrounding ECM and basement membranes being bound to heparan sulfate. Little is known about the regulation of the ECM component synthesis in adult heart .

In blood vessels, the media and the intima elaborate a complex and highly ordered ECM, the major constituents of which fibronectin, elastin, collagen type I and laminin, are produced by SMC [18]. A likely function of TGFß1 during the neointima formation is the stimulation of ECM synthesis by SMC [19,20].

Extracellular matrix and growth factors during cardiovascular ontogenic development.

There is now evidence that ECM and growth factors act as signals in epithelial-mesenchymental transformation that occurs during cardiogenesis (Review in [21]). Mesenchymal cells secrete fibrillar collagens and fibronectin and their membranes contain integrins. During developmental growth, collagens are believed to be continuously deposited into the extracellular matrix, which is increasingly stabilized by covalent cross-linking throughout life. There are marked age-related changes in the rates of collagen metabolism; it is still actively synthesized in old animals, but degradation rates increase from 5 to 96% with age so that the bulk of collagens produced in old rats is destined to be degraded [22].

The accumulation of FN mRNAs and the expression of the embryonic forms (EIIIA+ or EIIIB+) appear specifically regulated during the ontogenic development of the rat myocardium. At an early stage (11 d pc) FN mRNA levels are very high in the myocardium and progressively decrease afterwards. The 2 embryonic forms, FNEIIIA+ and FNEIIIB+, are abundant particularly in the endothelium, in vessels and in areas rich in non muscle cells (trabeculae) and almost absent within the ventricular wall during life *in utero*. After birth the 2 embryonic forms decrease rapidly and are undectable in 3 week-old animals [23,24]. Quantitation of the relative amounts of the 2 embryonic mRNAs confirms that both embryonic forms are highly expressed in fetus and progressively decrease with age to attain undetectable (FNEIIIB+) or very low levels (FNEIIIA+) in adult (Rappaport, unpublished data; [5]) The FN is particularly abundant at the crest of the developing interventricular septum [25] during the early stage of development. After birth, FNEIIIA+ that is poorly expressed in the rat myocardium and vessels may accumulate in the intima of human arteries [4]. Presumably changes in the expression of the ECM proteins, and the developmental regulations of ECM binding proteins, determine the adhesive preference of cardiomyocytes for ECM components; neonatal myocytes attach to collagen as well as other ECM proteins while adult cells do not attach to both collagen and fibronectin [26].

The synthesis of ECM proteins and processes of cell differentiation in cardiovascular systems may depend on growth factors as in other systems. Indeed a large body of evidence suggests that TGFßs are initiators of inductive interactions and of many cellular activities critical for morphogenesis (cell proliferation, migration, differentiation, ECM production), (reviews in [7,27]). TGFß has been shown to 1) activate directly the transcription of the collagen and fibronectin genes; stabilize some ECM mRNA, and increase synthesis and secretion of collagens, fibronectin, elastin, and proteoglycans; 2) increase the transcription, translation and processing of ECM receptors, and 3) decrease the synthesis of ECM-degrading enzymes and increase synthesis of protease inhibitors that block the activity of these enzymes [7,28]. The multiple levels at which TGFß acts suggest that the control interactions between ECM and cells may represent one of the principal mechanisms by which the peptide controls growth, differentiation and ultimately the function of mesenchymal cells. Both extracts of ECM and conditioned medium from myocardial cultures stimulate the formation of cardiac mesenchyme (review in [21]; mainly TGFß3 but also TGFß1 are found to be required for the mesenchymal induction (reviews in [7,21]). Moreover Armstrong and Armstrong [29] followed myocyte and mesenchymal cell segregation in tissue culture and demonstrated the role of both FN and TGFßs: the ECM composition elaborated by the cardiac mesenchyme exerts an important influence on the mutual organization of the two tissues: tissue segregation is promoted by a

FN-rich ECM, whereas a poor ECM development favors tissue invasion. Deposition of an ECM enriched by FN is stimulated by fetal serum or TGFß. During chicken heart development, TGFß1 is present at time and locations consistent with an inductive function at early stages and a function of up-regulation of fibronectin-rich ECM which then stimulates mesenchyme cell proliferation [21,30]. The ECM production appears as a sufficient stimulus for cell proliferation and would act as the adhesive support for cellular anchorage [30].

Beside myocardial morphogenesis, angiogenesis must also involve a high degree of regulation of ECM formation. In the mouse, mutations interfering with the collagen transcription yield a developmentaly lethal phenotype associated with impaired vascular integrity [31]. In the smooth muscle cells of the large arteries (aorta and coronary arteries) the accumulation of FGF is intense at early stages of development but becomes faint or negative with increasing cell differentiation (review in [8]) while FN-EIIIA and-EIIIB mRNAs level remain high until birth [24].

The expression of growth factors or ECM constituents during development of the cardiovascular system strongly suggests that the processes of cell proliferation, differentiation and migration depend on the composition of ECM, which is directly correlated to growth factor expressions and is regulated by the specific changes in the expression of various isoforms of both growth factors (TGFßs) and ECM proteins (FN, collagens).

Extracellular matrix and growth factors in pathological situations

Growth factors and ECM components appear to play also a major role in numerous pathological situations implicating repair of injuried tissues as well as neoangiogenesis and hypertrophy.

ECM and growth factors during angiogenesis and cardiac injury repair

After coronary occlusion in the rat, c-FN is synthetized and deposited in the zone of myocardial infarction, the accumulation of p-FN preceeding that of c-FN ([32,33]; the process is similar to that observed in any tissular healing. TGFß1 may play a role since it accumulates in the myocytes located at the border area of infarction [9] and in hypoperfused myocardial area [34] The changes implicating directly growth factors and ECM occur at the level of the vessels. Indeed

TGF-ß1 prevents cardiac injury secondary to ischemia, perhaps by alleviating vascular damages mediated by increases in circulating tumor necrosis factor [35]. TGF-ß may also act directly on ECM protein expression during angiogenesis since it modulates the FN alternative splicing by cultured endothelial cells which increase IIICS+ containing FN [36]. The peptide is also involved in modulating the attachment and migration of these cells [2]. bFGF, as an autocrine factor, may direct endothelial cells and fibroblasts at the site of neovascularization to break down the extracellular scaffolding -by increasing the release of ECM-degrading enzymes- in an effort to facilitate the formation of new vessels but eventually participate in the processes to stimulate tissular repair by stimulating collagen, FN and proteoglycan productions as well as the synthesis of inhibitors of ECM degradation (review in [8]). The switches of capillary endothelial cells between phases of growth, quiescence differentiation, or involution in the presence of a constant FGF concentration must depend upon the adhesivity or mechanical integrity of their extracellular matrix [37].

In injured rat carotid arteries smooth muscle cells (SMC) produce TGFß1 during neointima formation *in vivo*. The increase in TGFß-1 transcripts precedes and accompanies intimal thickening and is correlated with an increased expression of FN, and collagen I, and III genes [10]. TGFß1 could contribute to neointimal thickening after injury in two ways: (a) stimulation of SMC proliferation [38] and chemotaxis [19], possibly *via* local induction of other growth factor synthesis (PDGF-AA) and (b) stimulation of ECM accumulation [10]. Human atheromas accumulate also extracellular matrix proteins such as collagen types I and III. It is proposed that the formation of a neointima in injured arteries is related to the transition from contractile to synthetic SMC resulting in cell proliferation and production of a new ECM, both processes being under the dependence of growth factors.

ECM, growth factors and cardiac hypertrophy:

ECM components accumulate in myocardium and arteries of heart submitted to an increased arterial pressure [13,14,23,39,40]. Among the early responses of the myocardium to pressure overload is a prompt rise in the accumulation of FN and collagens I,III, IV mRNAs [23,41,42,43]. Both the expression of FN mRNA [41,42] and accumulation of the protein [13] precede the expression of mRNAs and accumulation of collagen I-III in ischemic areas. FN also accumulates in both the media and the adventitia of coronaries arteries, but not in the veins of animals with either spontaneously or induced hypertension suggesting the role of factors either mechanical or humoral induced by increased perfusion pressure [23]. The collagens accumulate mainly in the perivascular areas and the triggering event was proposed to be the rise in aldosterone level (review in [14]). Using cultured cardiac fibroblasts, Carver et al [44] demonstrated that cyclic mechanical stretch induces an increased accumulation of collagen III mRNA, however the synergistic role of endogeneous growth factors or hormones cannot be excluded. The pattern of expression of FN is unique in that FN-EIIIA+ and -EIIIB+ mRNA which are undectable in the adult heart, are reexpressed within arterial media (Figure 2) and ischemic ventricular areas where an important tissular remodeling occurs. Both forms are thus associated with medial hypertrophy and myocardial repair [23]. These increased expressions of collagens and FN are probably

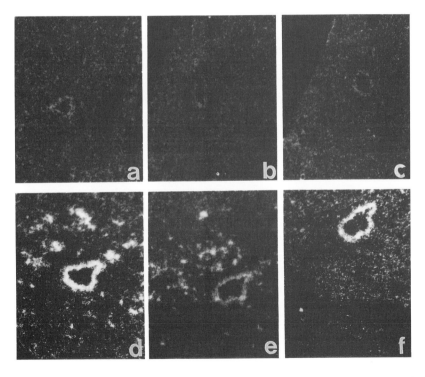

Figure 2. FN type I (a,d), -EIIIA+ (b,e), -EIIIB+ (c,f) mRNA accumulations within coronary arteries 24 h after aortic stenosis (d,e,f). Note the absence of signal in normal heart (a,b,c).

dependent on a TGF-ß activity since *in vivo* the marked increase in TGF-ß1 mRNA precedes the collagen and FN mRNA accumulations [41].

In vitro TGFß increase also the accumulation of procollagen mRNA in quiescent cultured rabbit cardiac fibroblasts but has no effect on the early gene expression, as the transcriptional regulator Egr-I, and the proto-oncogenes, c-fos and c-jun. Thus the increased TGF-ß1 level in the hypertrophying myocardium may have an important role in the regulation of collagen biosynthesis and the development of fibrosis, independently of the fibroblastic response to immediate growth enhancing events that accompany cardiac hypertrophy [45]. The TGF-ß treatment of cultured human fibroblasts preferentially increases the expression of the FN-EIIIB+ [46,47].Therefore, TGF-ßs control ECM composition and function, not only by increasing the accumulation of FN and collagens but also by modifying the relative amount of the different isoforms through the modulation of both FN pre-mRNA splicing and pre-mRNA encoding for other ECM proteins, with a consequent heigthened expression of isoforms which may have specific biological functions. It cannot be excluded that TGFßs modify also adhesive properties of cells since hypertrophied adult myocytes increase their collagen receptor number and then are able to attach to collagen type I and III [1].

Conclusions

The cardiac extracellular matrix provides a critical interface between a cell and its environment. There is a dynamic reciprocity between the extracellular matrix and the intracellular cytoskeleton and the nuclear matrix with each controlling the other [48,49]. Many growth factors are regulators of the formation and destruction of the ECM, and it is becoming clear that ECM can affect cell growth and differentiation not only by the direct attachment of its component molecules to receptors on the cell's surface, but also by binding and/or activating other molecules, like TGF-ß and bFGF (Review in [20]). FN interacts with many ECM molecules and is likely to contribute importantly to the structural organization of embryonic matrix, in addition to its role as a cell adhesion molecule (review in [2]). Laminin is a significant substratum for mesenchymal cell migration [50] and may together with collagen and fibronectin promote differentiation by mechanisms involving indirect effects on the cytoskeleton or direct effects on gene expression.

Peptide growth factors are critical determinants of almost every aspect of hypertrophying heart, tissular responses to injury and the ensuing processes that involve cell migration, angiogenesis and fibrosis. ECM proteins and particularly fibronectin modulate cell responsiveness to growth factors and one possible mechanism may be the altered adhesive interactions and subsequent tensile forces generated within intracellular cytoskeleton [48].

Acknowledgements

The authors wish to thank F Contard, F Faradian, F Marotte, P Oliviero and A Barrieux for their helpful participation. The work was supported by INSERM and CNRS.

References

1. Terracio L, TK Borg. Factors affecting cardiac cell shape. Heart Failure 1988; 4: 114-124
2. Hynes RO. In: Rich A. editor. Fibronectins. Berlin, Springer Verlag 1990; 1-545.
3. ffrench-Constant C, Hynes RO. Alternative splicing of fibronectin is temporally and spatially regulated in chicken embryos. Development 1989; 106:375-388.
4. Glukhova MA, Frid MG, Shekhonin BV, Vasilevskaya TD, Grunwald J, Saginati M, Koteliansky VE. Expression of extra domain A fibronectin sequence in vascular smooth muscle type is phenotype dependent. J Cell Biol 1989; 109: 357-363.
5. Magnuson VL, Young M, Schattenberg DG, Mancini MA, Chen D, Klebe RJ. The alternative splicing of fibronectin pre-mRNA is altered during aging and in response to growth factors. J Biol Chem 1991; 266:14654-14662.
6. ffrench-Constant C, Van De Water L, Dvorak HF, Hynes RO. Reappearance of an embryonic pattern of fibronectin splicing during wound healing in the adult rat. J Cell Biol 1989; 109: 903-914.
7. Roberts AB, Sporn MB. The transforming growth factor-ßs. In Peptide Growth Factors and their Receptors (MB Sporn and AB Roberts, eds) Springer Verlag NY; 1991,vol I, pp 419-472.
8. Baird A, Böhlen P. Fibroblast growth factors. In: Sporn MB, Roberts AB, editors. Peptide Growth Factors and their Receptors. Springer Verlag NY; 1991; 1: 369-418.

9. Thompson NL, Bazoberry F, Speir EH, Casscells W, Ferrans VJ, Flanders KC, Kondaiah P, Geiser AG, Sporn MB. Transforming growth factor beta-1 in acute myocardial infarction in rats. Growth Factors 1988; 1: 91-99.

10. Majesky MW, Lindner V, Twardzik DR, Schwartz SM, Reidy MA. Production of transforming growth factor ß1 during repair of arterial injury. J Clin Invest 1991; 88: 904-910.

11. Ignotz RA, Massague J. Transforming growth factor-ß stimulates the expression of fibronectin and collagen and their incorporation into extracellular matrix. J Biol Chem 1986; 261: 4337-4345

12. Kanemoto T, Reich R , Royce L, Greatorex D, Adler SH, Shiraishi N, Martin GR, Yamada Y, Kleinman HK. Identification of an amino acid sequence from the laminin A chain that stimulate metastasis and collagen IV production. Proc Natl Acad Sci USA 1990; 87: 2279-2283.

13. Contard F, Koteliansky V, Marotte F, Dubus I, Rappaport L, Samuel JL. Specific alterations in the distribution of extracellular matrix components within rat myocardium during the development of pressure overload. Lab Invest 1991; 64: 65-75.

14. Weber KT. Cardiac Interstitium: Extracellular Space of the myocarium. In: Fozzard HA. et al editors, The Heart and the Cardiovascular system. Raven Press NY 1992; 2: 1466-1480.

15. Eghbali M, Czaja M, Zeydel FR, Weiner MA, Zern S, Seifter S, Blumenfeld OO. Collagen chain mRNAs in isolated heart cells from young and adult rats. J Mol Cell Cardiol 1988; 20: 267-276.

16. Kardami E, Fandrich RR. Basic fibroblast growth factor in atria and ventricles of the vertebrate heart. J Cell Biol 1989; 109:1865-1873

17. Weiner HL, Swain JL. Acidic fibroblast growth factor mRNA is expressed by cardiac myocytes and the protein is localized to the extra cellular matrix. PNAS 1989; 86: 2683- 2687.

18. Snow AD, Bolender RP, Wight TN, Clowes AW. Heparin modulates the composition of the extracellular matrix domain surrounding arterial smooth muscle cells. Am J Pathol 1990; 137:313-330.

19. Liau G, Chan LM. Regulation of extracellular matrix RNA levels in cultured smooth muscle cells: relationship to cellular quiescence. J Biol Chem 1989; 261; 4337-4345.

20. Chen JK, Hoschi H, McKeehan WL. Transforming growth factors type ß specifically stimulates synthesis of proteoglycans in human adult arterial smooth muscle cells. Proc Natl Acad Sci USA 1987; 84: 5287-5391.

21. Hay ED. Collagen and other matrix glycoproteins in embryogenesis. In: Hay ED editor. Cell Biology of Extracellular Matrix. 2nd edition, Plenum Press NY 1991; 419-462.

22. May PK , Mcanulty RJ, Campa JS, Laurent GA. Age-related changes in collagen synthesis and degradation of newly synthetized collagen in regulating collagen production. Biochemical J 1991; 276: 307-314.

23. Samuel JL, Barrieux A, Dufour S, Dubus I, Contard F, Faradian F, Koteliansky V, Marotte F, Thiery JP, Rappaport L. Reexpression of a fetal pattern of fibronectin mRNAs during the development of rat cardiac hypertrophy induced by pressure overload. J Clin Invest ; 88: 1737-1746.

24. Faradhian F, Barrieux A, Marotte F, Dufour S, Thiery JP, Samuel JL, Rappaport L. Fibronectin mRNA localization in the rat myocardium during ontogenic development J Mol Cell Cardiol 1992; 24 (Sup I): S129

25. Ahumada GG, Rennard SI, Figueroa AE, Silver MH. Cardiac fibronectin: developmental distribution and quantitative comparison of possibles sites of synthesis. J Mol Cell Cardiol 1981; 13: 667-678.

26. Borg T K, Kristofer R, Lundgren E, Borg K, Obrink B. Recognition of extracellular matrix components by neonatal and adult cardiac myocytes. Dev Biol 1984; 104: 86-94.

27. Martin GR, Sank AC. Extracellular Matrices, cells and growth factors. In: Sporn MB, Roberts AB. editors. Peptide Growth Factors and their Receptors. Springer Verlag NY; 1991; 2: 463-477.

28. Penttinen RP, Kobayashi S, Bornstein P. Transforming growth factor ß increases mRNA for matrix proteins both in the presence and in the absence of changes in mRNA stability. Proc Natl Acad Sci USA 1988; 85: 1105-1108.

29. Armstrong PB, Armstrong MT. An instructive role for the interstitial matrix in tissue patterning: tissue segregation and intercellular invasion. J Cell Biol 1990; 110: 1439-1455.

30. Choy M, Amstrong MT, Amstrong PB. Transforming growth factor ß1 localized within the heart of chick embryo Anat Embryol 1991; 183: 345-52

31. Hartung S, Jaenisch R, Breindl M. Retrovirus insertion inactivates mouse $\alpha 1(I)$ collagen gene by blocking initiation of transcription. Nature 1986; 320: 365-367)

32. Shekhonin BV, Guriev SB, Irgashev SB, Koteliansky VE. Immunofluorescent identification of fibronectin and fibrinogen/ fibrin in experimental myocardial infarction. J Mol Cell Cardiol 1990; 22: 533-541.

33. Casscels W, Kimura H, Sanchez JA, Yu ZX, Ferrans VJ. Immunohistochemical study of fibronectin in experimental myocardial infarction. Amer J Pathol 1990; 137: 801-810

34. Wuensch M, Sharma HS, Markert T, Bernotat-Danielowski S, Schott RJ, Kremer P, Bleese N, Schaper W. In situ localization of transforming growth factor ß1 in porcine heart: Enhanced expression after chronic coronary artery constriction. J Mol Cell Cardiol 1991; 23: 1059-1062.

35. Lefer AM, Tsao P, Aoki N, Palladino MA. Mediation of cardio-protection by transforming growth factor-ß. Science 1990; 249: 61-63.

36. Kocher O, Kennedy SP, Madri JA. Alternative splicing of endothelial cell fibronectin mRNA in the IIICS region. Am J Pathol 1990; 137: 1509-1524

37. Ingber DE, Folkman J. Mechanochemical switching between growth and differentiation during fibroblast growth factor stimulated angiogenesis in vitro: role of extracellular matrix. J Cell Biol 1989; 109: 317-330.

38. Majack RA. Beta type transforming growth factors specifies organizational behavior in vascular smooth muscle cultures J Cell Biol 1987; 105; 465-472.

39. Contard F, Gluckova M , Marotte F, Chatz C, Pomies JP, Samuel JL, Guez D, Rappaport L. Expression of fibronectin EIIIA in the coronaries arteries of SHR-SP rat and comparative effects of indapamide and hydrochlorothiazide. J Mol Cell Cardiol 1992; 24 (Sup I): S79

40. Brilla, CG, Pick R, Tan LB, Janicki JS, Weber KT. Remodelling of the rat right and left ventricles in experimental hypertension. Circ Res 1990; 67: 1355-1364.

41. Villarreal FJ, Dillman WH. Cardiac hypertrophy-induced changes in mRNAs levels for TGF-ß1, fibronectin and collagen.Am J Physiol 1992; 262: H1861-H1866

42. Mamuya WS, Brecher P.1992 Fibronectin expression and hypertrophic rat heart. J Clin Invest 1992; 89:

43. Chapman D, Weber KT, Eghbali M. Regulation of fibrillar collagen types I and III and basement membrane type IV collagen gene expression in pressure overloaded rat myocardium. Circ Res 1990; 67: 787-794.

44. Carver W, Nagpal ML, Nachtigal M, Borg TK, Terracio L. Collagen expression in mechanically stimulated cardiac fibroblast. Circ Res 69: 116-122.

45. Eghbali M, Tomek R, Sukhatme VP, Woods C, Bhambi B. Differential expression of transforming growth factor ß1 and phorbol myristate acetate on cardiac fibroblast: Regulation of fibrillar collagen messengers RNA and early transcription factors Circ Res 1991; 69: 483-490.

46. Balza E, Borsi L, Allemani G, Zardi L. Transforming growth factor ß regulates the levels of different fibronectin isoforms in normal human cultured fibroblasts. FEBS Lett 1988; 228: 42-44

47. Borsi L, Balza E, Allemani G, Zardi L. Differential expression of the fibronectin isoform containing the ED-B oncofetal domain in normal human fibroblast cell lines originating from different tissues. Exp Cell Res 1992; 199; 98-105

48. Bissel MJ, Barcellos-Hof MH. The influence of extracellular matrix on gene expression; is structure the message? J Cell Sci 1987; Suppl 8: 327-343.

49. Samuel JL, Schiaffino S, Rappaport L. Myocardial cells: early changes in the expression and distribution of proteins or their mRNAs during the development of myocardial hypertrophy in the rat. In: Swynghedauw B. editor. Hypertrophy and heart failure. INSERM / J. Libbey , Paris-London 1990; 277-292.

50. Thiery JP, Duband JL, Dufour S. Adhesion system in morphogenesis and cell migration during avian embryogenesis. In: Edelman GM, Cunningham BA, Thiery JP. editors, Morphoregulatory Molecules. John Willey and Sons, New York 1990; 597-625.

4. Transforming growth factor-ß: localization and possible functional roles in cardiac myocytes

ANITA B. ROBERTS and MICHAEL B. SPORN

Introduction

Recently it has become appreciated that the myocardium produces several growth factors (cytokines) and that their expression is highly regulated not only in development but also in injury and disease [1]. One of these cytokines, transforming growth factor-ß (TGF-ß), a dimeric, multifunctional peptide [2], is expressed at high levels in the heart during both embryonic and adult life [3,4]. In this brief review, we will discuss the results of investigations directed at elucidating the role of TGF-ß in the heart with emphasis on its localization in the adult myocardium, its possible function in maintaining the rhythmic, contractile nature of cardiac tissue, and its role in response of the heart to injury and to ischemia.

Intracellular localization of TGF-ß in adult myocardium

Our original description of the biological activity of TGF-ß noted its presence in the rat heart [5]. Later, following the development of specific antibodies for the TGF-ß isoforms, intense intracellular staining of atrial and ventricular cardiac myocytes for TGF-ß1 was demonstrated in both neonatal and adult mice [3,4]; similar staining patterns have been observed for each of the three TGF-ß isoforms (K. Flanders, personal communication). Using a combination of light microscopic, electron microscopic, and cell fractionation techniques, we were able to demonstrate intracellular localization of TGF-ß1 in mitochondria of both rat and mouse cardiac myocytes [6]. Depending on the peptide antibody and the fixation procedure employed, staining could also be found in contractile filaments, suggesting that there might be multiple intracellular locations of the peptide, perhaps with different functional roles.

Although it is known that regulation of oxidative metabolism as well as calcium movements by mitochondria are critical to myocyte function, it is premature to speculate on any role of TGF-ß in these processes. Moreover, since mitochondrial DNA does not code for any of the TGF-ß's, mechanisms responsible for targeting TGF-ß to these organelles must also be identified. One possibility might involve a carrier function for the 135 kDa TGF-ß binding protein that is associated with latent TGF-ß and has several binding sites for Ca^{2+} [7,8]. Regardless of our limited understanding of the function of TGF-ß in either mitochondria or contractile filaments at the present time, these findings are certain eventually to reveal new roles for TGF-ß, possibly in coupling the activities of the mitochondria to the rest of the cell or in regulating the contractility of myocytes [6].

Altered expression of TGF-ß following experimental myocardial infarction

TGF-ß plays a central role in the repair of many tissues after injury [2]. Since the infarcted or ischemic heart can be viewed as an injured tissue, we examined the effects of TGF-ß in repair or modulation of cardiac tissue damage following ligation of the left coronary artery in rats. Studies on the immunohistochemical staining patterns of TGF-ß1 in the heart showed that staining was quickly lost in ischemic areas following experimental myocardial infarction [3]. However, certain cells around the margins of the infarct began staining intensely for TGF-ß1 approximately 24 to 48 hours after infarction, leading to the suggestion that TGF-ß might accelerate repair and restore function to these myocytes.

Expression of TGF-ß1 mRNA also increased in infarcted myocardium 48 hr after coronary ligation and was characterized by the appearance of an additional 1.9 kb TGF-ß1 mRNA. This smaller TGF-ß1 mRNA species is absent in normal heart tissue but elevated in a variety of tissues in response to injury [9]. Characterization of this 1.9 kb mRNA demonstrated that it has a unique 3'-untranslated region (UTR) and suggested that it also has a shortened 5'-UTR. Since sequences in the 5'-UTR of the more abundant 2.4 kb TGF-ß1 mRNA known to be inhibitory to translation [10] are deleted in the 1.9 kb transcript [9], it has been proposed that translation of TGF-ß1 might be facilitated under conditions of tissue injury and in subsequent repair processes [9].

TGF-ß administered systemically before or after experimental infarction has been shown to have cardioprotective effects [11,12]. Similar protective effects of TGF-ß have been demonstrated in a model of splanchnic ischemia-reperfusion injury [11]. These effects are discussed in detail elsewhere in this monograph and are thought to be mediated indirectly via the ability of TGF-ß to preserve and stabilize endothelial function and to inhibit endothelial adhesiveness for neutrophils [11,13]. This ability of TGF-ß to protect against infiltration of inflammatory cells and hence suppress release of pro-inflammatory cytokines such as interleukin-1ß (IL-1ß) and tumor necrosis factor-α (TNF-α) may ultimately result in its use in treatment of septic shock and as an adjunct to thrombolytic agents such as streptokinase or tissue plasminogen activator [14].

TGF-ß maintains the function of cultured neonatal cardiac myocytes

Recently, we have begun investigating direct effects of TGF-ß on cultured neonatal cardiac myocytes, which beat spontaneously. We have found that *exogenous* TGF-ß regulates the beating rate of neonatal rat myocytes cultured in serum-free medium and maintains both their regular rhythm and their rate of beating [15]. Each of the TGF-ß isoforms appears to function equivalently. More importantly, we have demonstrated that cultured myocytes secrete relatively high levels of TGF-ß (principally TGF-ß2) and that this *endogenous* TGF-ß acts in an autocrine fashion to sustain the beating rate of myocytes cultured in serum-free medium. These data are consistent with previous proposals that TGF-ß might promote repair and restore function to damaged areas of the myocardium [3].

Cytokine mediators of acute and chronic cardiac damage, such as IL-1ß and TNF-α, have been shown to have suppressive effects on myocyte function [16]. Again using the model of neonatal cardiac myocytes cultured in serum-free medium, we have shown that TGF-ß, added simultaneously, can antagonize the suppressive effects of IL-1ß on the beating rate [15], analogous to its ability to oppose many of the actions of IL-1 on other cell types [17-19]. Myocytes cultured in the presence of TGF-ß beat at a constant rate, while myocytes treated with IL-1ß beat more slowly in an irregular fashion characterized by pauses of different lengths of time. The suppressive effects of IL-1ß on the beating rate usually were apparent between 10-14 hr following cytokine addition. By 24 hr, myocytes treated with IL-1ß often ceased to beat, whereas those treated with either TGF-ß alone or TGF-ß and IL-1ß continued to beat at rates ranging from 25 to 80 percent of the original rate, depending on the concentration of TGF-ß added [15].

Nitric oxide plays a role in the antagonistic effects of TGF-ß and IL-1ß on cardiac myocytes

Nitric oxide (NO) is known to be a critical regulator of many physiological and pathological processes, and the enzymes catalyzing its production from L-arginine have now been characterized and cloned [20]. Recently, synthesis of NO has been implicated in regulation of cardiac contractility in several different model systems including isolated papillary muscles [21], myocardium following reoxygenation injury [22], myocardium of rats treated with endotoxin, and cultured adult rat cardiac myocytes [23]. We have now shown that the opposite effects described above for IL-1ß and TGF-ß on the spontaneous beating rate of cultured neonatal rat cardiac myocytes are also mediated, in part, by NO [24].

Our results have shown that IL-1ß stimulates neonatal myocytes to express an inducible form of NO synthase (iNOS) and to release NO, and that TGF-ß, added alone or together with IL-1ß, suppresses the release of NO by reducing the level of iNOS [24]. Bacterial lipopolysaccharide (LPS), present in the serum-free medium ITS+ supplement (Collaborative Research), was a co-inducer of NO secretion. The time required for induction of iNOS by IL-1ß correlated closely with that required for suppression of the beating rate. Treatment with IL-1ß, but not TGF-ß, also increased cellular cGMP, presumably by activation of guanylate cyclase by NO.

The effects of either IL-1ß or TGF-ß on synthesis of NO paralleled their effects on cGMP and were opposite to their effects on the beating rate of the cells [24]. Our observations that increased NO secretion resulted in suppression of the myocyte beating rate are consistent with previously described relaxant effects of NO in vascular smooth muscle cells [25]. Effects of IL-1ß on NO, cGMP, and the beating rate were all dependent on the presence of L-arginine in the medium and could be suppressed by the competitive inhibitor, N^G-monomethyl-L-arginine. Taken together, the data suggest that induction of the L-arginine-NO-cGMP pathway may play a critical role in suppression of myocyte contraction and rhythmicity. Our findings raise the possibility that TGF-ß itself, or local agents which induce its expression [26], could be useful adjuncts to combination therapies targeted to iNOS. Suppression of iNOS activity has been proposed for treatment of myocardial dysfunction in situations where NO might be generated in response to LPS or pro-inflammatory cytokines, as in some of the newer anti-tumor cytokine therapies, in inflammatory diseases of the heart, and in septic shock [27].

The mechanisms by which NO regulates the beating rate of the myocytes are unknown. However, it has been shown that elevation of cellular cGMP, resulting from activation of soluble guanylate cyclase by NO, can stimulate Na^+/Ca^{2+} exchange in vascular smooth muscle cells [28]. This has been proposed to lead to a reduction of intracellular Ca^{2+}, which in turn causes relaxation of these cells with consequent vasodilation. cGMP has also been shown to exert a negative inotropic effect on cardiac myocytes, presumably by activation of an endogenous cGMP-dependent protein kinase which regulates the Ca^{2+} channel current [29]. Preliminary experiments have demonstrated that TGF-ß stimulates and IL-1ß inhibits Ca^{2+} uptake by neonatal myocytes (T. Santa Coloma, personal communication), consistent with these mechanisms. However, it cannot yet be ruled out that other, as yet unidentified, key regulatory proteins, possibly including cytokines secreted by the myocytes, may also be targets for nitrosylation, resulting in alteration of their biological activity [30].

The effects of nitric oxide can be attenuated by culture conditions

Myocyte function in the intact myocardium is critically dependent on matrix architecture, and impairment of function in a variety of pathologic conditions is accompanied by alterations in or loss of the fibrillar collagen network [31]. In our initial experiments characterizing the effects of IL-1ß and TGF-ß on the beating rate of neonatal myocytes cultured in serum-free medium, it was observed that suppressive effects of IL-1ß on the beating rate were found only when the myocytes were co-cultured with cardiac fibroblasts or were grown on cardiac fibroblast matrix [15]. When the myocytes were plated on a coating of gelatin (denatured collagen), they maintained their initial beating rate, even in the presence of IL-1ß.

Subsequent experiments showed that production of NO and cGMP following treatment with IL-1ß were equivalent whether myocytes were cultured on native fibroblast matrix or on gelatin, demonstrating that induction of NO and cGMP represent but one set of multiple parameters involved in regulation of myocyte beating rate [24]. Since myocytes cultured on gelatin assume a distinctly different, more spread, flattened shape than myocytes cultured on fibroblast matrix, the possibility must be considered that the myocyte phenotype itself or growth factors bound to the native matrix [32] may modulate the cellular response to NO.

Another notable exception to the inverse correlation between the activity of iNOS and beating rate was the inability of high levels of NO, resulting from treatment with the combination of IL-1ß, IFN-γ, and TNF-α, to suppress the beating rate of myocytes cultured on either fibroblast matrix or gelatin [24]. Interestingly, whereas it has been shown that IL-1ß and TNF-α suppress myocardial contractility (16) and that TNF-α mimics the injury seen following myocardial ischemia-reperfusion (11), pretreatment of animals with either IL-1ß, TNF-α, or LPS was found to provide protection against subsequent damage following myocardial ischemia-reperfusion injury [33-35].

Since IL-1ß and TNF-α pretreatment have been shown to induce manganous superoxide dismutase [33], and LPS pretreatment to induce catalase [34], it has been suggested that consequent detoxification of superoxide anions might play a role in the protection. Accordingly, the paradoxical effects of treatment with combinations of these cytokines on the beating rate of cultured myocytes might result from a multiplicity of both early and later effects on gene expression and depend on relative contributions of reactive nitrogen and reactive oxygen intermediates [20].

Summary

From the foregoing it can be concluded that myocyte function can be regulated by both endogenous and exogenous TGF-ß. Although the mechanisms are not yet understood, the intracellular localization of TGF-ß in mitochondria and contractile filaments may be critical to maintaining the rapid calcium fluxes of myocytes and consequently their rhythmicity. In response to injury, inflammation, and sepsis, increased expression of TGF-ß by both myocytes and non-myocytes likely represents a defense mechanism to suppress NO production, thereby both limiting injury and promoting repair.

Acknowledgements

The authors thank Thomas Winokur, Kathleen Flanders, and

Tomas Santa-Coloma for helpful discussions, Nanette Roche for invaluable technical assistance, Alain Tedgui for suggestions regarding NO, and our collaborators Carl Nathan and Yoram Vodovotz for contributing their expertise in NO to this problem.

References

1. Schneider MD, Parker TD. Cardiac growth factors. Rec Prog Growth Factor Res 1991; 3:1-26.
2. Roberts AB, Sporn MB. The transforming growth factors-ß, In: Sporn MB, Roberts AB editors: Handbook of Experimental Pharmacology. Peptide Growth Factors and Their Receptors. Springer-Verlag, Berlin, 1990; 95: 419-472.
3. Thompson NL, Bazoberry F, Speir EH, et al. Transforming growth factor-ß1 in acute myocardial infarction in rats. Growth Factors 1988; 1: 91-99.
4. Thompson NL, Flanders KC, Smith JM, et al. Expression of transforming growth factor-ß1 in specific cells and tissues of adult and neonatal mice. J Cell Biol 1989; 108: 661-669.
5. Roberts AB, Anzano MA, Lamb LC, et al. New class of transforming growth factors potentiated by epidermal growth factor: isolation from non-neoplastic tissues. Proc Natl Acad Sci U S A 1981; 78: 5339-5343.
6. Heine UI, Burmester JK, Flanders KC, et al. Localization of transforming growth factor-ß1 in mitochondria of murine heart and liver. Cell Regulation 1991; 2: 467-477.
7. Dahlback B, Hildebrand B, Linse S. Novel type of very high affinity calcium-binding sites in ß-hydroxy-asparagine-containing epidermal growth factor-like domains in vitamin K-dependent proteins. J Biol Chem 1990; 265: 18481-18489.
8. Kansaki T, Olofsson A, Moren A, et al. TGF-ß1 binding protein: a component of the large latent complex of TGF-ß1 with multiple repeat sequences. Cell 1990; 61: 1051-1061.
9. Qian SW, Kondaiah P, Casscells W, et al. A second messenger RNA species of transforming growth factor-ß1 in infarcted rat heart. Cell Regulation 1991; 2: 241-249.
10. Kim S-J, Kim K-Y, Wakefield LM, et al: Post-transcriptional regulation of the human transforming growth factor-ß1 gene. J Biol Chem 1992; 267: 13702-13707.
11. Lefer AM, Tsao P, Aoki N, et al. Mediation of cardioprotection by transforming growth factor-ß. Science 1990; 249: 61-64.

12. Lefer AM. Mechanisms of the protective effects of transforming growth factor-ß in reperfusion injury. Biochem Pharmacol 1991; 42: 1323-1327.
13. Gamble JR, Vadas MA. Endothelial adhesiveness for blood neutrophils is inhibited by transforming growth factor-ß. Science 1988; 242: 97-99.
14. Roberts AB, Sporn MB. Physiological actions and clinical applications of transforming growth factor-ß (TGF-ß). Growth Factors 1992; in press.
15. Roberts AB, Roche NS, Winokur TS, et al. Role of TGF-ß in maintenance of function of cultured cardiac myocytes: autocrine action and reversal of damaging effects of interleukin-1. J Clin Invest 1992; in press.
16. Gulick T, Chung MK, Pieper SJ, et al. Interleukin 1 and tumor necrosis factor inhibit cardiac myocyte ß-adrenergic responsiveness. Proc Natl Acad Sci U S A 1989; 86: 6753-6757.
17. Heino J, Heinonen T. Interleukin-1 ß prevents the stimulatory effect of transforming growth factor-ß on collagen gene expression in human skin fibroblasts. Biochem J 1990; 271: 827-830.
18. Musso T, Espinoza-Delgado I, Pulkki K, et al. Transforming growth factor ß downregulates interleukin-1 (IL-1)-induced IL-6 production by human monocytes. Blood 1990; 76: 2466-2469.
19. Pfeilschifter J, Pignat W, Leighton J, et al. Transforming growth factor ß2 differentially modulates interleukin-1 ß and tumour-necrosis-factor-α-stimulated phospholipase A2 and prostaglandin E2 synthesis in rat renal mesangial cells. Biochem J 1990; 270: 269-271.
20. Nathan C. Nitric oxide as a secretory product of mammalian cells. FASEB J 1992; 6: 3051-3064.
21. Finkel MS, Oddis CV, Jacob TD, et al. Negative inotropic effects of cytokines on the heart mediated by nitric oxide. Science 1992; 257: 387-389.
22. Matheis G, Sherman MP, Buckberg GD, et al. Role of L-arginine-nitric oxide pathway in myocardial reoxygenation injury. Am J Physiol 1992; 262: H616-H620.
23. Schulz R, Nava E, Moncada S. Induction and potential biological relevance of a Ca^{2+}-independent nitric oxide synthase in the myocardium. Br J Pharmacol 1992; 105: 575-580.
24. Roberts AB, Vodovotz Y, Roche NS, et al. Role of nitric oxide in antagonistic effects of TGF-ß and IL-1ß on the beating rate of cultured cardiac myocytes. Molec Endocrinol 1992; in press.
25. Ignarro JJ. Biosynthesis and metabolism of endothelium-derived nitric oxide. Annu Rev Pharmacol Toxicol 1990; 30: 535-560.

26. Roberts AB, Sporn MB. Mechanistic interrelationships between two superfamilies: the steroid/retinoid receptors and transforming growth factor-ß. Cancer Surveys 1992; 14: 205-220.

27. Kilbourn RG, Griffith OW. Overproduction of nitric oxide in cytokine-mediated and septic shock. J Natl Cancer Inst 1992; 84: 827-831.

28. Furukawa K-I, Ohshima N, Tawada-Iwata Y, et al. Cyclic GMP stimulates Na^+/Ca^{2+} exchange in vascular smooth muscle cells in primary culture. J Biol Chem 1991; 266: 12337-12341.

29. Méry PF, Lohmann SM, Walter U, et al: Ca^{2+} current is regulated by cyclic GMP-dependent protein kinase in mammalian cardiac myocytes. Proc Natl Acad Sci U S A 1991; 88: 1197-1201.

30. Stamler JS, Simon DI, Osborne JA, et al. S-Nitrosylation of proteins with nitric oxide: Synthesis and characterization of biologically active compounds. Proc Natl Acad Sci U S A 1992; 89: 444-448.

31. Weber KT. Cardiac interstitium in health and disease: the fibrillar collagen network. J Am Coll Cardiol 1989; 13: 1637-1652.

32. Vukicevic S, Kleinman H, Luyten FP, et al. Identification of multiple active growth factors in basement membrane Matrigel suggests caution in interpretation of cellular activity related to extracellular matrix components. Exp Cell Res 1992; in press.

33. Eddy LJ, Goeddel DV, Wong GHW. Tumor necrosis factor-α pretreatment is protective in a rat model of myocardial ischemia-reperfusion injury. Biochem Biophys Res Commun 1992; 184: 1056-1059.

34. Brown JM, Grosso MA, Terada LS, et al. Endotoxin pretreatment increases endogenous myocardial catalase activity and decreases ischemia-reperfusion injury of isolated rat hearts. Proc Natl Acad Sci USA 1989; 86: 2516-2520.

35. Brown JM, White CW, Terada LS, et al. Interleukin-1 pretreatment decreases ischemia/reperfusion injury. Proc Natl Acad Sci U S A 1990; 87: 5026-5030.

5. Basic fibroblast growth factor in cardiac myocytes: expression and effects

ELISSAVET KARDAMI, RAYMOND R. PADUA, KISHORE
BABU S. PASUMARTHI, LEI LIU, BRADLEY W. DOBLE,
SARAH E. DAVEY and PETER A. CATTINI

Introduction

Ventricular myocytes of the adult mammalian myocardium are considered essentially incapable of regeneration. These cells cease dividing soon after birth and subsequent cardiac growth is brought about by increases in cellular size (hypertrophy) rather than cell number [1]. Following irreversible injury and death of cardiomyocytes, caused by a variety of factors such as ischemia, excess catecholamines or genetic defects, necrotic muscle becomes replaced by scar tissue. The remaining myocardium hypertrophies to meet the need for extra work but beyond a certain potential for adaptation, cardiac failure ensues. There is some evidence that ventricular myocytes may not have lost their proliferative potential irreversibly, since they can be stimulated to synthesize DNA in culture [2] and are apparently capable of a hyperplastic response in hypertrophic or ageing hearts [3].

Endogenous mechanisms responsible for regulation of cardiac proliferative and hence regenerative response are not known. Polypeptide growth factors provide the signals stimulating, directly or indirectly, the mitogenic response of cells. The heart expresses a variety of growth factors thought to act locally, in an autocrine or paracrine manner [4]. These factors include acidic and basic fibroblast growth factor (aFGF or FGF-1 and bFGF or FGF-2, respectively), transforming growth factor-beta (TGFß), and the insulin-like growth factors (IGFs) [4]. These factors are able to affect DNA synthesis in culture, and are likely to play a similar role in vivo.

Basic FGF is a 18-25 kDa protein, which binds heparin with high affinity and which has been detected to a variable extent in all tissues examined [5,6]. It belongs to a larger FGF family of growth factors, with which it shares 30-55% amino acid sequence homology [7]. Basic FGF is a mitogen but also affects differentiation, mesoderm formation, adhesion and migration of fibroblasts and endothelial cells. Basic FGF is found in the extracellular matrix [5,6]. Its mode of secretion, however, is not understood because of the absence of a signal peptide [8]. Cell injury results in bFGF release into the extracellular environment where it likely remains associated with heparin-like components [9]. Administration of bFGF promotes endothelial regeneration in denuded arteries, stimulates dermal wound healing as well as cartilage repair [10-12].

To understand the role and regulation of bFGF in the context of cardiac myocyte physiology and growth, we have studied its expression in development and in injury. In addition, we have examined the effects of bFGF on cultured cardiomyocytes. This chapter represents a review and discussion of some of our findings.

Effects of bFGF on cardiac myocytes

Proliferation

Cardiac myocytes divide slowly in culture and potential stimulatory effects of growth factors can be masked by fibroblast overgrowth. To overcome this problem we determined the ratio of myocytes (myosin-positive) to non-myocytes (myosin-negative cells) as well as the total cell number in chick embryo or neonatal rat cardiomyocyte cultures. In this manner a realistic estimate of myocyte numbers at any time point can be obtained [14]. Supplementation of culture media with bFGF (up to 20 ng/ml) resulted in a statistically significant stimulation of cardiomyocyte proliferation [14] (Figure 1). Similar results were obtained when DNA synthesis was assessed [14,15].

TGFß is also found in the heart and was shown to inhibit the stimulatory effects of bFGF on proliferation of several cell types [16]. Thus, we examined the effects of TGFß on myocyte cell division [14]. As shown in Figure1, TGFß reduced the bFGF-induced stimulation of cardiomyocyte proliferation, although there was no detectable effect on division when it was used alone. This observation may be of profound

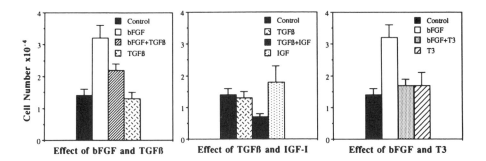

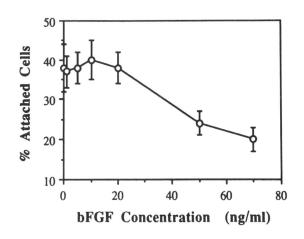

Figure 1 (top). Effect of endogenous growth factors on cardiac myocyte proliferation [14]. Embryonic chicken ventricular cardiomyocytes (20,000 cells/cm^2) were plated in the presence of 1% fetal bovine serum [14,15]. Growth factors (bFGF, 10 ng/ml; TGFß, 5 ng/ml; IGF, 20 ng/ml) or triiodothyronine (1 nM) were added every 48 hours, starting at 24 hours after plating. Myocyte numbers were determined 7 days after plating, as described [14]. Non-muscle cell contamination remained less than 10% throughout. Note stimulation of myocyte proliferation by bFGF and the inhibition of this stimulation by TGFß as well as thyroid hormone.

Figure 2 (bottom). Effect of bFGF on myocyte adhesion. Embryonic chicken ventricular myocytes (100,000 cells/cm^2) were plated on fibronectin coated dishes in the presence of 2% fetal bovine serum and increasing concentrations of bFGF. The percentage of myocytes which adhere to the substrate 6 h after plating is plotted as a function of bFGF concentration. Values shown represent the mean of four determinations. Note the decrease in the number of attached cells at higher bFGF concentrations.

physiological significance. Both of these factors are present in the heart [4], and both are increased after cardiac injury [17-19]. In addition to its effects on the bFGF response, TGFß cancels the IGF-induced stimulation of cardiomyocyte proliferation in culture (Fig.1). We have some evidence that endogenous or serum-derived TGFß interferes with myocyte proliferation in culture, since addition of TGFß neutralizing antibodies results in increased DNA synthesis (unpublished observations). It is possible that TGFß or similar proteins contribute to the inability of the cardiomyocyte to mount an effective regenerative response in vivo, despite the presence of bFGF and other stimulatory factors.

Another factor which may interfere with bFGF-induced stimulation of myocyte DNA synthesis is thyroid hormone, which promotes muscle differentiation and controls expression of contractile or sarcolemmal protein genes [20]. We examined the effects of thyroid hormone on myocyte proliferation. Thyroid hormone did not affect cell division on its own; it did, however, diminish the extent of bFGF-induced stimulation [14] (Figure 1). The mechanism of this inhibition is not known at present, although it may be of physiological significance. Levels of thyroid hormone increase dramatically after birth [21] and may blunt the ability of cardiac myocytes to respond to endogenous bFGF by cell division.

Adhesion

Cardiac myocytes were isolated from 7d chick embryo ventricles [14]. To examine attachment, cells were plated on fibronectin-coated dishes, in the presence of 2% fetal bovine serum and increasing concentrations of pure bovine bFGF. Attached cells were lifted by trypsinization and counted 6 h later. Results are shown in Figure 2. No appreciable effect on attachment was seen at bFGF concentrations below 20 ng/ml. At higher concentrations, however, bFGF inhibited attachment significantly (Figure 2). Inhibition of adhesion is likely the result of competition for cell-binding sites: Basic FGF contains two Asp-Gly-Arg (DGR) sequences [8] which represent the inverse of the RGD sequence (the cell-binding domain of cell-adhesive proteins) and which compete with adhesive proteins for integrin interaction [22]. Basic FGF present in the extracellular matrix might therefore influence myocyte-matrix or myocyte-myocyte adhesion in vivo.

Protection

Oxidative stress induced by hydrogen peroxide (H_2O_2) may contribute to the pathogenesis of ischemia-reperfusion injury in the heart. Addition of H_2O_2 to confluent cultures of rat cardiomyocytes causes lethal sarcolemmal disruption [23]. A preliminary series of experiments indicated that bFGF reduced the H_2O_2-induced myocyte injury (readily measured by lactate dehydrogenase, LDH, release) to a statistically significant extent (Figure 3). Basic FGF was also effective in reducing LDH release from myocytes in serum-starved cultures (Figure 3). Visual inspection of serum-starved or H_2O_2-treated cultures revealed some preservation of cellular morphology in the presence of bFGF. Continuous presence of the growth factor was necessary for this protection, since brief exposure of cells to bFGF did not have any effect. It is possible that bFGF (which possesses 4 thiol groups, usually in the reduced state) [24] may act as an anti-oxidant. Basic FGF is a trophic factor for neural cells [25] and likely acts on cardiomyocytes in a similar fashion. Extrapolation of these findings to the in vivo situation introduces the notion that bFGF may contribute to endogenous maintenance and protection mechanisms in the differentiated myocardium.

Expression of bFGF in the heart

Expression of bFGF has been examined mostly at the level of protein

60

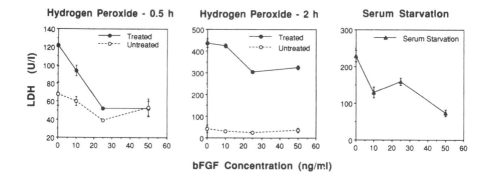

bFGF Concentration (ng/ml)

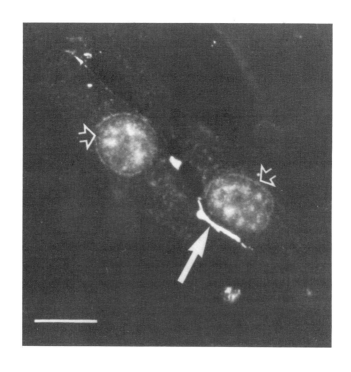

Figure 3 (top). Effect of bFGF on LDH release by H_2O_2-treated or serum-starved myocytes. Cardiac myocytes were obtained from the ventricles of 1 day old rat pups [14], and maintained in culture at confluent densities in the presence of 5% calf serum in DMEM medium. One week old myocyte cultures were rinsed and incubated without serum, in the presence or absence of 250 μM H_2O_2 and increasing concentrations of recombinant bFGF. Lactic dehydrogenase (LDH) activity was determined (SIGMA kit) at 0.5 and 2 h of incubation for myocytes treated with H_2O_2 and at 24 h for myocytes maintained in the absence of serum. Note the decrease in LDH release (and therefore cellular injury) induced either by H_2O_2 or starvation in the presence of increasing concentrations of bFGF.

Figure 4 (bottom). Localization of bFGF to cardiac intermyocyte junctions. Cardiac ventricular myocytes were obtained from 19 day old fetal rats and maintained in culture (40,000 cells/cm^2) for 48 h, in the presence of 5% calf serum. Cells were fixed with 1% paraformaldehyde, permeabilized with 0.5% Triton-X100 in PBS (30) and stained for bFGF using affinity purified anti-bFGF IgG (#S2) [29]. Fluorescein-conjugated anti-rabbit IgG was used to visualize antigen-antibody complexes. Note the strong labelling of cell-cell contacts, indicated by closed arrow. Labelling is also observed in association with the nucleus and nuclear envelope. (Bar, 20 μm).

accumulation and distribution in our laboratory. Because bFGF represents less than 0.0001% of total extracted protein, conventional biochemical purification and identification are not usually practical, especially when a large number of samples is examined. Combination of heparin-sepharose chromatography and western blotting with specific antibodies, however, allows detection and quantitation of nanograms of bFGF from small amounts of tissue (0.3 to 1 g wet weight) [26-28]. Good antibodies are crucial for these experiments. Several preparations of antibodies have been obtained, raised against residues 1-24 of the truncated (146 amino acids) bovine bFGF [8]. This region of the molecule is highly immunogenic, has negligible homology to the other members of the larger FGF family of growth factors [7] and consistently elicits antibodies specific for bFGF. Our anti-bFGF antibody preparations recognize native or denatured 18-25 kD bFGF and have been used extensively in western blots and immunolocalization studies [26-32].

Using indirect immunofluorescence and a collection of antibodies, bFGF has been localized to extracellular as well as intracellular sites of the myocyte, suggestive of an intimate and continuous involvement with physiological function. Specifically, bFGF was detected in association with basement membrane, intercalated discs, cytoplasm as well as

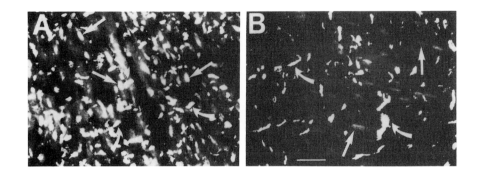

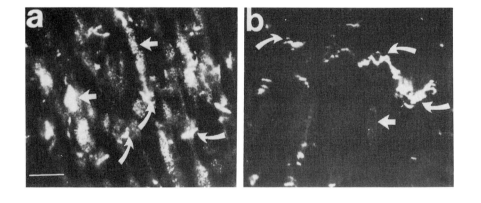

nucleus of cardiomyocytes [26-30,32]. The bFGF protein has been extracted from nuclear, cytoplasmic and extracellular fractions [33] in agreement with the immunolocalization studies. Localization of bFGF in intercalated discs [26,28] and in the cytoplasmic face of cardiac and astrocytic gap junctions [29,32] (see also Figure 4) is of particular interest. Basic FGF may play a role in gap junction-mediated intercellular communication. Alternatively, association with gap junctional membranes may render this factor unavailable for interaction with other sites. Numerous studies have pointed to an inverse relationship between abundance of functional gap junctions and stimulation of proliferation (34). It is therefore tempting to speculate that the association of bFGF with cardiac gap junctions may provide a means for growth control of the cardiomyocyte.

Regenarative potential and bFGF.

Because bFGF has been strongly implicated in tissue repair, its expression was compared between adult cardiac atria and ventricles, and between immature and adult cardiac ventricles. This was done as part of an effort to understand differences in the regenerative properties of cardiomyocytes. Neonatal ventricular myocytes, in contrast to their adult counterparts, are not fully differentiated and are still capable of DNA synthesis and cell division [1]. Adult atrial cardiomyocytes are still capable of DNA synthesis and possibly cell division and are considered

Figure 5 (top). Localization of bFGF in atria and ventricles. Frozen longitudinal sections fron adult rat heart atria (A) and ventricles (B) were examined for bFGF localization by indirect immunofluorescence, using affinity-purified anti-bFGF IgG, which preferentially recognizes epitopes within residues 15-24 of bovine bFGF in vivo [28]. Curved arrows point at intercalated discs. Straight arrows point at nuclei. Note the increased nuclear as well as cytoplasmic anti-bFGF labelling in atrial compared to ventricular myocytes. (Bar, 50 μm).

Figure 6 (bottom). Distribution of bFGF in the neonatal and adult rat heart ventricles. Frozen, longitudinal sections, obtained from the ventricles of, (a), neonatal (5 day old) or, (b), adult (5 week old) rats were probed for bFGF by indirect immunofluorescence using affinity-purified anti-bFGF IgG, which preferentially recognizes epitopes within res. 15-24 of bovine bFGF [28], in vivo. Curved or straight arrows denote position of intercalated discs or nuclei, respectively. Note the higher intensity of nuclear anti-bFGF staining in neonatal compared to adult ventricles. (Bar, 20 μm).

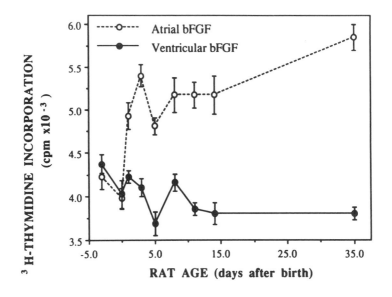

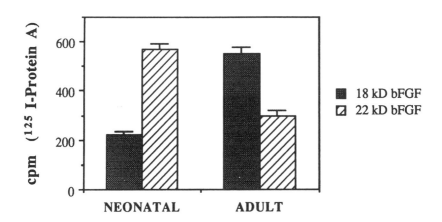

less differentiated than ventricular cells [35]. To localize bFGF, we made use of an affinity-purified antibody preparation which preferentially detects epitopes within residues 15-24 of bovine bFGF, and which does not recognize heparin-associated bFGF (28). Characteristic results are shown in Figure 5 (atrial versus ventricular myocytes) and Figure 6 (neonatal versus adult myocytes).Anti-bFGF labelling was observed in association with myocyte intercalated discs, but also with muscle nuclei, as reported previously [26,28]. Atrial myocytes displayed stronger nuclear as well as cytoplasmic anti-bFGF staining compared to their ventricular counterparts (Figure 5). Similarly, nuclear as well as cytoplasmic anti-bFGF staining was more intense in neonatal compared to adult ventricular cardiomyocytes (Figure 6). In contrast, the intensity of anti-bFGF immunostaining associated with basement membrane/extracellular matrix was comparable between neonatal and adult rat myocytes (unpublished observations). Therefore, atrial and neonatal ventricular myocytes, which represent more immature and proliferative cells, display increased intracellular bFGF compared to fully differentiated adult ventricular myocytes.

Bioassays were also used to obtain an assessment of bFGF content as a function of developmental stage in rat atrial and ventricular extracts. The mitogenic activity of heparin-binding fractions was tested on embryonic chicken skeletal myoblasts, a system highly dependent on bFGF for DNA synthesis [26,36], and results are shown in Figure 7. Basic FGF activity increased steadily with age in atrial extracts. In

Figure 7 (top). Basic FGF activity in immature or adult vertebrate hearts. Extracts were obtained from cardiac atria and ventricles of several species, at different developmental stages and fractionated by heparin-sepharose chromatography, as described [26]. Heparin-binding peptides from equivalent amounts of extracts were tested for bFGF activity (stimulation of DNA synthesis, as assessed by ^{3}H-thymidine incorporation) using a cell culture system (embryonic chicken skeletal myoblasts) highly sensitive to bFGF [36]. Incorporation of ^{3}H-thymidine is shown as a function of age. Values shown represent the mean of six determinations. Note the increase in bFGF activity in atrial extracts.

Figure 8 (bottom). HIigh and low molecular mass bFGF in development. Equivalent amounts of extracts from 1 day and 5 week old rat ventricles were analyzed for bFGF by western blotting and autoradiography (^{125}I-protein A) [19,37]. Radioactive bFGF bands were excised and counted in a gamma counter, and radioactive counts associated with the 18 or 22 kD bFGF are shown as a function of developmental stage. Note the prevalence of 22 kD or 18 kD bFGF in neonatal or adult hearts, respectively.

contrast, bFGF activity decreased somewhat with age in ventricular extracts; this decrease was more noticeable between embryonic and neonatal ventricles. Atrial and ventricular extracts had comparable levels of bFGF activity before birth, while atrial activity was higher compared to ventricular at all postpartum points. Increased concentration of bFGF in atrial compared to ventricular extracts has also been documented independently by western blotting [26].

We have shown that bFGF in adult cardiac ventricles consists predominantly of an 18 kD species and trace amounts of higher molecular mass forms (21.5-22 kD) [18,19,37,38]. Different forms suggest different functions. The larger bFGF species have been implicated in nuclear localization and the proliferative response [39]. We therefore compared bFGF content as well as composition between immature (1 day old) and adult (5 week old) ventricles. This was done by western blotting [19,37], followed by autoradiography, excision and quantitation of radioactivity of immunoreactive bands. A characteristic set of results is shown in Figure 8. Interestingly, although the overall bFGF levels were similar, bFGF composition was clearly different between neonatal and adult ventricles. Neonatal bFGF was composed primarily of an 22 kD species, the relative concentration of which decreased significantly with age [19,37]. In contrast, the 18 kD bFGF actually increased in more differentiated muscle. Accumulation of the 22 or 18 kD bFGF, therefore, correlated with a hyperplastic or hypertrophic phenotype, respectively, in ventricular cardiomyocytes. Higher molecular mass, N-terminal extended forms of bFGF are the result of translation from non-conventional leucine (CUG) start sites, found upstream of the classical methionine AUG start codon in the bovine, human and rat sequences [40,41]. The N-extension of human bFGF contains a nuclear targeting signal, resulting in nuclear localization of bFGF [42]. Consequently, predominance of the 22 kD rat bFGF (Figure 7) and increased nuclear anti-bFGF staining (Figure 6) would support a nuclear localization for the 22 kD bFGF in neonatal cardiomyocytes in vivo.

To determine subcellular localization of the various forms of rat bFGF, we introduced modified rat bFGF cDNAs directed by the Rous Sarcoma Virus promoter (RSVp) in cultured cardiac myocytes, by gene transfer [43,44]. The following hybrid genes were used: RSVp.*met*FGF, which contains the AUG site but no upstream CUG codons, and RSVp.δ*met*FGF, which contains the upstream CUG site but the AUG codon was removed. Production of low (18 kD) and high (22 kD) molecular mass bFGF by RSVp.*met*FGF and RSVp.δ*met*FGF, respectively, was confirmed in transfected tumor cells [43]. Transfected cardiomyocytes were stained simultaneously for myosin (for

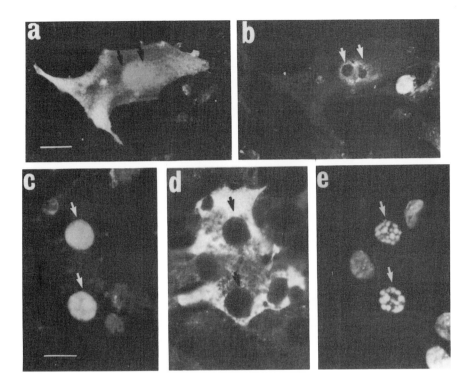

Figure 9. Over-expression of 18 or 22 Kd bFGF in ventricular cardiomyocytes in culture. (a) and (b): Double-immunofluorescence staining for bFGF and striated muscle myosin, respectively. (c), (d) & (e): Triple-fluorescence staining for bFGF, myosin and nuclear DNA, respectively. Cardiomyocyte cultures shown in (a) and (b) have been transfected with constract RSVp.metFGF, producing the 18 kD form of rat bFGF. Myocyte cultures shown in (c), (d) and (e), have been transfected with constract RSVp.δmetFGF, producing the 22 kD form of rat bFGF. Arrows indicate position of myocyte nuclei. Space bar in (a) or (c), 50 μm or 20 μm, respectively. Note the cytoplasmic as well as nuclear localization of the 18 kD bFGF, and the nuclear localization of the 22 kD bFGF. (Bar, 20 μM).

identification), bFGF, and nuclear DNA. Representative results are shown in Figure 9: Myocytes overexpressing the 18 kD bFGF displayed cytoplasmic, as well as nuclear staining. In contrast, myocytes overexpressing the 22 kD bFGF displayed strong nuclear anti-bFGF staining. It was concluded therefore that while the 18 kD rat bFGF is localized to the nucleus as well as the cytoplasm, the 22 kD species is preferentially targeted to the nucleus.

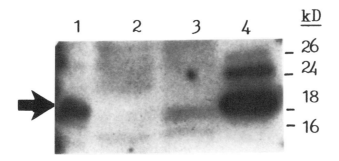

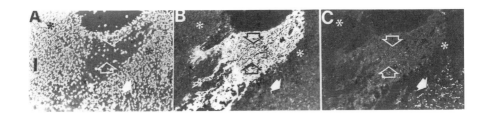

Interestingly, counter-staining with Hoechst 33342 revealed that nuclear DNA was fragmented or condensed in discrete packets in nuclei which contained high levels of the 22 kD bFGF (Figure 9). These DNA "packets" were different morphologically from prophase chromosomes (which are more elongated and "worm-like"). Furthermore the cells shown in Figure 9 (c,d,e) are clearly not in prophase, since the anti-bFGF or anti-myosin staining (sharply confined to a nuclear or cytoplasmic compartment, respectively) indicated presence of intact nuclear envelope. This pattern of nuclear staining was never seen in any of the myocytes overexpressing the 18 kD bFGF, despite the nuclear localization of the latter. It would appear therefore that overloading of the nucleus with the 22 kD bFGF induced fragmentation or condensation of chromatin. Although it is too early to appreciate the physiological significance of this observation, these data show that the 18 and 22 kD bFGFs have different properties in the cardiomyocyte nucleus, and therefore they are likely to contribute to different functions.

Presence of bFGF in the nucleus was first suggested based on immunolocalization studies [26]. Subsequently bFGF was extracted from the nuclei of several cell types [33]. Nuclear extracts from bovine ventricles were also found to contain a 18 kD bFGF (Figure 10). While nuclear targeting of the N-extended forms of FGF-like growth factors has been implicated in stimulation of proliferation (39), the potential function of the 18 kD bFGF in the nucleus appears related to differentiation.

Figure 10 (top). Identification of bFGF in the nucleus. Nuclear protein extracts were obtained from bovine heart ventricles. Heparin-binding peptides from these extracts were probed for bFGF by western blotting. Lane 1: Heparin-bound fraction from 50 μg nuclear protein. Lane 2: 20 μg nuclear protein after heparin-sepharose chromatography. Lane 3: 20 μg nuclear protein, before heparin-sepharose chromatography. Lane 4: Bovine pituitary bFGF (20 ng) used as positive control. Arrow indicates the 18 kD bFGF.

Figure 11 (bottom). Basic FGF in cardiac infarcts Triple-fluorescence labelling for (A), nuclei, (B), bFGF, and, (C), desmoplakin. Infarction was induced to male SD rats (200 g) by coronary occlusion [46]. Transverse sections from infarcted ventricles were examined by immunofluorescence 48 h after surgery. Large open arrows denote centre of infarct. Full arrows point at viable myocardium. Asterisks mark areas of intense cellular infiltration. Note the stronge anti-bFGF label of the infarct (B). (Bar, 50 μm).

Cardiac myocyte injury and bFGF

We examined bFGF accumulation and localization in three distinct models of cardiac injury: a genetic model (the mdx mouse model of muscular dystrophy) [27], in catecholamine-induced cardiomyopathy [18,19], and in cardiac infarction induced by coronary occlusion (Figure 11). Evidence from all three models is consistent with a participation of bFGF in the short as well as long-term response of the heart to trauma. A typical set of results is shown in Figure 11. Two days after induction of infarction [46], cardiac ventricular sections were examined by triple-fluorescence staining for localization of bFGF, desmoplakin and nuclear DNA (Figure 10). Anti-desmoplakin staining of intercalated discs identified viable cardiomyocytes, and nuclear DNA staining provided an assessment of cellular infiltration [18,19,27]. Viable myocardium can be discerned in the lower right half of the section in the field shown in Figure 11. Desmoplakin staining is either totally absent or diminished in the remaining area (Figure 11,C), which represents the infarcted region. High cellular density is observed mainly at the periphery of the infarct (Figure 11,A). Necrotic myocytes at the central region of the infarct stain intensely for bFGF (Figure 11,B).

In all three models of injury examined, myocytes undergoing irreversible injury displayed intense cytoplasmic anti-bFGF labelling, an observation which, in conjunction with higher bFGF concentrations in extracts from injured hearts, indicated increased levels of bFGF in association with the lesions [18,19,27]. In all three models, the increase in myocyte cytoplasmic bFGF occured prior to cellular infiltration. It is probable that bFGF is important for the repair response that does take place in the heart, promoting for instance infiltration and proliferation of motile cells. It is also plausible that bFGF is responsible for the sluggish attempt made by the cardiomyocytes at the injury site to initiate a regenerative response [45]. Other local factors such as TGFß which increases after ischemic injury [17] may counteract the bFGF-induced effect on the myocytes, as is the case in vitro [14]. Elucidating the relationship between the effects of various endogenous growth factors on the myocytes and non-muscle cells populating areas of injury may provide an avenue for improving the myocardial regenerative response.

Concluding remarks

The myocardium does not regenerate, yet it expresses in relative abundance bFGF, a multifunctional molecule implicated strongly in tissue regeneration and, as our data suggest, cardiac repair processes.

Myocytes of the viable myocardium, therefore, have either lost the ability to respond timely to bFGF after injury (by not expressing the appropriate bFGF receptors for instance), or they are prevented from doing so by other local or humoral factors. We have presented here an overview of our work which points to TGFß and thyroid hormone as such potential "blockers" of cardiomyocyte regenerative reponse to extracellular bFGF. We have also obtained further data, not presented here, which suggest that thyroid status determines the relative levels of 18 or 22 kD bFGF in the heart [38]. It is interesting that transient hypothyroidism has been reported for victims of heart attack [47)] Since a drop in thyroid hormone levels might remove the inhibition of bFGF-induced stimulation of DNA synthesis in myocytes, we hypothesize that this response may represent an endogenous self-defense mechanism.

Study of bFGF in the context of cardiac growth and physiology is still in its infancy. Several important questions remain unanswered. How is the activity of bFGF regulated in vivo? Do immature or differentiated cardiomyocytes express functional bFGF receptors, and if so, which ones? Are these receptors linked to a signalling pathway leading to mitogenic stimulation and/or hypertrophy ? What is the role of cytoplasmic and especially nuclear or gap junction-associated bFGF? What are the functional differences between 18 and 22 kD bFGF? And last, but not least, can differentiated cardiomyocytes be induced to divide by bFGF in vivo? Answering these questions will improve our understanding of mechanisms regulating cardiomyocyte growth and response to injury and may lead to new strategies in the treatment of myocardial disease.

Acknowledgements

The technical assistance of Robert R. Fandrich is gratefully appreciated. Work reviewed here was supported by grants from the Heart and Stroke Foundation of Canada, the Medical Research Council (MRC) of Canada and the Manitoba Health Research Council. E.K and P.A.C. are MRC Scholars. L.L., R.R.P. and S.K.B.P. hold studentships from the Manitoba Health Research Council.

References

1. Zak R: Factors controlling cardiac growth. In: Zak R, editor. Growth of the Heart in Health and Disease. Raven Press, New York, NY. 1984; 165-185.
2. Claycomb WC, Moses RL. Growth factors and TPA stimulate DNA synthesis and alter the morphology of cultured terminally differentiated adult rat cardiac muscle cells. Devel Biol 1988; 127: 257-265.
3. Anversa P, Fitzpatrick D, Argani S, Capasso JM. Myocyte mitotic division in the aging mammalian rat heart. Circ Res 1991; 69: 1159-1164.
4. Parker TG, Schneider MD. Growth factors, protooncogenes, and plasticity of the cardiac phenotype. Ann Rev Physiol 1991; 53: 179-200.
5. Rifkin DB, Moscatelli D. Recent developments in the cell biology of basic fibroblast growth factor. J Cell Biol 1989; 109: 1-6.
6. Burgess WH, Maciag T. The heparin-binding (fibroblast) growth factor family of proteins. Ann Rev Biochem 1989; 58: 575-606.
7. Coulier F, Ollendorff V, Marics I, Rosnet O, Batoz M, Planche J, Marchetto S, Pebusque M-J, deLapeyriere O, Birnbaum D. The FGF6 gene within the FGF multigene family. Ann NY Acad Sci 1991; 638: 53-62.
8. Esch F, Baird A, Ling N, Ueno N, Hill L, Klepper R, Gospodarowicz D, Bohlen P, Guillemin R. Primary Structure of bovine pituitary basic fibroblast growth factor (FGF) and comparison with the amino-terminal sequence of bovine brain acidic FGF. Proc Natl Acad Sci USA 1985; 82: 6507-6511.
9. Muthukrishnan L, Warder E, McNeil PL. Basic fibroblast growth factor is efficiently released from a cytosolic storage site through plasma membrane disruptions of endothelial cells. J Cell Physiol 1991; 48: 1-16.
10. Lindner V, Majack RA, Reidy MA. Basic fibroblast growth factor stimulates endothelial regrowth and proliferation in denuded arteries. J Clin Invest Year 1990; 85, 2004-2008.
11. Hebda PA, Klingbeil CK, Abraham JA, Fiddes JC. Basic fibroblast growth factor stimulation of epidermal wound healing in pigs. J Invest Dermatol 1990; 95: 626-631.
12. Cuevas P, Burgos J, Baird A. Basic fibroblast growth factor promotes cartilage repair in vivo. Biochem Biophys Res Commun 1988; 156: 611-618.
13. Morisson RS, Sharma A, de Velis J, Bradshaw RA. Basic fibroblast growth factor suppports the survival of cerebral cortical neurons in primary culture. Proc Natl Acad Sci USA 1986; 83: 7537-7541.
14. Kardami E. Stimulation and inhibition of cardiac myocyte proliferation in vitro. Mol Cell Biochem 1990; 92: 124-134.

15. Kardami E, Fandrich RR. Heparin-binding growth factors in cardiac compartments. In: Cell and Molecular Biology of Muscle Development, UCLA Symposia Series, Alan R Liss, Inc, New York, 1989; 315-325.

16. Roberts AB, Sporn MB. The transforming growth factor betas. In: Sporn M, Roberts AB, editors. Peptide Growth Factors and Their Receptors. Heidelberg: Springer-Verlag 1990; 421-472.

17. Thomson NL, Bazoberry F, Speir E, Casscells W, Ferrans VJ, Flanders K, Kondaiah P, Geiser AG, Sporn MB. Transforming growth factor beta-1 in acute myocardial infarction in rats. Growth Factors 1988; 1: 91-99.

18. Padua RR, Kardami E. Increased basic fibroblast growth factor accumulation and distinct patterns of localization in isoproterenol-induced cardiomyocyte injury. 1992 (Submitted).

19. Padua RR, Doble BW, Kardami E. Basic fibroblast growth factor in development and after isoproterenol-induced injury in the rat heart. J Mol Cell Cardiol 1991; 23 (suppl.III): S90.

20. Mahdavi V, Izumo S, Nadal-Ginard B. Developmental and hormonal regulation of sarcomeric myosin heavy chain gene family. Circ Res 1987; 60: 804-814.

21. Dubois JD, Dussault JH. Ontogenesis of thyroid function in the neonatal rat. Thyroxine (T4) and triiodothyronine (T3) production. Endocrinology 1977; 101: 435-441.

22. Akiyama SK, Yamada KM. Synthetic peptides competitively inhibit both direct binding to fibroblasts and functional biological assays for the purified cell-binding domain of fibronectin. J Biol Chem 1985; 260: 10402-10405.

23. Janero DR, Hreniuk D, Sharif HM. Hydrogen peroxide-induced oxidative stress to the mammalian heart-muscle cell (cardiomyocyte): Lethal peroxidative membrane injury . J Cell Physiol 1991; 249: 347-364.

24. Thomson SA. The disulfide structure of bovine pituitary basic fibroblast growth factor. J Biol Chem 1992; 267: 2269-2273.

25. Eckenstein FP, Shipley GD, Nishi R. Acidic and basic fibroblast growth factors in the nervous system: distribution and differential alteration of levels after injury of central versus peripheral nerve. J Neurosci 1991; 11: 412-419.

26. Kardami E, Fandrich RR. Basic fibroblast growth factor in atria and ventricles of the vertebrate heart. J Cell Biol 1989; 109: 1865-1875.

27. Anderson J, Liu L, Kardami E. Distinctive basic fibrolast growth factor distribution in regenerating and degenerating dystrophic (mdx) striated muscle. Dev Biol 1991; 147: 96-109.

28. Kardami E, Murphy L, Liu L, Padua RR, Fandrich RR. Characterization of two preparations of immunoglobulins to basic fibroblast growth factor which exhibit distinct patterns of localization. Growth Factors 1990; 4: 69-80.

29. Kardami E, Stoski RM, Doble BW, Yamamoto T, Herzberg EL, Nagy JI. Biochemical and ultrastructural evidence for the association of basic fibroblast growth factor with cardiac gap junctions. J Biol Chem 1991; 266: 19551-19558.

30. Kardami E, Liu L, Doble BW. Basic fibroblast growth factor in cultured cardiac myocytes. Ann NY Acad Sci 1991; 638: 244-255.

31. Doble BW, Fandrich RR, Liu L, Kardami E. Calcium protects pituitary basic FGF from proteolysis by copurifying proteases. Biochem Biophys Res Commun 1990; 173: 1116-1122.

32. Brigstock DR, Sasse J, Klagsbrun M. Subcellular distribution of basic fibroblast growth factor in human hepatoma cells. Growth Factors 1991; 4: 189-196.

33. Yamamoto T, Kardami E, Nagy JI. Basic fibroblast growth factor in rat brain: localization to glial gap junctions correlates with connexin 43 distribution. Brain Res 1991; 554: 336-343.

34. Eghbali B, Kessler JA, Reid LM, Roy C, Spray DC. Involvement of gap junctions in tumorigenesis: Transfection of tumor cells with connexin 32 cDNA retards growth in vivo. Proc Natl Acad Sci USA 1991; 88: 10701-10705.

35. Rumyanchev PP. Interrelations of the proliferation and differentiation processes during cardiac myogenesis and regeneration. Int Rev Cytol 1977; 51:187-273.

36. Kardami E, Spector D, Strohman RC. Myogenic growth factor present in skeletal muscle is purified by heparin affinity chromatography. Proc Natl Acad Sci USA 1985; 82: 8044-8047.

37. Liu L, Doble BW, Kardami E. Perinatal phenotype and hypothyroidism are associated with elevated levels of basic fibroblast growth factor (bFGF) in cardiac ventricles. Submitted.

38. Liu L, Doble BW, Fandrich RR, Kardami E. Hypothyroidism favours tissue-specific accumulation of high molecular weight basic fibroblast growth factor. J Cell Biol 1991; 115: 417a.

39. Amalric F, Baldin V, Bosc-Bierne I, Bugler B, Gouderc B, Guyader M, Patry V, Prats H, Roman AM, Bouche G. Nuclear translocation of basic fibroblast growth factor. Ann NY Acad Sci 1991; 638: 127-138.

40. Florkiewicz RZ, Sommer A. Human basic fibroblast growth factor gene encodes four polypeptides: Three initiate translation from non-AUG codon. Proc Natl Acad Sci USA 1989; 86: 3978-3981.

41. Powell PP, Klagsbrun M. Three forms of rat basic fibroblast growth factor are made from a single mRNA and localize to the nucleus. J Cell Physiol 1991; 148: 202-210.

42. Quarto N, Finger FP, Rifkin D. The NH2-terminal extension of high molecular weight bFGF is a nuclear targeting signal. J Cell Physiol 1991; 147: 311-318.

43. Pasumarthi SKB, Doble B, Liu L, Bock M, Kardami E, Cattini PA. (1992). Overexpression of basic fibroblast growth factor in cardiac myocytes is associated with nuclear fragmentation. FASEB J 1992; 6: A1078.

44. Cattini PA, Kardami E, Eberhardt NL. Effect of butyrate on thyroid hormone-mediated gene expression in rat pituitary tumour cells. Mol Cell Endocrinol 1988; 56: 263-270.

45. Rumyantsev P. Regenerative possibilities of the ventricular myocardium of adult mammals. In: Carlson BM, editor. Growth and hyperplasia of cardiac muscle cells. Cardiology Soviet Medical Reviews Supplement Series, Harwood Academic Publishers 1991; 3: 194-209.

46. Fishbein MC, Maclean D, Maroko PR. Experimental myocardial infarction in the rat. Qualitative and quantitative changes during pathologic evolution Am J Pathol 1977; 90: 57-70.

47. Wiersinga WM, Lie KI, Touber JL. Thyroid hormones in acute myocardial infarction. Clin Endocrinol 1981; 14: 367.

6. Growth factor signal transduction in the cardiac myocyte: functions of the serum response element

MICHAEL D. SCHNEIDER, THOMAS BRAND, ROBERT J. SCHWARTZ and W. ROBB MACLELLAN

Introduction

Historically, the question of whether cardiac muscle cells might be targets for the action of polypeptide growth factors was prompted, in equal measure, by analogy and incrimination: proof for the paramount role of growth factors in the skeletal muscle lineage as regulators of myogenesis [1, 2] and differentiation [3-7], and evidence that growth factor-like activity accumulates in myocardium after experimental aortic constriction, promoting amino acid incorporation into recipient cardiac tissue [8]. Despite more recent, specific clues as to the potential identity of myocardial growth factors [9]—isolation from myocardium or detection of several already-familiar peptide growth factors, [10-13], detailed mapping of growth factor expression within the heart by immunocytochemical methods and in situ hybridization [14-16], association of increased growth factor expression with certain mechanical or pharmacological models of hypertrophy [17-20]—there have been surprisingly few direct attempts to test the promising hypothesis that growth factors might modulate or govern critical aspects of the cardiac phenotype. One regrettable truism, which often is cited to help account for this paucity of information, alludes to the technical limitations commonly associated with, if not inherent to, primary cell culture, especially primary culture of ventricular myocytes. These experimental obstacles include dedifferentiation [21], heterogeneity of cell types [22], and logistical constraints arising from a relatively modest cell yield, compared to that achievable with immortalized cell lines or cells such as fibroblasts, with greater potential for proliferation in vitro. Ironically, several impediments have been in large part overcome through the use of culture media that contain non-mitogenic concentrations of serum or by the development of chemically defined media for cardiac cells that are free of exogenous growth factors [23]. Furthermore, the assumption that permanent cell lines necessarily model growth and gene expression with greater fidelity than newly dissociated cells has undergone increased scrutiny. For example, by comparison with skeletal muscle itself, many myogenic cell lines in widespread use express discrepant sets of myosin heavy chain isoforms [24], growth factor receptors [25], or muscle determination genes of the MyoD family [26, 27]. The two points of emphasis for the present review will be a survey of the growth factors that control a broad array of myocardial genes—notably, members of the heparin-binding, "fibroblast" growth factor (FGF) and type ß transforming growth factor (TGFß) superfamilies—followed by a more intricate account of growth factor signal transduction in the case of a single gene, encoding the skeletal muscle isoform of α-actin, representative of a battery of genes associated jointly with early cardiac development and with myocardial hypertrophy. Other aspects of growth factor function in cardiac muscle cells such as contractile function and growth itself, along with additional information concerning the TGFß and FGF families, are detailed in contributions by Drs. Sporn and Kardami elsewhere in this volume.

Fibroblast and Type ß transforming growth factors induce a fetal program of cardiac gene expression resembling the consequences of mechanical load

Important early indications that serum components, apart from thyroid hormone or adrenergic agonists, might modulate the cardiac phenotype included ventricular myocytes' progression through increasingly differentiated states under mitogen-free conditions [23], and serum induction of hypertrophy [28] or hyperplasia [23], depending on the experimental conditions. Indeed, over the course of prolonged growth factor withdrawal, re-introducing serum successively elicited proliferative growth, DNA synthesis uncoupled from cell division, or neither growth response [23]. These phenomena correspond to the three phases of declining growth capacity observed in ventricular muscle in vivo, binucleation or tetraploidy being characteristic of mammalian ventricular myocytes even shortly after birth [29]. Concurrent effects on gene expression were also contingent on the duration of serum withdrawal. Serum caused downregulation of both the skeletal and cardiac α-actin genes in cells competent to undergo proliferation, after 48 hrs in a serum-free milieu, yet selectively upregulated skeletal α-actin (SkA) in the cells lacking an obvious growth response, after two weeks of withdrawal [23]. These investigations establish that growth factor withdrawal enhances differentiation in cultured cardiac myocytes and lead to the inference that serum growth factors can regulate cardiac growth and gene expression, at least at the stage of development captured in this in vitro model.

To ascertain more specifically whether cardiac muscle cells are targets for the action of peptide growth factors and to determine whether growth factor control over myocardial genes duplicates or departs from the global suppression of tissue-specific genes produced in skeletal muscle, neonatal rat ventricular muscle cells were challenged with growth factors and were analyzed for expression of seven developmentally regulated cardiac genes [30, 31]. Genes selected for investigation included four which, especially in small mammals, are expressed at higher abundance in the embryonic ventricle than the adult: ß-myosin heavy chain (ßMHC), atrial natriuretic factor (ANF), SkA, and smooth muscle α-actin, the earliest α-actin expressed during cardiac development [32]. Among these, ßMHC [33], ANF [34, 35], and SkA [35, 36] were known to be upregulated in adult ventricular muscle as hallmarks of pressure-overload hypertrophy in vivo. Conversely, two additional genes, αMHC [33] and the slow/cardiac Ca^{2+}-ATPase of sarcoplasmic reticulum (SR) [37], which are more abundantly expressed in adult myocardium than in the embryo, are downregulated by load.

Finally, a seventh gene, cardiac α-actin, had been shown to be relatively unaffected by mechanical [36] or pharmacological [38] interventions causing hypertrophy. TGFß1 and basic FGF resulted in a continuum of coexisting inhibitory and stimulatory responses: partial suppression of genes encoding aMHC and the SR Ca^{2+}-ATPase, no effect on cardiac α-actin, and selective up-regulation of all four genes associated with embryonic myocardium [30, 31]. Thus, each of these growth factors preferentially induced, in the absence of load, an array of fetal cardiac genes that are characteristic of myocardial hypertrophy. Basic FGF increased protein content in the cardiac myocyte cultures, whereas TGFß1 did not, indicating that the fetal program of gene expression can be evoked independently of hypertrophic growth [30].

Disparities and even a dichotomy in the actions of acidic versus basic FGF illustrate a second distinction from growth factor control over skeletal muscle cells [3]. Like basic FGF, acidic FGF produced reciprocal changes in the abundance of α and ßMHC mRNA, down-regulation and up-regulation, respectively, notwithstanding the presence of thyroxine in the medium [30]. Furthermore, again resembling basic FGF, acidic FGF inhibited expression of the SR Ca^{2+}-ATPase gene, while up-regulating ANF [31]; these two events are convincingly associated not only with rodent models of hypertrophy but also with end-stage heart failure in humans [39, 40]. Nonetheless, acidic FGF inhibited expression of cardiac α-actin (which was not affected by TGFß or by basic FGF) and even diminished the expression of SkA (which, contrarily, was up-regulated by TGFß1 or basic FGF) [30]. Of the three growth factors investigated, only acidic FGF was a mitogen for cardiac muscle cells [30]. In the presence of supplemental serum factors, basic FGF also has been reported to cause proliferation in neonatal cardiac myocytes [11].

All three peptide growth factors stimulated the smooth muscle a-actin gene [30]. At the time of these initial cell culture studies, it was unknown whether smooth muscle α-actin could be reactivated in vivo by aortic banding like other transcripts associated with embryonic myocardium, a potentially novel aspect to plasticity, predicted by the general "fetal" phenotype following load and implied by autocrine or paracrine concepts of hypertrophy. As shown subsequently, expression of the smooth muscle α-actin gene indeed is evoked by coarctation, even more consistently than SkA: smooth muscle α-actin is a molecular marker of the presence and extent of ventricular hypertrophy, whose induction is tightly correlated with the degree of ventricular growth [41]. Thus, transforming and fibroblast growth factors selectively up-regulate a broad and representative ensemble of the genes associated with myocardial hypertrophy in vivo.

The proximal skeletal α-actin promoter suffices for tissue-specific expression and transcriptional control by three peptide growth factors

Necessary steps towards defining the molecular basis for growth factor control of cardiac gene expression were to ascertain whether exogenous α-actin promoters could be transcribed appropriately in neonatal rat cardiac muscle, and to delineate what specific portions of the gene might be required for basal and regulated expression in a cardiac background. With increasing knowledge of the cis-acting DNA motifs responsible for cardiac- and skeletal muscle-restricted transcription of genes shared in common by the striated muscle lineages, two general cases are emerging. For a subset of genes, identical cis-acting domains mediate transcription in both cell types (for example, ße2 and ße3 elements of the ßMHC enhancer) [42]; for others, activation in cardiac versus skeletal muscle requires elements that are distinct. Examples of this latter class include cardiac troponin C [43], cardiac troponin T [44], and muscle creatine kinase [45], indicating that, for these genes, transcription activation pathways differ between the two striated muscle lineages.

Efficient tissue-specific transcription and accurate responsiveness to all three peptide growth factors required only short proximal segments of the avian skeletal and cardiac α-actin promoters (nucleotides -202 to -11 and -318 to +18, respectively) [31]. In ventricular muscle cells, these regions of the skeletal and cardiac α-actin promoters were both highly expressed, relative to a constitutive viral control, in agreement with co-expression of the endogenous skeletal and cardiac α-actin genes under the experimental conditions used. Neither a 2-fold nor a 10-fold larger fragment of the SkA promoter was expressed more efficiently than this proximal -202/-11 domain. In agreement with these results, chick SkA promoters were truncated from 2000 to 200 nucleotides with little or no loss of transcriptional activity in rat L8 myotubes [46] or chick primary myocyte cultures [47]. A proximal fragment of the human skeletal actin promoter proximal to -153 likewise was sufficient for maximal expression in L8 cells [48], and more distal sequences of this promoter contribute relatively little to basal activity in cardiac muscle [49]. By contrast, in cardiac fibroblasts, the skeletal and cardiac α-actin promoters were expressed at minute levels, similar to a promoterless control. The avian α-actin promoters also possess appropriate tissue-specificity and developmental regulation in transgenic mice [50, 51], similar to results obtained using the rat α-actin gene [52].

In exact concordance with the effects of each growth factor on the endogenous SkA gene, activity of the SkA promoter was increased 3-fold by TGFß1 or basic FGF, relative to vehicle-treated cells, yet was decreased by acidic FGF by 60%. Thus, the reciprocal effects of basic and acidic FGF on SkA RNA abundance depend upon antithetical effects of these highly related growth factors on SkA transcription. In addition, showing fidelity comparable to that of the SkA promoter for expression of the corresponding endogenous gene, the transfected cardiac α-actin promoter was inhibited exclusively by acidic FGF; basic FGF and TGFß had little or no effect on cardiac α-actin transcription. Together with constitutive expression of an SV40 control during growth factor stimulation, this selective impact on the skeletal versus cardiac α-actin promoter ensures that the growth factor effects are not merely global changes in total transcription or spurious properties of the reporter construct. As copurifying factors, notably other heparin-binding growth factors, might confound the interpretation of results obtained with acidic FGF, basic FGF, or both, recombinant FGFs were utilized as a means to verify that the dichotomous effects of basic and acidic FGF on SkA transcription were inherently divergent actions, not misleading artifacts of contaminant proteins.

In short, these experiments established that the proximal SkA promoter provides the information necessary in cardiac muscle for all four of the transcriptional functions that were investigated: efficient tissue-specific expression, activation by TGFß1, activation by basic FGF, and suppression by acidic FGF. However, detailed mutagenesis of the promoter was required to identify the exact cis-acting sequences responsible for basal expression and to determine whether regulation by disparate growth factors involved a final common pathway.

Binding sites for serum response factor mediate lineage-specific transcription of the skeletal α-actin promoter in cardiac and skeletal muscle

The SkA promoter encompasses three repeats, spaced precisely 45 nucleotides apart, of a palindromic motif, $CC(A/T)_6GG$ or CArG box (for CC-A/T-rich-GG), present within other muscle-specific promoters or enhancers, including cardiac α-actin [53], myosin light chain 1/3 [54], ventricular myosin light chain-1 [55], cardiac myosin light chain 2 [56], cardiac troponin T [57], muscle creatine kinase [58], dystrophin [59], and myogenin [60]. Among these, the functional importance of CArG boxes varies but has been established unequivocally for transcription of cardiac [61, 62] and skeletal [63, 64] α-actin in skeletal myocytes. CArG boxes also are found as regulatory elements in a significant subset of genes induced with immediate-early kinetics following trophic signals, including cytoskeletal ß-actin [65], Egr-1/zif268 [66], and the c-*fos* proto-oncogene [67]. The canonical serum response element (SRE) in the c-*fos* promoter is activated by mitogenic signals [67], peptide growth factors including FGF [68], and postulated components of the growth factor signal transduction cascade such as *ras* [69], protein kinase C [70], *raf*-1 kinase [71], and casein kinase II [72]. In cardiac muscle cells, this element also is thought to mediate induction of *fos* by mechanical stress [73] (S. Izumo, personal communication).

First isolated as a sequence-specific DNA-binding protein that recognizes the c-*fos* SRE [74], serum response factor (SRF) now is understood, through the detailed mapping of promoters summarized above, to mediate tissue-specific transcription of certain muscle genes as well. One critical clue in establishing this concept was appreciation that the principal CArG box-binding protein for the sarcomeric actin promoters was indistinguishable from SRF, by a host of biochemical and immunological criteria [75], a conclusion later substantiated with the availability of recombinant reagents [76-79]. As shown for the *fos* SRE itself, mutations that disrupt SRF binding likewise extinguish activity of the skeletal [60, 63, 76] and cardiac [80, 81] α-actin promoters in differentiated skeletal muscle cells. Conversely (and perhaps counter-intuitively), SREs isolated either from α-actin promoters [60, 63, 80, 82] or the c-*fos* promoter [82] confer tissue-specific expression to minimal, neutral promoters in skeletal muscle; furthermore, the *fos* SRE can substitute for the cardiac α-actin proximal SRE to direct muscle-specific activation in developing *Xenopus* embryos [80]. Alternatively, it has also been concluded in the case of the cardiac α-actin promoter that intact binding sites for SRF are necessary yet not sufficient, and that SRF acts in concert with the muscle determination protein MyoD and the activator protein Sp1 to drive transcription of the gene [81]; see ref. [83]. Together these investigations have substantiated the obligatory role for SRF in skeletal muscle expression of both striated α-actin genes but have also suggested the possibility that its activity may require collaboration with lineage-specific and ubiquitous factors.

The molecular cloning of SRF [84] revealed critical aspects of its structure—a basic region of amino acids for high-affinity DNA binding and adjacent dimerization interface—similar to DNA-binding domains of the yeast regulatory proteins MCM1 [85, 86] and ARG80 [87] and the plant homeotic factors agamous [88] and deficiens [89, 90], collectively, the MADS box family [91, 92]. MCM1 is expressed in haploid cells of *Saccharomyces cerevisiae* having either of the two mating phenotypes, **a** or α, and provides an exceptionally well characterized example of multifunctionality that is conferred by accessory proteins (93). MCM1 directly binds a dyad symmetry element, or P box, for activation of **a**-specific genes in **a** cells. Conversely, in the α cell background, MCM1 binds this site cooperatively with the alpha-specific factor α 2, to repress the **a** gene set. Third, MCM1 cooperates with another α-specific factor, α 1, to activate α-specific genes. Thus, the SRF homologue MCM1 functions as a transcriptional activator (unassisted), a cell-specific activator (with α1), or cell-specific repressor (with α 2) [93].

With this as background, to define sites within the first 200 5'-flanking nucleotides of the SkA promoter that might mediate transcription in ventricular myocytes, cardiac muscle cells were transfected with a series of deletion-gap and linker-scanning mutations, with emphasis on the previously identified positive and negative elements that contribute to expression in skeletal muscle [64, 76]. Relative to the wild-type promoter used for mutagenesis, spanning nucleotides -424 to +24, excisions overlying the upstream (-175; SRE3), central (-130; SRE2), and downstream (-85; SRE1) SREs yielded residual CAT activity of 45, 24, and 9%, respectively. Deletion of the GC-rich motif between SRE2 and SRE1, a potential Sp1/*Egr*-1 site, did not alter basal expression though this region functions as a negative regulator in skeletal myocytes (64). Thus, under these experimental conditions (with relatively high SkA expression even in vehicle-treated cardiac cells), promoter regions containing all 3 SREs contribute to basal expression, particularly SRE1. In agreement with this latter conclusion, a 5'Æ3' deletion retaining nucleotides -107 to -11, but eliminating sequences upstream of SRE1, yielded roughly one-third the activity of the wild-type promoter.

Despite the utility of internal deletions for selectively ablating large as well as small promoter regions—illustrated by removal of proximal SREs from the cardiac α-actin promoter, relocating distal SREs to the proximal position [94]—potential distortion of axial and rotational relationships between elements adjacent to the gap complicates the analysis of results obtained by this means. Such a requirement for precise spacing to optimize phase relations exists in skeletal muscle for SRE3 and SRE2, and for SRE2 versus SRE1 [95]. Consequently, to obviate this concern and establish with greater certainty the role of the proximal elements, cardiac myocytes were transfected with block-substitution mutations of the SkA promoter. Site-directed mutagenesis of SRE3, SRE2, and SRE1 corroborated the overall conclusions obtained by internal deletion [96]. The preferential dependence of cardiac myocytes on the most proximal SRE for SkA transcription was even more apparent in ventricular myocytes purified further by Percoll density gradient centrifugation and plated with reduced concentrations of fetal serum (W. R. MacLellan, T.-C. Lee, R. J. Schwartz, and M. D. Schneider, unpublished data). In skeletal muscle, by contrast, mutagenesis at all three SREs impaired promoter function equivalently [64].

To test the implication that SRE1 could function in the absence of distal SREs to drive expression of the SkA promoter in cardiac muscle cells, and to explore, further, the possibility that it might mediate cardiac-specific expression in the absence of other actin sequences entirely, a 28 bp oligonucleotide, centered on the SRE1 and inserted upstream from a neutral promoter (mouse c-*fos*, nucleotides -56 to +109), was transfected into neonatal rat cardiac myocytes [96]; cf. ref. [60, 63]. Basal expression of a chloramphenicol acetyltransferase reporter gene driven by the -202/-11 SkA promoter was not significantly different from that of the constitutive viral control, pSV2CAT. In agreement with the promoter truncated at -107, lacking all elements distal to SRE1, SRE1 itself produced up to one-third the CAT activity found with the -202/-11 promoter and was 25-fold greater than a negative control, comprising the vector, c-*fos* core promoter, and a mutation of SRE1 that cannot bind SRF. Thus, the plasmid sequences alone have no spurious intrinsic activity in ventricular muscle cells, and transcription of the reporter gene depends specifically on the inserted SRE motifs. Since neither SRE was expressed in cardiac fibroblasts, basal activity of the skeletal α-actin SRE1 and *fos* SRE in cardiac myocyte cultures is not confounded by contaminating non-muscle cells and reflects tissue-specific transcription of these isolated elements.

The proximal serum response element of the skeletal α-actin promoter mediates induction by basic FGF or TGFß1 and discriminates between signals generated in cardiac cells by basic and acidic FGF

In cardiac myocytes, basic and acidic FGF have antithetical effects on transcription of the exogenous SkA promoter, or on steady-state expression of the endogenous SkA gene, yet, as illustrated earlier, these two prototypes of the FGF family have qualitatively identical effects on five other cardiac-restricted genes (suppression of α MHC and the SR Ca^{2+}-ATPase; up-regulation of ANF, ßMHC, and smooth muscle α-actin). Furthermore, acidic and basic FGF both up-regulate the immediate-early response genes c-*fos*, c-*jun*, and *jun*B in cardiac myocyte cultures (T. G. Parker and M. D. Schneider, unpublished data). Among other mechanisms suggested by this finding is the possibility that the SkA SRE1 might differ inherently from the c-*fos* SRE in its regulation by FGFs. To examine this hypothesis directly, cardiac myocytes were transfected with reporter genes driven by the SkA SRE1 versus the *fos* SRE, detailed earlier, and were then exposed to recombinant basic FGF or acidic FGF, as described for the full-length promoter constructs. Basic FGF up-regulated transcription of both elements, whereas, surprisingly, acidic FGF increased activity of the *fos* SRE alone [96]. Thus, sequence differences between these two related sites are sufficient to enable the SkA SRE1 to distinguish between the effects of basic and acidic FGF; however, precisely which nucleotides confer this selectivity is not known. Furthermore, the failure of acidic FGF to influence transcription of the SkA SRE1 deviates from the repressive effect shown for acidic FGF with the larger SkA promoter or endogenous SkA gene. Whether a discrete negative regulatory element for acidic FGF exists elsewhere in the promoter or, as one alternative, inhibition requires cooperative interaction between SRE1 and other sites remains to be ascertained.

The SkA SRE1 also mediates induction by TGFß1 (W. R. MacLellan, R. J. Schwartz, and M. D. Schneider, unpublished data). This differs from previously identified mediators for TGFß-dependent signals, including *fos* and *jun* [97, 98], CTF/NF-I [99], the bHLH protein USF, and factors that bind a GC-rich element of the *myc* proto-oncogene promoter [100].

SRF and muscle-specific transcription

On the face of it, the finding of cardiac and skeletal muscle-restricted transcription mediated by SRF is paradoxical. How can a ubiquitous transcription factor cause cardiac-restricted expression? It should be reiterated, however, that this observation concurs with the reported specificity of skeletal alpha-actin [60, 63], cardiac α-actin [80, 82)] and even c-*fos* SREs [82] in skeletal muscle as well. One potential explanation could be the coexistence of unrelated, unrecognized regulatory motifs even within these narrowly delimited fragments of the promoter. For example, 3' to the *fos* SRE core there exists a potential E-box for basic-helix-loop-helix (bHLH) transcription factors (CCATATTAGGACATCTG). Although neither MyoD itself, nor any of the related muscle determination proteins has been detected in cardiac muscle cells at any stage of cardiac development, the likelihood of cardiac homologues has been inferred from investigations of the human cardiac α-actin promoter by Sartorelli et al.: mutation of the MyoD binding site at -56/-51 reduces expression to that of the basal promoter, promoter activation in cardiac myocytes is partially repressed by co-transfection with Id, the inhibitor of bHLH transcription factors, and certain bHLH proteins may be enriched in cardiac muscle cells [101]. Thus, apart from a priori considerations there also is credible circumstantial evidence to favor the notion that cardiac muscle both expresses and utilizes bHLH factors analogous to MyoD. The information available at present does not distinguish, however, between two interpretations, whose implications differ: the presence of hypothetical cardiac-restricted proteins or, rather, ubiquitous E2A gene products known to be expressed in the heart [102].

Furthermore, bHLH proteins seem unlikely to reconcile the tissue-specific transcription of the isolated SREs. First, the nominal E-box adjoining the *fos* SRE deviates from the consensus motifs defined for MyoD and *myc*-like bHLH transcription factors by PCR-mediated binding site selection [103, 104] and the c-*fos* SRE interacts with MyoD and myogenin poorly if at all (K. Walsh, personal communication). Second, even smaller constructs centered on the SRE but lacking this sequence confer tissue-specific expression in C2 myocytes versus L cells [82], and muscle versus non-muscle regions of *Xenopus* embryos [80]. Third, no E-box is associated with the skeletal α-actin SRE1, and, as expected, this element does not directly bind MyoD or myogenin [60].

Another potential basis for SREs to account for lineage-specific patterns of transcription proposes the falsehood of a long-standing assumption. Typically, SRF has been regarded as ubiquitous or constitutive, a generalization supported by reasonable and convincing data. For instance, no differences in SRE binding activity were seen among logarithmically growing, serum-starved, or serum-stimulated HeLa cells [67], nor were significant differences apparent between HeLa cells, other non-myogenic cells, and myoblasts or myotubes of three muscle cell lines [105]. However, the counter-examples are worth noting. The SRF gene itself is highly induced by serum factors [84], and SRE binding activity increases after EGF stimulation of A431 cells [106]. During *Xenopus* development, SRF RNA up-regulates at least 50-fold [77], and SRF is distributed with some limited regional specificity, enriched in the somites versus neurectoderm [107]. Of direct relevance here, increased accumulation of SRF was recently shown to accompany or precede differentiation in primary cultures of embryonic chick muscle cells and to be suppressed by 5-bromodeoxyuridine [79], an inhibitor of myogenesis [108]. Consequently, measurements of SRF abundance in cardiac muscle have become highly germane. A final possibility related to SRF itself is the potential for lineage-specific post-translational modifications.

Srf-related and SRF-associated proteins

Myocyte-specific enhancer factor 2 (MEF2)

Alternatively, hypothetical SRE-binding proteins have been envisaged, similar but not identical to SRF [80, 105]. This model is logically sound and has substantive basis in a recently identified family of mammalian factors related to SRF (RSRFs), cloned by low stringency hybridization with a DNA fragment spanning the DNA-binding domain of SRF [92] or by screening cardiac and skeletal muscle expression libraries (109) with concatemers of an A/T-rich site in the MCK enhancer that binds the myocyte-specific factor, MEF2 [110]. The diversity of MEF2 proteins results both from the existence of multiple genes for this family and from alternative mRNA splicing. MEF2 transcripts are ubiquitous, with increased abundance in skeletal muscle, heart, and brain; some spliced variants of MEF2, as well as transcripts of a second gene, xMEF2, are even more highly specific for these tissues [109]. The distributions of MEF-2 DNA-binding activity and immunoreactive MEF-2 protein—in differentiated cardiac and skeletal muscle but not cardiac fibroblasts or undifferentiated myoblasts—correspond to the presence of tissue-specific MEF2 transcripts rather than ubiquitous forms (109).

The importance of RSRF binding sites to muscle-specific transcription was suggested by mutational analysis of the MCK [110] and myosin light chain 1/3 [111] enhancers and the cardiac myosin light chain 2 promoter [56], and by the ability of isolated MEF2 sites derived from these genes to confer tissue-specificity to various minimal promoters. The consensus sequence for cloned RSRFs derived from binding site selection in vitro, $CTA(A/T)_4TAG$ [92], concurs well with the canonical MEF2 site in the muscle creatine kinase enhancer (CTAAAAATAA) [110]. However, one gap in the information provided by Pollock and Treisman in their initial description of mammalian SRF-related proteins was the lack of direct proof for trans-activation by cloned RSRFs, using cotransfection. More recently, Nadal-Ginard, Mahdavi, and their co-workers have succeeded in demonstrating that cloned RSRFs trans-activate transcription mediated by the MCK MEF2 site or a related A/T rich promoter sequence of the embryonic skeletal muscle MHC gene [109]. Like SREs, RSRF binding sites also exist in the promoters for a variety of immediate early response genes including N10/*nur*77 and c-*jun*. It is plausible to speculate that RSRFs, like SRF itself, might regulate both muscle-specific and growth factor-dependent transcription. In support of this prediction, the N10 and c-*jun* sites bind RSRFs [92) and the N10 element mediates transactivation by the cloned transcription factors [109]. Although these SRF-related factors bind DNA as dimers, they do not form dimers with SRF or bind to SRE motifs in vitro [92, 109].

Ternary complex factor

A number of other proteins, however, associate with SREs, indirectly [112, 113] or directly [60, 63, 76, 78, 79]. Proteins related to the *ets* proto-oncogene form a ternary complex involving SRF itself at a CAGGA sequence 5' to the c-*fos* SRE [112, 113] and mediate activation of the *fos* gene by protein kinase C-dependent signals [70]. Cardiac muscle contains a relatively high level of ternary complex factor (W. R. MacLellan, R. J. Schwartz, and M. D. Schneider, unpublished data); however, the skeletal α-actin SRE1 lacks this contiguous site and does not interact with this class of SRF accessory proteins from cardiac or skeletal muscle; see also ref. [60].

90

YY1, a competitive inhibitor of SRF

On the basis of electrophoretic mobility-shift assays, DNA-binding factors have been reported which directly but asymmetrically bind the SkA SRE1, c-*fos* SRE, or both. The relationship, if any, among the binding activities designated F-ACT1 [76, 79], MAPF1 [60, 63], p62^{DBF} [114] and common factor/CF1 [115] was uncertain until recently. By the criteria of DNA-binding specificity, methylation interference footprints, apparent mass during sodium dodecyl sulfate-polyacrylamide gel electrophoresis, zinc-dependence, and immunological cross-reactivity, these SRE-binding proteins are identical to YY1 [78, 79], a multifunctional C_2H_2 zinc finger protein of the GLI-Krüppel family with very widespread tissue distribution [116-120]. The methylation interference footprint for YY1 overlaps that of SRF, and recombinant YY1 and SRF compete for binding to both the SkA SRE1 and c-*fos* SRE in vitro [78]. The functional importance of this mechanism in vivo was verified by transfection into skeletal muscle [78, 79], YY1 represses transcription of the *fos* SRE and SkA SRE1, as anticipated, an effect which can be overcome by overexpression of exogenous SRF. In embryonic skeletal muscle, expression of YY1 binding activity shows reciprocity with SRF, diminishing with differentiation and increasing markedly with BrdU [79].

The authors have begun to correlate a mutational analysis of SkA promoter activity in cardiac cells with defined changes in DNA-protein recognition (W. R. MacLellan, T.-C. Lee, R. J. Schwartz, and M. D. Schneider, unpublished data). SRF and YY1 coexist in nuclear extracts of Percoll-purifed cardiac myocytes and are the predominant cardiac proteins that contact either SRE. Sequence-specificity was shown using a 100-fold excess of unlabeled SRE1, whereas a MEF1 site competes neither for SRF nor F-ACT-1. As expected, the c-*fos* SRE prevents SRF binding to SRE1 but interacts YY1 with lower affinity; see [76, 78]. The identity of SRF was corroborated further with a "supershift" by mouse antiserum to SRF, provided by R. Prywes. Despite their distinctly different contributions to basal transcriptional activity of the SkA promoter, SRE1, SRE2, and SRE3 exhibit virtually equivalent affinity for SRF in cardiac nuclear extracts. Site-directed mutations of SRE1 that prevent recognition by SRF and YY1 or by SRF alone virtually abolish tissue-restricted transcription of the SkA promoter in cardiac cells, as well as TGFß1-dependent activity. By contrast, a mutation within the 3' arm of SRE1 selectively replaces the site for YY1, the putative inhibitor of SRF binding, and, as predicted, increases both basal and TGFß-dependent expression. These results concur with the increased activity of the YY1 mutation observed in cardiac non-muscle cells and substantiate the postulated role of YY1 as a negative regulator of SRF effects. Quantitative differences exist in the levels of SRF and YY1 binding activities in ventricular myocytes, cardiac fibroblasts, and HeLa cells, yet the observed discrepancies between cardiac muscle and non-muscle cells are relatively minor and cannot be easily reconciled with 1000-fold greater expression of the SkA promoter in a cardiac muscle background.

Summary

TGFß1 and basic FGF each modify the expression of at least six cardiac-restricted genes. In the aggregate, these effects conform to the selective up-regulation of fetal cardiac genes seen with mechanical load, and provide evidence for the plausibility of autocrine and paracrine mechanisms in the context of hypertrophy. Although the proximal serum response element appears to be the principal target for transcriptional control of the SkA promoter by both TGFß1 and basic FGF, the corresponding classes of growth factor receptors differ fundamentally in their cytoplasmic signalling domains (serine/threonine kinase activity versus tyrosine kinase activity). The point or points of the transduction cascade at which these signals converge is conjectural at present. Moreover, it is unknown whether TGFß1 and FGFs act upon the SkA promoter through altered abundance of SRF, altered SRF binding activity, or events subsequent to sequence recognition. In the case of transactivation by myogenin, the mechanism for repression by TGFß occurs distal to DNA binding, whereas other serum factors inhibit the DNA-binding properties of myogenin, possibly by inducing the HLH inhibitor Id [121]. A related complexity for SRF as well is the obvious possibility that binding and transactivation could be modulated indirectly, through YY1 or other accessory proteins, as proven for MCM1, the SRF-like protein in yeast. Each of these suggested mechanisms also could contribute, in principle, to the tissue-restrictedtranscription of the SkA promoter and to resolving the paradox that isolated SREs are transcribed preferentially in cardiac and skeletal muscle.

Genetic screens in yeast have been utilized in efforts to identify accessory factors, such as the homeodomain protein Phox [122], that potentiate transactivation by SRF. During embryogenesis, the murine homologue of Phox is found in lateral mesoderm, visceral arches, limb bud, and dorsal aorta [123]. Together these findings suggest a role for Phox or related homeodomain proteins in collaboration with SRF for mesoderm development and mesodermal gene transcription. This notion draws particular support from the molecular synergy between MCM1 and a homeodomain protein, the mating cell type-specific factor α 2 [124]. Whether Phox itself cooperates with SRF in vivo and, more generally, whether biochemical properties of YY1 or putative SRE accessory proteins correctly predict biological actions, might best be resolved by genetic means [125], using gain-of-function and loss-of-function mutants—transgenic animals and "knock-out" mutations—to substantiate the role played by these transcription factors in myocardial development and growth factor control of the cardiac phenotype.

Acknowledgments

The authors are grateful to Drs. Ken Walsh, Roger Breitbart, and Seigo Izumo for discussions of their work prior to publication, and to Dr. Brent French for comments on the manuscript.

This research was supported by grants to T. B. from the Deutsche Forschungsgemeinschaft, Germany, to W. R. M. from the Medical Research Council of Canada; to R. J. S. from the National Institutes of Health (R01 HL45476, P50 HL42267), and to M. D. S. from the National Institutes of Health (R01 HL39141, R01 HL47567, T32 HL07706) and American Heart Association (91009790). M. D. S. is an Established Investigator of the American Heart Association.

References

1. Kimelman D, Kirschner M. Synergistic induction of mesoderm by FGF and TGF-beta and the identification of an mRNA coding for FGF in the early Xenopus embryo. Cell 1987; 51: 869-877.

2. Slack JM, Darlington BG, Heath JK, Godsave SF. Mesoderm induction in early Xenopus embryos by heparin-binding growth factors. Nature 1987; 326: 197-200.

3. Clegg CH, Linkhart TA, Olwin BB, Hauschka SD. Growth factor control of skeletal muscle differentiation: Commitment to terminal differentiation occurs in G1 phase and is repressed by fibroblast growth factor. J Cell Biol 1987; 105: 949-956.

4. Massagué J, Cheifetz S, Endo T, Nadal-Ginard B. Type beta transforming growth factor is an inhibitor of myogenic differentiation. Proc Natl Acad Sci USA 1986; 83: 8206-8210.

5. Olson EN, Sternberg E, Hu JS, Spizz G, Wilco C. Regulation of myogenic differentiation by type beta transforming growth factor. J. Cell Biol 1986; 103: 1799-1805.

6. Caffrey JM, Brown AM, Schneider MD. Ca^{2+} and Na^+ currents in developing skeletal myoblasts are expressed in a sequential program: Reversible suppression by transforming growth factor beta-1, an inhibitor of the myogenic pathway. J Neurosci 1989; 9: 3443-3453.

7. Florini JR, Ewton DZ, Magri KA. Hormones, growth factors, and myogenic differentiation. Annu Rev Physiol 1991; 53: 201-216.

8. Hammond GL, Wieben E, Markert CL. Molecular signals for initiating protein synthesis in organ hypertrophy. Proc Natl Acad Sci USA 1979; 76: 2455-2459.

9. Schneider MD, Parker TG. Cardiac growth factors. Progr Growth Factor Res. 1991; 3: 1-26.

10. Quinckler WM, Maasberg M, Bernotat-Danielowski S, Luthe N, Sharma HS, Schaper W. Isolation of heparin-binding growth factors from bovine, porcine and canine hearts. Eur J Biochem 1989; 181: 67-73.

11. Kardami E, Fandrich RR. Basic fibroblast growth factor in atria and ventricles of the vertebrate heart. J Cell Biol 1989; 109: 1865-1875.

12. Sasaki H, Hoshi H, Hong Y-M, Suzuki T, Kato T, Sasaki H, Saito M, Youki, Karube K, Konno S, Onodera M, Saito T, Aoyagi S. Purification of acidic fibroblast growth factor from bovine heart and its localization in the cardiac myocytes. J Biol Chem 1989; 264: 17606-17612.

13. Weiner HL, Swain JL. Acidic fibroblast growth factor mRNA is expressed by cardiac myocytes in culture and the protein is localized to the extracellular matrix. Proc Natl Acad Sci USA 1989; 86: 2683-2687.

14. Joseph-Silverstein J, Consigli SA, Lyser KM, Ver Pault C. Basic fibroblast growth factor in the chick embryo: Immunolocalization to striated muscle cells and their precursors. J Cell Biol 1989; 108: 2459-2466.

94

15. Thompson NL, Flanders KC, Smith, JM Ellingsworth LR, Roberts AB, Sporn MB. Expression of transforming growth factor-beta 1 in specific cells and tissues of adult and neonatal mice. J Cell Biol 1989; 108: 661-669.

16. Akhurst RJ, Lehnert SA, Faissner A, Duffie E. TGF beta in murine morphogenetic processes: the early embryo and cardiogenesis. Development 1990; 108: 645-656.

17. Komuro I, Katoh Y, Hoh E, Takaku F, Yazaki Y. Mechanism of cardiac hypertrophy and injury: Possible role of protein kinase C activation. Japan Circ J 1991; 55: 1149-1157.

18. Villarreal FJ, Dillmann WH. Cardiac hypertrophy-induced changes in messenger RNA levels for TGF-beta1, fibronectin, and collagen. Am J Physiol 1992; 262: H1861-H1866.

19. Chiba M, Sakai S, Nakata M, Toshima H. The role of basic fibroblast growth factor in myocardial hypertrophy. Circulation 1990; 82: III-761 (Abstr.).

20. Wahlander H, Isgaard J, Jennische E, Friberg P. Left ventricular insulin-like growth factor I increases in early renal hypertension. Hypertension 1992; 19: 25-32.

21. Eppenberger-Eberhard TM, Flamme I, Kurer V, Eppenberger HM. Re-expression of alpha-smooth muscle actin isoform in cultured adult rat cardiomyocytes. Dev Biol 1990; 139: 269-278.

22. Long CS, Henrich CJ, Simpson PC. A growth factor for cardiac myocytes is produced by cardiac nonmyocytes. Cell Regul 1991; 2: 1081-1095.

23. Ueno H, Perryman MB, Roberts R, Schneider MD. Differentiation of cardiac myocytes following mitogen withdrawal exhibits three sequential stages of the ventricular growth response. J Cell Biol 1988; 107: 1911-1918.

24. Miller JB. Myogenic programs of mouse muscle cell lines: Expression of myosin heavy chain isoforms, Myod1, and myogenin. J Cell Biol 1990; 111: 1149-1159.

25. Werner S, Duan D, Devries C, Peters KG, Johnson DE, Williams LT. Differential splicing in the extracellular region of fibroblast growth factor receptor-1 generates receptor variants with different ligand-binding specificities. Mol Cell Biol 1992; 12: 82-88.

26. Braun T, Bober E, Busch-hausen-Denker G, Kotz S, Grzeschik K-H, Arnold HH. Differential expression of myogenic determination genes in muscle cells: Possible autoactivation by the Myf gene products. EMBO J 1989; 8: 3617-3625.

27. Rhodes SJ, Konieczny SF. Identification of MRF4: A new member of the muscle regulatory factor gene family. Genes Dev 1989; 3: 2050-2061.

28. Simpson P, McGrath A, Savion S. Myocyte hypertrophy in neonatal rat heart cultures and its regulation by serum and by catecholamines. Circ Res 1982; 511: 787-801.

29. Clubb FJ Jr, Bishop SP. Formation of binucleated myocardial cells in the neonatal rat: an index for growth hypertrophy. Lab Invest 1984; 50: 571-577.

30. Parker TG, Packer SE, Schneider MD. Peptide growth factors can provoke "fetal" contractile protein gene expression in rat cardiac myocytes. J Clin Invest 1990; 85: 507-514.

31. Parker TG, Chow K-L, Schwartz, RJ, Schneider MD. Differential regulation of skeletal a-actin transcription in cardiac muscle by two fibroblast growth factors. Proc Natl Acad Sci USA 1990; 87: 7066-7070.

32. Ruzicka DL, Schwartz RJ. Sequential activation of α-actin genes during avian cardiogenesis: vascular smooth muscle α-actin gene transcripts mark the onset of cardiomyocyte differentiation. J Cell Biol 1988; 107: 2575-2586.

33. Izumo S, Lompre AM, Matsuoka R, Koren G, Schwartz K, Nadal-Ginard B, Mahdavi V. Myosin heavy chain messenger RNA and protein isoform during cardiac hypertrophy: Interaction between hemodynamic and thyroid hormone-induced signals. J Clin Invest 1987; 79: 970-977.

34. Lee RT, Bloch KD, Pfeffer JM, Pfeffer MA, Neer EJ, SeidmanCE. Atrial natriuretic factor gene expression in ventricles of rats with spontaneous biventricular hypertrophy. J Clin Invest 1988; 81: 431-434.

35. Izumo S, Nadal-Ginard B, Mahdavi V Proto-oncogene induction and reprogramming of cardiac gene expression produced by pressure overload. Proc Natl Acad Sci USA 1988; 85: 339-343.

36. Schwartz K, de la Bastie D, Bouveret P, Oliviero P, Alonso S, Buckingham M. alpha-Skeletal muscle actin mRNAs accumulate in hypertrophied adult rat hearts. Circ Res 1986; 59: 551-555.

37. Nagai R., Zarain-Herzberg A, Brandl CJ, Fujii J, Tada JM, MacLennan DH, Alpert NR, Periasamy M. Regulation of myocardial Ca2+-ATPase and phospholamban mRNA expression in response to pressure overload and thyroid hormone. Proc Natl Acad Sci USA 1989; 86: 2966-2970.

38. Bishopric N, Simpson PC, Ordahl CP. Induction of the skeletal α-actin gene in α1-adrenoreceptor-mediated hypertrophy of rat cardiac myocytes. J Clin Invest 1987; 80: 1194-1199.

39. Mercadier JJ, Samuel JL, Michel JB, Zongazo MA, Delabastie D, Lompre AM, Wisnewsky C, Rappaport L, Levy B, Schwartz K. Atrial natriuretic factor gene expression in rat ventricle during experimental hypertension. Am J Physiol 1989; 257: H979-H987.

40. Saito Y, Nakao K, Arai H, Nishimura K, Okumura K, Obata K, Takemura G, Fujiwara H, Sugawara A, Yamada T, Itoh H, Mukoyama M, Hosoda K, Kawai C, Ban T, Yasue H, Imura H. Augmented expression of atrial natriuretic polypeptide gene in ventricle of human failing heart. J Clin Invest 1989; 83: 298-305.

41. Black FB, Packer SE, Parker TG, Michael LH, Roberts R, Schwartz RJ, Schneider MD. The vascular smooth muscle alpha-actin gene is reactivated during cardiac hypertrophy produced by load. J Clin Invest 1991; 88: 1581-1588.

42. Thompson WR, Nadal-Ginard B, Mahdavi V. A MyoD1-independent muscle-specific enhancer controls the expression of the beta-myosin heavy chain gene in skeletal and cardiac muscle cells. J Biol Chem 1991; 266: 22678-22688.

43. Parmacek MS, Vora AJ, Shen TL, Barr E, Jung F, Leiden JM. Identification and characterization of a cardiac-specific transcriptional regulatory element in the slow/cardiac troponin C gene. Mol Cell Biol 1992; 12: 1967-1976.

44. Ianello RC, Mar JH, Ordahl CP. Characterization of a promoter element required for transcription in myocardial cells. J Biol Chem 1991; 266: 3309-3316.

45. Hauschka SD, Amacher SL, Apone S, Buskin JN, Donoviel DB, Shields MA, Templeton TJ, Wenderoth MP. In: Kelly AM, Blau HM editors. Neuromuscular Development and Disease. Raven Press, New York 1992; 73-86.

46. Nudel U, Greenberg D, Ordahl CP, Saxel O, Neuman S, Yaffe D. Developmentally regulated expression of a chick muscle-specific gene in stably transfected rat myogenic cells. Proc Natl Acad Sci USA 1985; 85: 3106-3109.

47. Bergsma DJ, Grichnik JM, Gossett LM, Schwartz RJ. Delimitation and characterization of cis-acting DNA sequences required for the regulated expression and transcriptional control of the chicken skeletal alpha-actin gene. Mol Cell Biol 1986; 6: 2462-75.

48. Muscat GE, Kedes L. Multiple 5′ flanking regions of the human alpha skeletal actin synergistically modulate muscle specific expression. Mol Cell Biol 1987; 7: 4089-4099.

49.   Bishopric NH, Kedes L. Adrenergic regulation of the skeletal α–actin gene promoter during myocardial cell hypertrophy. Proc Natl Acad. Sci USA 1991; 88: 2132-2136.

50.   Petropoulos CJ, Rosenberg MP, Jenkins NA, Copeland NG, Hughes SH. The chicken skeletal α-actin promoter is tissue-specific in transgenic mice. Mol Cell Biol 1989; 9: 3785-3792.

51.   Lee TC, French B, Moss J, Sands A, Schwartz R. In: Kelly AM, Blau HM editors. Neuromuscular Development and Disease. Raven Press, 1185 Ave of the Americas, New York, NY 10036. 1992; 87-105.

52.   Einat P, Bergman T, Yaffe D, Shani M. Expression in transgenic mice of two genes of different tissue specificity integrated into a single chromosomal site. Genes Dev 1987; 1: 1075-84.

53.   Mint A, Kedes L. Upstream regions of the human cardiac actin gene that modulate transcription in muscle cells: presence of an evolutionarily conserved repeated motif. Mol Cell Biol 1986; 6: 2125-2136.

54.   Ernst H, Walsh K, Harrison CA, Rosenthal N. The myosin light chain enhancer and the skeletal actin promoter share a binding site for factors involved in muscle-specific gene expression. Mol Cell Biol 1991; 11: 3735-44.

55.   Kurabayashi M, Komuro I, Shibasaki Y, Tsuchimochi H, Takaku F, Yazaki Y. Functional identification of the transcriptional regulatory elements within the promoter region of the human ventricular myosin alkali light chain gene. J Biol Chem 1990; 265: 19271-8.

56.   Zhu H, Garcia AV, Ross RS, Evans SM, Chien KR. A conserved 28-base pair element (HF-1) in the rat cardiac myosin light chain-2 gene confers cardiac-specific and α-adrenergic-inducible expression in cultured neonatal rat myocardial cells. Mol Cell Biol 1991; 11: 2273-2281.

57.   Mar JH, Antin PB, Cooper TA, Ordahl CP. Analysis of the upstream regions governing expression of the chicken cardiac troponin T gene in embryonic cardiac and skeletal muscle cells. J Cell Biol 1988; 107: 573-585.

58.   Sternberg EA, Spizz G, Perry WM, Vizard D, Weil T, Olson EN. Identification of upstream and intragenic regulatory elements that confer cell-type restricted and differentiation-specific expression on the muscle creatine kinase gene. Mol Cell Biol 1988; 8: 2896-2909.

59.   Klamut HJ, Gangopadhyay SB, Worton RG, Ray PN. Molecular and functional analysis of the muscle-specific promoter region of the Duchenne muscular dystrophy gene. Mol Cell Biol 1990; 10: 193-205.

60.   Santoro IM, Walsh K. Natural and synthetic DNA elements with the CArG motif differ in expression and protein-binding properties. Mol Cell Biol 1991; 11: 6296-6305.

61. Miwa T, Boxer LM, Kedes L. CArG boxes in the human cardiac α-actin gene are core sites for positive trans-acting regulatory factors. Proc Natl Acad Sci USA 1987; 84: 6702-6706.

62. Mohun TJ, Taylor MV, Gurdon GN, Gurdon JB. The CArG promoter sequence is necessary for muscle-specific transcription of the cardiac actin gene in Xenopus embryos. EMBO J 1989; 8: 1153-61.

63. Walsh K. Cross-binding of factors to functionally different promoter elements in c-fos and skeletal actin. J Biol Chem 1989; 9: 2191-2201.

64. Chow KL, Schwartz RJ. A combination of closely associated positive and negative cis-acting promoter elements regulates transcription of the skeletal alpha-actin gene. Mol Cell Biol 1990; 10: 528-538.

65. Liu ZJ, Moav B, Faras AJ, Guise KS, Kapuscinski AR, Hackett P. Importance of the CarG box in regulation of beta-actin-encoding genes. Gene 1991; 108: 211-217.

66. Christy B, Nathans D. Functional serum response elements upstream of the growth factor-inducible gene zif268. Mol Cell Biol 1989; 9: 4889-4895.

67. Treisman R. Identification of a protein-binding site that mediates transcriptional response of the c-fos gene to serum factors. Cell 1986; 46: 567-574.

68. Sheng M, Dougan ST, McFadden G, Greenberg ME. Calcium and growth factor pathways of c-fos transcriptional activation require distinct upstream regulatory sequences. Mol Cell Biol 1988; 8: 2787-2796.

69. Gauthier-Rouviere C, Fernandez A, Lamb NJ. ras-induced c-fos expression and proliferation in living rat fibroblasts involves C-kinase activation and the serum response element pathway. EMBO J 1990; 9: 171-80.

70. Graham R, Gilman M. Distinct protein targets for signals acting at the c-fos serum response element. Science 1991; 251: 189-92.

71. Jamal S, Ziff E. Transactivation of c-fos and beta-actin genes by raf as a step in early response to transmembrane signals. Nature 1990; 344: 463-6.

72. Gauthier-Rouviere C, Basset M, Blanchard JM, Cavadore JC, Fernandez A, Lamb NJC. Casein kinase-II induces c-fos expression via the serum response element pathway and p67SRF phosphorylation in living fibroblasts. EMBO J 1991; 10: 2921-2930.

73. Komuro I, Katoh Y, Kaida T, Shibazaki Y, Kurabayashi M, Hoh E, Takaku F, Yazaki Y. Mechanical loading stimulates cell hypertrophy and specific gene expression in cultured rat cardiac myocytes. Possible role of protein kinase C activation. J Biol Chem 1991; 266: 1265-1268.

74. Treisman R. Identification and purification of a polypeptide that binds the c-fos serum response element. EMBO J 1987; 6: 2711-2717.

75. Boxer LM, Prywes R, Roeder RG, Kedes L. The sarcomeric actin CArG-binding factor is indistinguishable from the c-fos serum response factor. Mol Cell Biol 1989; 9: 515-522.

76. Lee TC, Chow KL, Fang P, Schwartz RJ. Activation of skeletal alpha-actin gene transcription: The cooperative formation of serum response factor-binding complexes over positive cis-acting promoter serum response elements displaces a negative-acting nuclear factor enriched in replicating myoblasts and nonmyogenic cells. Mol Cell Biol. 1991; 11: 5090-5100.

77. Mohun TJ, Chambers AE, Towers N, Taylor MV. Expression of genes encoding the transcription factor SRF during early development of Xenopus laevis: identification of a CArG box-binding activity as SRF. EMBO J 1991; 10: 933-940.

78. Gualberto A, LePage D, Pons G, Mader SL, Park, K Atchison ML, Walsh K. Functional antagonism between YY1 and the serum response factor. Mol Cell Biol 1992; 12: 4209-4214.

79. Lee T-C, Shi Y, Schwartz RJ. Displacement of BrdU-induced YY1 by SRF activates skeletal α-actin gene transcription in embryonic myoblasts. Proc Natl Acad Sci USA 1992; In press.

80. Taylor M, Treisman R, Garrett N, Mohun T. Muscle-specific (CArG) and serum-responsive (SRE) promoter elements are functionally interchangeable in Xenopus embryos and mouse fibroblasts. Development 1989; 106: 67-78.

81. Sartorelli V, Webster KA, Kedes L. Muscle-specific expression of the cardiac alpha-actin gene requires MyoD1, CArG-box binding factor, and Sp1. Genes Dev 1990; 4: 1811-1822.

82. Tuil D, Clergue N, Montarras D, Pinset C, Kahn A, Phan DTF. CC Ar GG boxes, cis-acting elements with a dual specificity. Muscle-specific transcriptional activation and serum responsiveness. J Mol Biol 1990; 213: 677-86.

83. Taylor MV, Gurdon JB, Hopwood ND, Towers N, Mohun TJ. Xenopus embryos contain a somite-specific, MyoD-like protein that binds to a promoter site required for muscle actin expression. Genes Dev 1991; 5: 1149-1160.

84. Norman C, Runswick M, Pollock R, Treisman R. Isolation and properties of cDNA clones encoding SRF, a transcription factor that binds to the c-fos serum response element. Cell 1988; 55: 989-1003.

85. Passmore S, Maine GT, Elble R, Christ, C Tye BK. A Saccharomyces cerevisiae protein involved in plasmid maintenance is necessary for mating of MATa cells. J Mol Biol 1988; 204: 593-606.

86. Passmore S, Elble R, Tye BK. A protein involved in minichromosome maintenance in yeast binds a transcriptional enhancer conserved in eukaryotes. Genes Dev 1989; 3: 921-35.

87. Dubois E, Bercy J, Messenguy F. Characterization of two genes ARGRI and ARGRIII required for specific regulation of arginine metabolism in yeast. Mol Gen Genet 1987; 207: 142-8.

88. Yanofsky MF, Ma H, Bowman JL, Drews GN, Feldman KA, Meyerowitz EM. The protein encoded by the Arabidopsis homeotic gene agamous resembles transcription factors. Nature 1990; 346: 35-39.

89. Sommer H, JBeltran JP, Huijser P, Pape H, Lonnig WE, Saedler H, Schwarz SZ. Deficiens, a homeotic gene involved in the control of flower morphogenesis in Antirrhinum majus: the protein shows homology to transcription factors. EMBO J 1990; 9: 605-13.

90. Ma H, Yanofsky MF, Meyerowitz EM. AGL1-AGL6, an Arabidopsis gene family with similarity to floral homeotic and transcription factor genes. Genes Dev 1991; 5: 484-95.

91. Schwarz-Sommer Z, Huijser P, Nacken W, Saedler H, Sommer H. Genetic control of flower development by homeotic genes in antirrhinum majus. Science 1990; 250: 931-936.

92. Pollock R, Treisman R. Human SRF-related proteins: DNA-binding properties and potential regulatory targets. Genes Dev 1991; 5: 2327-2341.

93. Jarvis EE, Clark KL, prague GF Jr. The yeast transcription activator PRTF, a homolog of the mammalian serum response factor, is encoded by the MCM1 gene. Genes Dev 1989; 3: 936-945.

94. Pari G, Jardine K, McBurney MW. Multiple CArG boxes in the human cardiac actin gene promoter required for expression in embryonic cardiac muscle cells developing in vitro from embryonal carcinoma cells. Mol Cell Biol. 1991; 11: 4796-803.

95. Chow KL, Hogan ME, Schwartz RJ. Phased cis-acting promoter elements interact at short distances to direct avian skeletal alpha-actin gene transcription. Proc Natl Acad Sci USA 1991; 88: 1301-1305.

96. Parker TG, Chow KL, Schwartz RJ, Schneider MD. Positive and negative control of the skeletal alpha-actin promoter in cardiac muscle: A proximal serum response element is sufficient for induction by basic fibroblast growth factor (FGF) but not for inhibition by acidic FGF. J Biol Chem 1992; 267: 3343-3350.

97. Kim SJ, Angel P, Lafyatis R, Hattori K, Kim KY, Sporn MB, Karin M, Roberts AB. Autoinduction of transforming growth factor beta 1 is mediated by the AP-1 complex. Mol Cell Biol 1990; 10: 1492-1497.

98. Keeton MR, Curriden SA, Van ZAJ, Loskutoff DJ. Identification of regulatory sequences in the type 1 plasminogen activator inhibitor gene responsive to transforming growth factor beta. J Biol Chem 1991; 266: 23048-23052.

99. Rossi P, Karsenty G, Roberts AB, Roche NS, Sporn MB, de Crombrugghe B. A nuclear factor 1 binding site mediates the transcriptional activation of a type I collagen promoter by transforming growth factor-beta. Cell 1988; 52: 405-14.

100. Pietenpol JA, Munger K, Howley PM, Stein RW, Moses HL. Factor-binding element in the human c-myc promoter involved in transcriptional regulation by transforming growth factor beta1 and by the retinoblastoma gene product. Proc Natl Acad Sci USA 1991; 88: 10227-10231.

101. Sartorelli V, Hong NA, Bishopric NH, Kedes L. Myocardial activation of the human cardiac α-actin promoter by helix-loop-helix proteins. Proc Natl Acad Sci USA 1992; 89: 4047-4051.

102. Nelson C, Shen LP, Meister A, Fodoer E, Rutter WJ. Pan: a transcriptional regulator that binds chymotrypsin, insulin, and AP-4 enhancer motifs. Genes Dev 1990; 4: 1035-1043.

103. Blackwell TK, Weintraub H. Differences and similarities in DNA-binding preferences of MyoD and E2A protein complexes revealed by binding site selection. Science 1990; 250: 1104-10.

104. Blackwell TK, Kretzner L, Blackwood EM, Eisenman RN, Weintraub H. Sequence-specific DNA binding by the c-Myc protein. Science 1990; 250: 1149-51.

105. Gustafson TA, Miwa T, Boxer LM, L. Kedes L. Interaction of nuclear proteins with muscle-specific regulatory sequences of the human cardiac alpha-actin promoter. Mol Cell Biol 1988; 8: 4110-4119.

106. Prywes R, Roeder R. Inducible binding of a factor to the c-fos enhancer. Cell 1986; 47: 777-784.

107. Taylor MV. A family of muscle gene promoter element (CArG) binding activities in Xenopus embryos: CArG/SRE discrimination and distribution during myogenesis. Nucleic Acids Res 1991; 19: 2669-75.

108. Tapscott SJ, Lassar AB, Davis RL, Weintraub H. 5-bromo-2'-deoxyuridine blocks myogenesis by extinguishing of MyoD1. Science 1989; 245: 532-6.

109. Yu Y-T, Breitbart RE, Smoot LB, Lee Y, Mahdavi V, Nadal-Ginard B. Human myocyte-specific enhancer factor 2 comprises a group of tissue-restricted MADS box transcription factors. Genes Dev 1992; 6: 1783-1798.

110. Gossett LA, Kelvin DJ, Sternberg EA, Olson EN. A new myocyte-specific enhancer-binding factor that recognizes a conserved element associated with multiple muscle-specific genes. Mol Cell Biol 1989; 9: 5022-5033.

111. Donoghue M, Ernst H, Wentworth B, Rosenthal N, Rosenthal NGB. A muscle-specific enhancer is located at the 3' end of the myosin light-chain 1/3 gene locus. Genes Dev 1988; 2: 1779-1790.

112. Hipskind RA, Rao VN, Mueller CG, Reddy ES, Nordheim A. Ets-related protein Elk-1 Is homologous to the c-fos regulatory factor p62TCF. Nature 1991; 354: 531-534.

113. Dalton S, Treisman R. Characterization of SAP-1, a protein recruited by serum response factor to the c-fos serum response element. Cell 1992; 68: 597-612.

114. Ryan WAJ, Franza BRJ, Gilman MZ. Two distinct cellular phosphoproteins bind to the c-fos serum response element. EMBO J 1989; 8: 1785-92.

115. Riggs K J, Merrell KT, Wilson G, Calame K. Common factor 1 is a transcriptional activator which binds in the c-myc promoter, the skeletal alpha-actin promoter, and the immunoglobulin heavy-chain enhancer. Mol Cell Biol 1991; 11: 1765-1769.

116. Shi Y, Seto E, Chang ELS, Shenk T. Transcriptional repression by YY1, a human GLI-Krüppel-related protein, and relief of repression by adenovirus E1A protein. Cell 1991; 67: 377-88.

117. Seto E, Shi Y, Shenk T. YY1 is an initiator sequence-binding protein that directs and activates transcription in vitro. Nature 1991; 354: 241-245.

118. Flanagan JR, Ennist DL, Gleason SL, Driggers PH, Levi BZ, Appella E, Ozato K. Cloning of a negative transcription factor that binds to the upstream conserved region of Moloney murine leukemia virus. Mol Cell Biol 1992; 12: 38-44.

119. Hariharan N, Kelley DE, Perry RP. Delta, a transcription factor that binds to downstream elements in several polymerase II promoters, is a functionally versatile zinc finger protein. Proc Natl Acad Sci USA 1991; 88: 9799-803.

120. Park K, Atchison ML. Isolation of a candidate repressor/activator, NF-E1 (YY-1, delta), that binds to the immunoglobulin kappa 3' enhancer and the immunoglobulin heavy-chain mu E1 site. Proc Natl Acad Sci USA 1991; 88: 9804-9808.

121. Brennan TJ, Edmondson DG, Li L, Olson EN. Transforming growth factor-beta represses the actions of myogenin through a mechanism independent of DNA binding. Proc Natl Acad Sci. USA 1991; 88: 3822-3826.

122. Grueneberg DA, Natesan S, Alexandre C, Gilman MZ. Human and drosophila homeodomain proteins that enhance the DNA-binding activity of serum response factor. Science 1992; 257: 1089-1095.

123. Cserjesi P, Lilly B, Bryson L, Wang Y, Sassoon DA, Olson EN. Mhox: a mesodermally-restricted homeodomain protein that binds an essential site in the muscle creatine kinase enhancer. Development 1992; 115: 1087-1101.

124. Smith DL, Johnson AD. A molecular mechanism for combinatorial control in yeast: MCM1 protein sets the spacing and orientation of the homeodomains of an alpha 2 dimer. Cell 1992; 68: 133-142.
125. Rossant J, Hopkins N. Of fin and fur: Mutational analysis of vertebrate embryonic development. Genes Dev 1992; 6: 1-13.

7. Effects of growth factors on human cardiac myocytes

BRUCE I. GOLDMAN and JOHN WURZEL

Introduction

This review will summarize current knowledge regarding the effects of peptide growth factors on human cardiac myocytes in vitro and, when known, in vivo. Excellent reviews on this general topic which include studies of animal experimentation exist elsewhere [1,2], and thus this chapter will confine itself to human studies only.

In vitro culture of human cardiac myocytes is essential to understanding the effects of growth factors on human heart muscle cells, because some properties of human cells differ substantially from those of rodents. The effects of serum or fibroblast growth factor (FGF) on actin isoform expression in cultured human fetal ventricular cardiac myocytes differ from those reported in neonatal rat cardiac cells, as do the effects of insulin-like growth factor I (IGF-I) on myocyte DNA synthesis [3]. Developmental regulation of both sarcomeric actin [4,5].and myosin heavy chain [6] isoform expression in humans also differs from that in rats.

To develop a human heart muscle cell culture system, initial studies employed passaged (expanded) human fetal cardiac myocytes. Dissociated ventricular cells expanded in mitogen-rich growth medium (containing 20% fetal bovine serum, 1% chick embryo extract, multiplication-stimulating activity [MSA; rat IGF-II] and bovine pituitary [basic] FGF) did not appreciably express cardiac myocyte markers such as cardiac actin mRNA, sarcomeric myosin heavy chain, or atrial natriuretic factor until switched to medium containing 4% horse serum [7,8]. These cultures, which were prepared without enrichment for myocytes, could be passaged through multiple generations and maintained the ability to express cardiac-specific markers after withdrawal of growth medium. They did not contain cells which morphologically resembled primary cultured cardiac myocytes, however, and did not spontaneously beat. Beating is typical of cultured fetal and neonatal ventricular myocytes [9].

These findings suggested that passaged human fetal cardiac myocytes were capable only of limited differentiation in vitro, and raised questions concerning the role of peptide growth factors on growth and differentiation of cultured human fetal ventricular cells. Factors present in growth medium both promoted proliferation and inhibited differentiation of cardiac myocytes, inducing an apparently undifferentiated "myoblast-like" phenotype. This interpretation is based on the knowledge that true cardiac myoblasts (i.e. determined but phenotypically undifferentiated cardiac muscle cell precursors) do not persist in the heart much after the formation of the primitive heart tube [10]. The failure to observe induction of a typical myocyte phenotype after a change to differentiation medium also indicated that other factors were necessary for differentiation of human ventricular cardiac myocytes in vitro. For the purposes of this review, "cardiac differentiation" refers to induction of sarcomeric protein expression and/or the development of spontaneous contractions.

Growth medium as initially formulated included serum, bFGF, and IGFs. These substances thus are likely candidates for regulators of proliferation and differentiation of human cardiac myocytes in vitro, and this chapter will largely concern itself with a review of their effects. As will be seen, however, the components of growth medium which inhibit differentiation in vitro remain to be defined. Preliminary data regarding the effects of epidermal growth factor (EGF) have some bearing on this question and also will be presented.

Effects of serum

Serum, which contains nutrients, attachment factors, and multiple growth factors, has long been an essential, convenient omponent of many cell culture media. A review of previous studies employing primary cultures of human cardiac muscle cells [11-18] affords information about the effects of serum on the growth and differentiation of human cardiac cells in vitro.

These studies are similar in that all use serum-supplemented media, although sources (fetal bovine, calf, human) and amounts (10%-30%) vary. Two observations are of particular note. First, nearly all studies, including one of myocytes from 5-7 year-old ventricles [16], document myocyte proliferation or DNA synthesis, indicating that serum is mitogenic for human cardiac myocytes in vitro. Second, serum itself does not inhibit cardiac differentiation. Even in the presence of fetal bovine serum at high concentration, all studies describe a differentiated myocyte phenotype, which included spontaneous beating in fetal cell cultures [11-13,15,17].

Fibroblast growth factors

Acidic and basic fibroblast growth factors (aFGF and bFGF) are structurally related 16 kD heparin-binding peptides which are mitogenic for multiple mesenchymal and neuroectodermal cell types [19]. Both aFGF and bFGF have been isolated from adult human cardiac tissues, and bFGF has been localized to cardiac myocytes [20]. Expression of other genes in the FGF family has not been systematically studied in the human heart, but data to date suggest that such expression is unlikely [20].

As mentioned above, initial studies which included bFGF in growth medium showed enhanced propagation of human fetal cardiac myoblast-like cells [7,8]. A subsequent combined autoradiographic / immunocytochemical study [3] showed that bFGF strongly induced DNA synthesis in cardiac myocytes expressing sarcomeric myosin heavy chain (MHC). FGF did not inhibit induction of differentiation occurring after serum withdrawal. Cultures in which bFGF was added to serum-free medium at the onset of serum withdrawal actually showed a slight increase over control in the absolute number of MHC-positive myocytes present 9 days later, a result consistent with a mitogenic effect of bFGF. Similar results have been observed in experiments using recombinant human bFGF instead of the bovine preparation (unpublished observations).

Insulin and insulin-like growth factors

Insulin, IGF-I, and IGF-II are small peptides with similar amino acid structures and overlapping biological activities (reviewed in [21-24]). All three circulate, but the IGFs are bound to high molecular weight binding proteins which modulate their activities. Many organs and tissues produce IGFs; their local paracrine and autocrine actions may be more significant than their endocrine activities. Multiple factors, including hormones and growth factors, nutritional status, cell type, and developmental stage, affect IGF production and secretion. Growth hormone (GH) is thought to be the major regulator of IGF-I production in most tissues.

The human fetal heart contains IGF-I and IGF-II mRNAs [25]. Claycomb et al. [14] found that the amount of IGF-II mRNA present in freshly isolated human fetal ventricular myocytes was similar to that in left ventricular tissue, but the amount in myocytes declined after five days in culture.

The IGFs and insulin are mitogens for skeletal myoblasts; unlike FGFs and TGFß, they stimulate myogenic differentiation as well [26]. In most cells, the actions of insulin and the IGFs in promoting proliferation or differentiation are mediated by the IGF-I receptor [21]. Of the three peptides, IGF-I has the highest affinity for the IGF-I receptor, while insulin has the lowest. Therefore, the amount of insulin required to induce proliferation (or in the case of skeletal myoblasts, differentiation) is often orders of magnitude greater than the dose required to induce metabolic affects mediated by the insulin receptor.

Effects of IGFs in vivo

In vivo effects of insulin and the IGFs on human heart muscle may be inferred from observations in patients with clinical disorders of insulin and/or IGF action, including acromegaly, GH deficiency, and diabetes mellitus (DM).

In acromegaly, increased plasma levels of GH and IGF-I are associated with cardiomegaly and interstitial fibrosis, with or without asymmetrical ventricular hypertrophy (reviewed in [27]. Although cardiac hypertrophy in acromegaly may in part be attributable to the presence of hypertension and/or accelerated atherosclerosis, evidence has been presented supporting direct effects of GH and/or IGF-I on human heart muscle [28].

Frustaci et al. [29] have described reversible dilated cardiomyopathy in a patient with post-partum GH deficiency. Cardiac function at the time of presentation was severely impaired, with an ejection fraction of 15%. Endomyocardial biopsies showed markedly subnormal amounts myofibrils. A return to normal structure and function followed administration of recombinant human GH. This "experiment of nature" suggests that GH and/or IGF-I activity is essential to the maintenance of normal human cardiac structure and function.

Neonates born to women with uncontrolled DM sometimes have a syndrome which resembles hypertrophic cardiomyopathy, but which resolves spontaneously after birth [30]. It has been proposed that supranormal levels of circulating insulin and/or IGF-II in the fetal circulation cause this reversible neonatal cardiomyopathy.

In adults DM is associated with an increased incidence of heart failure (reviewed in [27]). Some data suggest the existence of a "diabetic cardiomyopathy " due to factors other than atherosclerosis and/or microvascular disease [27, 31]. Cardiomyopathy may in part reflect alterations in cardiac gene expression seen in diabetes [32]. Studies of the direct effects of diabetes on human heart muscle cells have not been described.

Effects of IGFs in vitro

High concentration (i.e., micromolar) insulin in serum-free medium does not appreciably induce DNA synthesis in cultured human fetal ventricular myocytes [3]. However, insulin markedly enhances differentiation of human ventricular cardiac myocytes expanded in

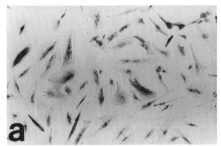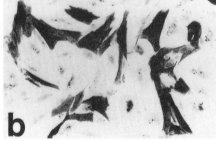

Figure 1. Effects of insulin on myosin heavy chain immunoreactivity in cultured human cardiac myocytes stained with monoclonal antibody MF20, specific for sarcomeric MHC [33]. (a) Cells expanded in growth medium and switched to differentiation medium DMEM plus 4% horse serum and antibiotics) for 7 days show few scattered immunoractive cells (dark cytoplasm). (b) Parallel cultures differentiated in identical medium containing added insulin (10 ug/ml) show an increase in the number and size of stained muscle cells. (alkaline phosphatase/anti-alkaline phosphatase, original magnification 37.5x)

growth medium and switched to serum-free medium or medium containing 4% horse serum (Figure 1). Increased differentiation is seen as an increase in the number and size of cells expressing sarcomeric proteins, as an increase in cardiac actin mRNA expression, and as induction of spontaneous beating. The induction of spontaneous beating occurs more quickly and reliably in medium containing 4% horse-serum than in serum-free medium, implying the presence of additional serum factors which promote cardiac differentiation in vitro.

Insulin at 10 nM, a concentration which primarily activates the insulin receptor, is equally effective in inducing spontaneous beating after changing to differentiation medium (unpublished observation). However, myocyte size, the cardiac α-actin/β actin mRNA ratio, and the intensity of cytoplasmic immunostaining with the anti-sarcomeric myosin antibody MF-20 [33] all are less at the lower insulin concentration (unpublished observation and [3]) . This dose-response relationship may reflect differing, additive effects of the insulin and IGF-I receptors on cardiac differentiation.

Insulin or MSA added to growth medium does not induce spontaneous beating or otherwise appreciably increase the degree of cardiac differentiation of cultured human ventricular myocytes (unpublished observation). Both withdrawal of growth medium and the addition of insulin are required for optimal expression of cardiac-specific properties.

Does the increase in myocyte size and in expression of muscle-specific markers (e.g., contractile proteins) by insulin and/or IGFs reflect differentiation-- a developmentally-regulated process-- or induction of hypertrophy, which is by definition an adaptive change? These processes are morphologically similar in vitro, but can be expected to differ significantly in terms of patterns of gene expression and cellular function [34]. Additional study of biochemical and functional changes mediated by IGFs in human cardiac myocytes are needed to answer this question.

Other growth factors

From the above discussion, it is evident that the neither serum, bFGF, nor the IGFs produce the inhibition of cardiac differentiation seen in human ventricular myocytes propagated and maintained in growth medium. TGFß similarly has no effect on this process [3]. In order to identify the components of growth medium which inhibit cardiac differentiation in vitro, recent studies have used the experimental design

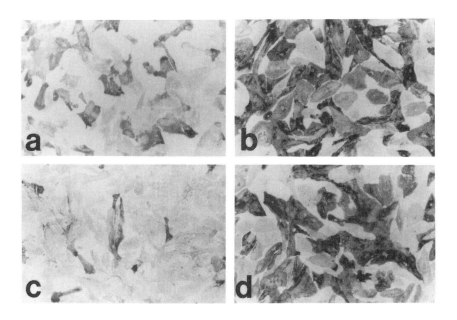

Figure 2. Effects of peptide growth factors on sarcomeric actin immunoreactivity in cultured human cardiac myocytes stained with monoclonal antibody 5C5, specific for sarcomeric actins [35]; Sigma Chemical Co., St. Louis MO.) (a) Cells cultured in growth medium, fixed at day 0. Scattered myocytes with immunostained cytoplasm are seen. (b) Parallel culture 7 days after switching to serum-free medium (DMEM/M199, transferrin 6.25 ug/ml, 0.1% bovine albumin, antibiotics) containing insulin, 10 ug/ml. The number and size of stained muscle cells are significantly increased. (c) Cells cultured as in (b) but in medium containing added EGF 25 ng/ml (Collaborative Research, Waltham MA). The number of stained cells is lower than in (a), but the overall number of cells has increased. (d) Cells cultured as in (b), but in serum-free medium containing PDGF 20 ng/ml. No effects of PDGF on proliferation or differentiation is seen (avidin/biotin/alkaline phosphatase complex-hematoxylin, original magnification 37.5x).

described above for bFGF to examine the effects of other peptide growth factors on induction of differentiation in cultured human fetal ventricular myocytes.

In myocyte-enriched cultures from a 10 week human fetal cardiac ventricle, expansion in growth medium (DMEM plus 20% FBS, 1% chick embryo extract) followed by a change to serum-free medium containing 10 ug/ml insulin produced a significant increase in the number and size of myocytes, identified by expression of immunoreactive sarcomeric actin (Figures 2a and 2b). Addition of 20 ng/ml platelet-derived growth factor (PDGF;[36]) from human platelets did not affect this increase (Figure 2d.). However, 25 nM human recombinant epidermal growth factor (EGF; [37]) significantly decreased the number of cells expressing sarcomeric actin, while increasing total cell density over that seen with serum-free medium alone (Figure 2c). The number of sarcomeric actin-positive myocytes following exposure to EGF in serum-free medium plus insulin actually was significantly lower than that at day 0 in growth medium. Quantification of these effects of EGF are seen in Table 1.

Although preliminary, these observations suggest that EGF inhibits or reverses cardiac differentiation in cultured human fetal ventricular muscle cells. EGF plus insulin may promote their proliferation as well, although this remains to be proved. EGF is mitogenic for other mesenchymal cell types. Its effects have been

Table 1: **Effects of EGF on proliferation and differentiation of cultured human fetal ventricular myocytes**

Measurement	Day 0 GM	Day 9 SFMI	Day 9 SFMI + EGF
Cells/mm^2	75 ± 12	73 ± 2.3[a]	107 ± 4.3[a]
Myocytes/mm^2*	35 ±3.1[b]	54 ± 1.3[b]	18 ± 6.4[b]

*Myocytes are identified by cytoplasmic immunostaining with monoclonal antibody 5C5, specific for sarcomeric actins [35]
Results shown are mean + S.D. for microscopic cell counts in a minimum of 5 -150x fields (1.13 mm^2/field)
[a] $p<0.5$ by one way ANOVA and Newman-Keuls multiple comparison testing
[b] $p<0.5$ by one way ANOVA and Newman-Keuls multiple comparison testing
GM=growth medium; SFMI=serum-free medium plus 10 ug/ml insulin

primarily characterized in epithelial tissues, where it induces differentiation or metaplasia (reviewed in [38]). The response of cultured human ventricular myocytes to EGF is unlike that of skeletal muscle cells. With the exception of inhibition of differentiation in BC3H1 cells, EGF has no effect on skeletal myoblasts [26].

Summary

Clinical and experimental evidence demonstrates significant regulatory effects of peptide growth factors on growth, development, and function of human cardiac myocytes. FGF, insulin and the IGFs, and EGF have differing effects on human fetal ventricular myocytes in vitro: bFGF promotes myocyte proliferation without inhibiting expression of contractile proteins; IGFs promote cell growth, increase contractile protein expression, and promote spontaneous beating without inducing DNA synthesis; EGF appears both to inhibit expression of muscle-specific proteins and induce myocyte proliferation as well.

The demonstration of these effects prompts additional questions regarding the mechanisms whereby peptide growth factors influence human cardiac growth, development and function:

(1) Do the effects of these peptide growth factors on human fetal ventricular cells in vitro reflect direct actions of growth factors on myocytes, or are they indirect paracrine effects mediated by co-cultured non-muscle cell contaminants?

(2) Are the effects of insulin on cardiac myocytes mediated through the insulin receptor, the IGF-I receptor, or both? To what degree do the effects of insulin on differentiation relate to its general anabolic effects and to what degree to activation of muscle-specific gene expression?

(3) How do the signal transduction pathways of the receptors for these peptides, all of which have cytoplasmic tyrosine kinase domains, differ in human cardiac myocytes? How do these differences result in the differing growth responses produced by each peptide?

From a broader standpoint, it is striking that these peptide growth factors produce patterns of growth and differentiation in cultured human ventricular cells which are characteristic of the three principle phases of muscle cell development occurring in mammalian cardiomyogenesis (reviewed in [39,40]). EGF inhibits contractile protein expression, producing a phenotype similar to that of cardiac precursor cells; bFGF promotes proliferation of contractile myocytes, characteristic of embryonal and fetal hearts; and IGFs promote differentiation and

114

growth by hypertrophy, typical of post-natal, terminally-differentiated cardiac muscle cells. An intriguing question then is whether the effects of EGF, bFGF, and IGFs on cultured human fetal cardiac muscle cells reflect regulatory mechanisms which control the developmental program in vivo.

Many fundamental questions remain regarding the role of these peptide growth factors in the regulation of human cardiac growth, development, and function. Through continuing refinements in cell culture methods and assay techniques, in vitro study of human cardiac muscle cells should afford additional important data not available in any other experimental system. It is hoped that such information will provide us with novel strategies for the prevention, diagnosis, and/or treatment of human heart disease.

Acknowledgments

This work was in part supported by grants-in-aid from the American Heart Association, Southeastern Pennsylvania Affiliate. We thank Dr. Pia Pollack for critical reading of the manuscript. Monoclonal antibody MF-20 was obtained from the Developmental Studies Hybridoma Bank maintained by the Department of Pharmacology and Molecular Sciences, Johns Hopkins University School of Medicine, Baltimore, MD, and the Department of Biology, University of Iowa, Iowa City, IA, under contract N01-HD-6-2915 from the NIHCD.

References

1. Parker TG, Schneider MD. Growth factors, proto-oncogenes, and plasticity of the cardiac phenotype. Ann Rev Physiol 1991; 53: 179-200.
2. Schneider MD, Parker TG. Cardiac myocytes as targets for the action of peptide growth factors. Circulation 1990; 81: 219-233.
3. Goldman B, Wurzel J. Effects of subcultivation and culture medium on differentiation of human fetal heart muscle cells in vitro. In Vitro Cell Dev Biol 1992; 28A: 109-119.
4. Goldman B, Wurzel J: Cardiac but not skeletal actin is expressed in human fetal heart muscle cells in vivo and in vitro (abstract). J Cell Biochem 1991; Suppl. 15C:161.

5. Boheler KR, Carrier L, de la Bastie D, Allen PD, Konajda M, Mercadier J-J, Schwartz K. Skeletal actin mRNA increases in the human heart during ontogenic development and is the major actin isoform of control and failing human heart. J Clin Invest 1991; 88:323-330.
6. Swynghedauw B. Developmental and functional adaptation of contractile proteins in cardiac and skeletal muscles. Physiol Rev 1986; 66: 710-771.
7. Kohtz DS, Dische MR, Inagami T, Goldman B. Growth and partial differentiation of presumptive human cardiac myoblasts in culture. J Cell Biol 1989; 108: 1067-1078.
8. Kohtz DS, Goldman B. Induction of ANF expression is an early event marking the differentiation of human cardiac myoblasts in culture. In: Kedes L, Stockdale F editors, Cellular and Molecular Biology of Muscle Development, UCLA Symposia on Molecular and Cellular Biology, Alan R. Liss, Inc., New York, 1989.
9. Jacobson SL, Banfalvi M, Schwarzfeld TA. Long term primary cultures of adult human and rat cardiocytes. Basic Res Cardiol 1985; 80 (Suppl. 1): 79-82.
10. Manasek F. Histogenesis of the embryonic myocardium. Am J Cardiol 1970; 25: 149-168.
11. Chang TD, Cumming TR. Chronotropic responses of human heart tissue cultures. Circ Res 1972; 30: 628-633.
12. Halbert SP, Bruderer R, Thompson A. Growth of dissociated beating human heart cells in tissue culture. Life Sci 1973; 13: 969-975.
13. Kandolf R, Canu A, Hofschneider PH. Coxsackie B3 virus can replicate in cultured human fetal heart cells and is inhibited by interferon. J Mol Cell Cardiol 1985; 17: 167-181.
14. Claycomb WC, Delcarpio JB, Guice SE, Moses RL. Culture and characteization of fetal human atrial and ventricular cardiac muscle cells. In Vitro Cell Dev Biol 1989; 25: 1114-1120.
15. Nair RR, Kartha CC. A simplified method for culture of human fetal heart tissue. Ind J Exp Biol 1989; 27: 934-938.
16. Li R-K, Mickle DAG, Weisel RD, Tumiati LC, Jackowski G, Wu T-W, Williams WG. Effect of oxygen tension on the anti-oxidant enzyme activities of tetratology of Fallot ventricular myocytes. J Mol Cell Cardiol 1989; 21: 567-585.
17. Wang Y-C, Hershkowitz A, Gu L-B, Kanter K, Lattougf O, Sell KW, Ahmed-Ansari A. Influence of cytokines and immunosuppressive drugs on major histocompability complex class I/II expression by human cardiac myocytes in vitro. Hum Immunol 1991; 31: 123-133.
18. Smith DA, Golver JL, Townsend LE, Maupin DE. A method for the harvest, culture and characterization of human adult atrial myocardial cells: correlation with age of donor. In Vitro Cell Dev Biol 1991; 57: 914-920.

19. Gospodarowicz D, Ferrara N, Schweigerer L, Neufeld G. Structural characterization and biological function of fibroblast growth factor. Endocr Rev 1987; 8: 95-114.

20. Casscells W, Speir E, Sasse J, Klagsbrun M, Allen P, Lee M, Calvo B, Chiba M, Haggroth L, Folkman J, Epstein SE. Isolation, characterization, and localization of heparin-binding growth factors in the heart. J Clin Invest 1991; 85: 443-441.

21. Rechler MM, Nissley SP: The nature and regulation of the receptors for insulin-like growth factors. Ann Rev Physiol 1985; 47: 425-442.

22. Daughaday WH, Rotwein P. Insulin like growth factors I and II. Peptide, meesenger ribonucleic acid and gene structures, serum and tissue concentrations. Endocrine Rev 1989; 10: 68-91.

23. Froesch ER, Schmid C, Schwander CSJ, Zapf J. Actions of insulin-like growth factors. Ann Rev Physiol 1985; 47: 443-467.

24. Sara VR, Hall K. Insulin-like growth factors and their binding proteins. Physiol Rev 1990; 70: 591-614.

25. Han VKM, Lund PK, Lee DC, D'Ercole AJ. Expression of somatomedin/insulin-like growth factor messenger ribonucleic acids in the human fetus: identification, characterization, and tissue distribution. J Clin Endocrinol and Metab 1988; 66: 422-429.

26. Florini JR, Ewton DZ, Magri KA. Hormones, growth factors, and myogenic differentiation. Ann Rev Physiol 1991; 53: 201-216.

27. Klein I, Ojamaa K. Cardiovascular manifestations of endocrine disease. J Clin Encrinol Metab 1992; 75: 339-342.

28. Jonas EA, Aloia JF, Lane FJ. Evidence of subclinical heart muscle dysfunction in acromegaly. Chest 1975; 67: 190-194.

29. Frustaci A, Perrone GA, Gentiloni N, Russo M. Reversible dilated cardiomyopathy due to growth hormone deficiency. Am J Clin Pathol 1992; 97: 503-511.

30. Gutgesell HP, Speer ME, Rosenberg HS. Characterizaton of the cardiomyopthy in infants of diabetic mothers. Circulation 1980; 61: 441-450.

31. Regan TJ. Cardiac decompensation in diabetes mellitus. Cardiovasc Rev Reports 1985; 6: 1117-1126.

32. Dillman WH. Diabetes mellitus induced changes in the concetration of specific mRNAs and proteins. Diabetes/Metab Rev 1988; 4: 789-797.

33. Bader D, Masaki T, Fischman DA. Immunochemical analysis of myosin heavy chain during avian myogenesis in vivo and in vitro. J Cell Biol 1982; 95: 763-770.

34. Schneider MD, Roberts R, Parker TG. Modulation of cardiac genes by mechanical stress: the oncogene signalling hypothesis. Mol Biol Med 1991; 8: 167-183.

35. Skalli O, Gabbiani G, Babai F, Seemayer TA, Pizzolato G, Schurch W. Intermediate filament proteins and actin isoforms as markers for soft tissue tumor differentiation and origin II: rhabdomyosarcomas. Am J Pathol 1988; 130: 515-531.
36. Ross R. Platelet-derived growth factor. Lancet 1989; 1: 1179-1182 .
37. Cohen S. Isolation of a mouse submaxillary gland protein accelerating incisor eruption and eyelid opening in the newborn animal. J Biol Chem 1962; 237: 1555-1562.
38. Carpenter C, Goodman L, Shaver L: The physiology of epidermal growth factor. In: Kahn P, Graf T editors, Oncogenes and Growth Control, Springer Verlag, New York, 1986; 65-69.
39. Zak, R. Factors controlling cardiac growth. In: Zak R. editor, Growth of the Heart in Health and Disease. Raven Press, New York, 1984; 165-185.
40. Litvin J, Montogomery M, Gonzalez-Sanchez A, Bisaha JG, Bader D. Commitment and differentiation of cardiac myocytes. Trends Cardiovasc Med 1992: 2: 27-32.

8. Growth factors and development of coronary collaterals

HARI S. SHARMA and RENE ZIMMERMAN

Introduction

The existence of coronary collaterals in the heart and their potential role in salvaging the ischemic myocardium is well described. In experimental animals as well as in humans during ischemic heart disease, slowly developing occlusion of a large epicardial coronary artery leads to the formation of a collateral circulation [1,3,4]. This compensatory growth (collateralization) is able to prevent myocardial infarction and these alternate routes of blood supply to the jeopardized myocardium arise both from preformed and newly formed collateral vessels [1)] Over the past 25 years, studies from our group have shown that in the pig heart, collaterals are tiny vascular channels of < 20 μm in diameter and that they develop in response to ischemia usually in the sub-endocardial regions as a network interconnected with one another as well as with epicardial coronary arteries and their branches [1-4]. In canine heart, epicardial vessels increase from an initial diameter of 40 μm to an average diameter of 80 μm [1,4,5,31]. Hence, it can be stated that progressively slow coronary artery stenosis favours the induction of blood vessel growth, a phenomenon called angiogenesis. Angiogenesis in the heart could be of two types; sprouting angiogenesis, when collateral vessels develop from an existing capillary and non-sprouting angiogenesis, when collateral vessels develop as a tubular structure from pre-existing arterioles.

Endothelial cells, smooth muscle cells and pericytes are the major cell types which constitute a blood vessel [6]. The genetic information to form tubes, branches and the whole capillary network is usually carried by these vascular cells. Under normal physiological conditions the proliferation of endothelial cells is strictly controlled and they maintain a quiescent state. However, certain conditions such as corpus luteum formation, wound healing, psoriasis, diabetic retinopathy and tumor vascularization are associated with rapid endothelial cell growth [6-8]. The mechanisms involved in the process of angiogenesis have been studied using in vivo and in vitro models. Angiogenesis initiates with the activation of endothelial cells which can be characterized by an increase in the number of cell organelles and followed by the degradation of basement membrane involving the activity of certain proteases [8-10].

Angiogenesis being a complex multistep biological process is undoubtly regulated by a number of factors. In the last decade various angiogenic growth factors and inhibitors have been discovered [for recent reviews see: 6,7,10,11]. Their biological properties as well as their role in angiogenesis in vitro have been described, very little is known about their physiological significance in vivo and in particular during coronary angiogenesis. We have recently demonstrated that the potent mitogenic polypeptide growth factors like acidic fibroblast growth factor (aFGF), vascular endothelial growth factor (VEGF) and transforming growth factor-β1 (TGF-β1) are expressed in the porcine myocardium and their expression can be provoked by ischemia [12-14,22]. These findings suggest that polypeptide growth factors contribute in coronary angiogenesis but at the same time several questions are raised; e.g, why does normal adult myocardium express mitogenic growth factors? what is the time course of growth factors expression during myocardial ischemia? where are they localized in the heart? In this chapter, we summarize the state of art on a variety of angiogenic growth promoting peptides in the heart and their possible participation in ischemia induced coronary collateralization.

Cardiac growth factors

A landmark was the discovery by Schaper and DeBrabander [15] more than 20 years ago when they found that endothelial and smooth muscle cell proliferation and DNA synthesis was the basis of myocardial collateralization. The obvious implication of these findings was to search for the stimulus of vascular growth in the heart. In 1983, Kumar et al [16] isolated an angiogenic growth factor from the infarcted human heart. This low molecular weight growth factor was found to be similar to a human tumor derived angiogenic growth factor [16]. Recent investigations demonstrated that the adult heart produces a number of growth promoting poly-peptides which are well characterized to be angiogenic in vitro and in vivo [12-14,17,20-22]. Quinkler and coworkers from our institute have isolated and characterized heparin binding peptide mitogens from normal adult bovine, porcine and canine hearts [17]. Amino acid analysis of these poly-peptide mitogens showed a very high degree of homology to the previously known acidic and basic fibroblast growth factors isolated from other tissues [19,44,45]. Following our report on these cardiac growth factors, Cassells et al (20) and Sasaki et al [21] have also purified and characterized on the basis of western blotting, heparin binding growth factors identical to acidic and basic FGF.

Recently, our group and others have shown the TGF-β 1 expression in normal and ischemic myocardium of different species [22-24]. Using applications of reverse transcriptase-polymerase chain reaction (RT-PCR), we specifically amplified DNA fragments encoding VEGF, tumor necrosis factor-α (TNF-α), transforming growth factor-β1 (TGF-β1) and aFGF from the adult porcine heart [25,32]. Results depicted in Figure 2-8 (see below) demonstrate that a variety of potent peptide mitogens, aFGF, bFGF, VEGF, TNF-α, IGF-II, TGF-β1 and IL-6 are expressed in the normal adult porcine heart and their respective mRNAs of known size can be detected by Northern hybridization. Furthermore, using human specific cDNA inserts in Northern hybridization technique, we attempted to investigate other growth factors like platelet derived growth factor (PDGF), platelet derived endothelial cell growth factor (PD-ECGF), transforming growth factor-α (TGF-α) and transforming growth factor-β2 (TGF-β2). We could not demonstrate the expression of above growth factors in the myocardial tissue. The existence of potent angiogenic growth factors in the adult heart, where practically no angiogenesis occurs under normal physiological conditions raises questions. However, one may predict certain roles like, maintenance of normal vascular permeability and vascular repair (for VEGF, TGF-β1) and/or they are vital for the normal survival of terminally differentiated cardiac cells (for FGF).

Experimental models of ischemia induced myocardial angiogenesis

Using coronary artery occlusion leading to myocardial ischemia, various methods of collateralization in different species have been described in the literature. These methods are based on: acute coronary artery occlusion, stenosis of coronary artery by a fixed known degree, progressively slow coronary artery occlusion until complete stenosis, repeated short coronary occlusions, microembolization, chronic coronary vasodilation by severe anemia and drugs etc [26-30]. The diagnostic and verification techniques used to study collateralization, include radioactive tracers scanning, angiography, histology, ultrastructure and cell biology. Various groups used dogs for the study of collateral vessel development but some others have used pigs also. Species difference exist between mammals, however, from an anatomic point view, the pigs coronary and collateral circulation is closest to that of the human heart [26].

Porcine models of myocardial angiogenesis

In recent years, our group has mainly investigated the myocardial angiogenesis in pigs by inducing regional ischemia by an ameroid constrictor or by injecting 15-25 μm microspheres in the left circumflex (Lcx) coronary artery. Both models are well established and described in previous reports [1,3,33,34].

Ameroid constrictor model of collateralization

The principle of ameroid constrictor model is that the hygroscopic plastic material on formalin based casein swells by absorbing the tissue fluid and compresses the coronary artery slowly [3]. In our experiments, a series of pigs (mini pigs and German landrace pigs), were implanted with a hygroscopic ameroid constrictor around the Lcx. Stenosis or occlusion of a coronary artery and collateralization were verified by in vivo angiography after 2-4 weeks of ameroid implantation. At more than 90% of LCx stenosis, pigs were sacrificed, the hearts were removed quickly and rinsed in ice-cold saline. Small tissue pieces from the LCx region (macroscopically examined to exclude any infarcted tissue) and normally perfused interventricular septum were excised and snap frozen in liquid nitrogen and stored at -80°C until analysed. Myocardial tissues from an infarcted and from normally perfused areas from a pig were also collected for analysis. Using molecular biological techniques, we examined the expression of various angiogenic growth factors viz., aFGF and bFGF, VEGF, TGF-β1 and TNF-α in the tissues mentioned above.

Microembolization model of collateralization

Details of the surgical procedures have been described previously [34].

Briefly, male mixed-breed Landrace type domestic pigs, were sedated with azaperone and then anesthetized with pentobarbital. The electocardiogram from standard limb leads was monitored through out the procedure. Under sterile conditions, 25 μm non radioactive polystrene microspheres (NEN-TRAC, Du Pont, USA) were injected into the left circumflex coronary artery (Lcx) either with or without subsequent thoracotomy. After successful microspheres embolization, the pericardium was sutured and the chest was closed in layers. In case of embolization without thoracotomy, a 7F modified multipurpose catheter (Cordis Europa) was introduced via the exposed carotid artery and microspheres were injected through the catheter into the Lcx. The pigs were reanesthetized and sacrificed at different time points (6h, 12h, 24h, 72h or 7 days) of microembolization, heart was exposed through a midline thoracotomy and excised quickly. Myocardial tissue samples were collected from non-ischemic (control) and the Lcx perfused ischemic embolized (experimental) region in liquid nitrogen and stored at -80° C until analysed. One sham catheterized pig served as control. We examined the expression pattern of different growth factors, cytokines and components of plasminogen activators/plasmin system (PAs/P).

Characterization of mitotic activity in the ischemic myocardium

It is well described that in progressive coronary artery occlusion, pre-existing collateral vessels respond with growth by DNA synthesis, mitosis and proliferation of endothelial cells and smooth muscle cells (2,15). In our experimental models myocardial tissue, which was angiographically verified for the collateralization was further analysed by in situ hybridization with a radioactive histone-H3 cRNA probe. Enhanced mRNA expression for histone H3 in a particular cell indicates cell division and can be used as a marker of cells in S phase (35). A significantly higher labelling of vascular cells was found in the ischemic myocardium (where the collateralization was documented by in vivo angiography) compared to normally perfused myocardium (Figure 1).

Myocardial ischemia alters growth factor expression

Myocardial regional ischemia induced either by an ameroid constrictor or by microembolization in the porcine heart leads to numerous phenotypic alterations in the expression of angiogenic growth factors

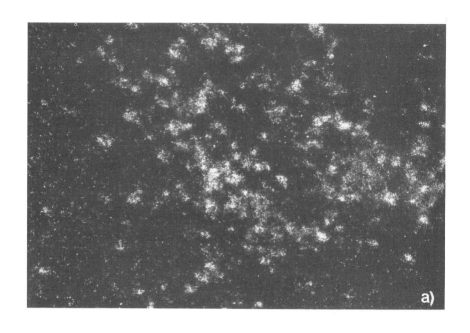

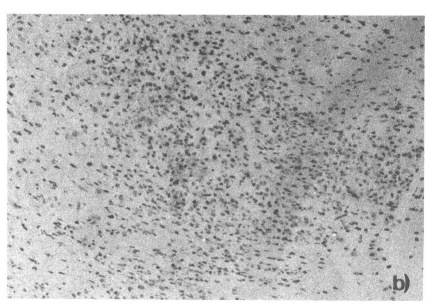

Figure 1. In situ hybridization for histone-H3 mRNAs in the collateralized myocardium. 5 μm tissue sections were hybridized with histone-H3 antisense cRNA probe (provided by Dr. D.T. Wong) and washed under stringent conditions. a) Darkfield microphotograph depicting high density silver grains focally distributed over the nuclei of endothelial and other cells in the necrotic area. b) Bright field micrograph of the ischemic collateralized region (above tissue section) showing a micronecrotic area with the accumulation of inflammatory cells and endothelial cells nuclei.

genes which can be summarized as follows:

Vascular endothelial growth factor

Vascular endothelial growth factor (VEGF) is a heparin binding, highly glycosylated cationic homodimeric protein of 46 kD [36]. VEGF, also called as vasculotropin is very similar to vascular permeability factor which contains a 24 amino acids insertion [37]. VEGF cDNA has been cloned and analysis of its nucleotide sequence suggests that it is a member of the platelet derived growth factor (PDGF) family with 21-24% amino acid homology [36,38]. VEGF may exist by alternative splicing of mRNA as four different molecular forms with 121, 165, 189 and 206 amino acids polypeptides. The two shorter forms are secreted proteins, whereas, the longer ones seem to be cell associated [37]. VEGF has been isolated from a number of normal and tumor cells and its expression has been shown in the corpus luteum and developing brain and kidney [40,41]. It is a highly specific peptide mitogen for endothelial cells derived from small and large vessels and is a potent angiogenic factor in vivo [36, 38].

We examined the expression of VEGF in normal and collateralized myocardium. As a diagnostic search, we performed RT-PCR on cDNA templates from normal and collateralized tissues and amplified a VEGF specific DNA fragment from both tissues. Amplified PCR product was verified by Southern hybridization using radiolabelled internal oligonucleotide primer. Furthermore, the PCR product was cloned into a plasmid vector and sequenced which showed high homology (94%) with the human cDNA sequence [42]. Using a porcine specific cDNA probe encoding VEGF, we detected two mRNAs of 3.9 (major) and 1.7 kb (minor) in the normal and collateralized myocardium (Figure 2). The expression pattern of VEGF revealed an overall enhanced expression in the collateralized tissue as compared to the normally perfused tissue. In the pig, where we observed infarction, expression of VEGF was significantly reduced indicating the myocytes as a major contributor of

VEGF [32]. The tissue distribution of VEGF showed maximal expression of its mRNA in the heart as compared to other organs in the pig [42].

By in situ hybridization, VEGF mRNA could be localized predominantly in normal cardiac myocytes. Berse et al [93] have shown very recently the tissue distribution of VEGF where they have also localized VEGF mRNA transcripts in cardiac myocytes. In the ischemic tisssue, significant labelling was seen in the granulation tissue and in the viable myocytes somewhat remote from fibrotic regions of ischemic myocardium [32]. These results indicate a potential role of VEGF in the collateral vessel development in response to progredient chronic ischemia. Enhanced expression of VEGF in the collateralized myocardial tissue could also contribute to the enhanced permeability of endothelial cells. In a porcine model of myocardial stunning with two cycles of 10 min ischemia and 30 min reperfusion, we observed significantly enhanced VEGF expression in the stunned tissue as compared to the control [14]. The rapid induction of VEGF in the ischemic myocardium may suggest its properties as an intermediate molecule which may be needed to induce other genes like proteases which are involved in the extracellular matrix degradation. Pepper et al. [43] have very recently shown that the VEGF induces tissue- and urokinase-type plasminogen activators (uPA and tPA) and their potential inhibitor PAI-1 in isolated microvascular endothelial cells in culture. Presumably, VEGF is involved in the induction of uPA and tPA as well as their inhibitor PAI-1 in the ischemic myocardium for a regulated extracellular matrix degradation, an essential component of angiogenesis.

Acidic and Basic Fibroblast Growth Factor

Acidic FGF is a heparin binding anionic peptide mitogen of 18 kD with pI of 5. aFGF shares an absolute sequence identity to bFGF with more than 53% [44]. Basic FGF is a cationic (pI 9.6) polypeptide mitogen which may exist as higher molecular weight form (> 18 kD) due to initiation of synthesis at CUG rather than AUG start codon [7,45]. Both aFGF and bFGF lack the signal sequence for direct secretion from the cell and seem to be cell associated [5,7,45]. They bind to low affinity cell surface receptors which appear to be heparan sulfate proteoglycans [46]. Endothelial cells synthesize substantial amounts of bFGF which is found to be stored in the extracellular matrix [7,47]. Various oncogenic peptides like *int*-2 (27 kD), *hst* (23 kD), K-*fgf* and FGF-5 (29 kD) have been described to be 40-50% homologous to aFGF and bFGF [7,46,48,49]. It is well documented that aFGF and bFGF are mitogenic

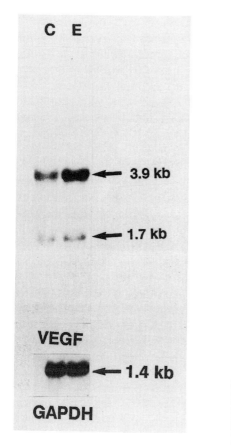 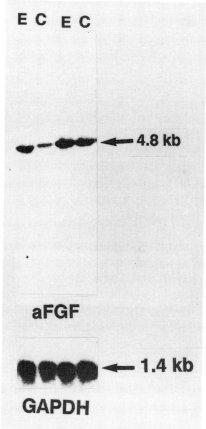

Figure 2 (left) . VEGF expression in the normal (C) and collateralized (E) swine myocardium. Northern blot analysis with a porcine specific cDNA probe was performed as described in the text. One major (3.9 kb) and one minor (1.7 kb) mRNAs are expressed in both regions. The expression of VEGF mRNAs is drastically induced in the E as compared to the C. GAPDH mRNA (1.4 kb) was used as a reference.

Figure 3: (right). Expression of aFGF mRNA in the porcine myocardium in relation to ischemia. Northern blot analysis was performed by hybridizing similar amounts of total cellular RNA isolated from the collateralized (E) and normally perfused (C) myocardium with a radiolabelled human cDNA probe encoding aFGF. A single dominant band (4.8 kb) specific for aFGF was expressed in the E region whereas, a faint signal was seen in the C. In another pig without collateralization, no difference in the aFGF expression pattern was ssen (right panel). Bottom panel shows GAPDH expression of 1.4 kb mRNA confirming the quality and quantity of the RNA loaded on the gel.

in vitro for cells of vascular, connective and muscle tissue origin [44,45] and induce complete angiogenic response in vivo [11]. aFGF promotes neurite outgrowth and under specific conditions it may act as differentiating and maintenance factor for nerves [50]. It is not clear how FGF mediates angiogenesis in vivo, however, it is proposed that they are released during cell injury from their store site and later stimulate the connective tissue growth and angiogenesis [7]. The pre-requisite of FGF release after cell injury does not appear to be a natural act and needs further possible explanations.

We investigated the expression of mRNAs encoding aFGF in the ischemic collateralized porcine myocardium. By RT-PCR we amplified a DNA fragment of 472 bp encoding aFGF from a normal myocardium, verified by Southern hybridization with a radiolabeled internal oligo-nucleotide probe and sequencing [13,51]. By Northern blotting, we detected a dominant band of 4.8 kb encoding aFGF in the collateralized myocardium, whereas, a faint signal corresponding in size (4.8 kb) was seen in the normal myocardium (Figure 3, left panel). In pigs with less than 90% of coronary stenosis and no collateralization, aFGF expression was not altered in the ischemic as compared to normally perfused myocardial regions (Figure 3, right panel). However, in a pig with ameroid constrictors and visible infarction, aFGF expression was drastically decreased in the experimental area [32]. Studying the tissue distribution of aFGF, we found that the heart is a major source of aFGF as compared to other porcine tissues [42]. Porcine normal and collateralized tissue sections were hybridized with a [35S] labelled cDNA probe encoding human aFGF (provided by Dr. T. Maciag) in order to localize the aFGF mRNA transcripts. aFGF transcripts were mainly seen in the vascular wall cells presumably in the endothelial and smooth muscle cells [52]. Previously it was shown by immunohistochemical methods that aFGF is localized in viable cardiac myocytes in the zone surrounding focal necrosis and no aFGF staining was seen in the normally perfused myocardial tissue sections with the exception of the Purkinje-fibres [53]. Weiner and Swain [54)]have also shown that cultured neonatal myocytes produce aFGF as they could detect the mRNA and Spier et al [94] showed the immunoreactive aFGF in the isolated adult rat heart myocytes. Enhanced expression of aFGF in collateralized porcine tissue in our experimental models points to its role in ischemia induced myocardial angiogenesis.

Using a bovine specific cDNA probe (provided by Dr. J. Abraham) in Northern hybridization, we detected two mRNA species of 6.5 and 3.7 kb encoding bFGF in the porcine myocardium after several days of exposure of blots and they appear to be unchanged during collateralization (Figure 4). bFGF has been shown to be present in the

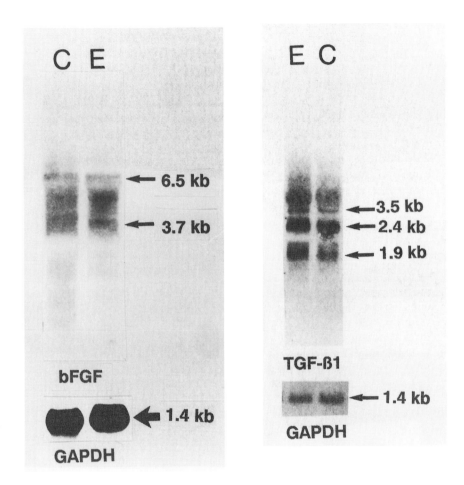

Figure 4 (left). bFGF expression in the ischemic and normal myocardium. Northern hybridization was performed from total isolated from C and E using a 1.4 kb EcoRI insert from a bovine cDNA clone encoding bFGF. Two mRNA species of 6.5 and 3.7 kb were detected in the porcine heart which were not altered in two (C and E) myocardial tissues. Lower panel shows the 1.4 kb GAPDH mRNA used as reference.
Figure 5 (right). Expression of TGF-β1 in the collateralized and normally perfused myocardium. 20 μg of total RNA from Collateralized (E) and Normally perfused (C) tissue was separated on a 1% agarose gel, transferred to a nylon membrane and hybridized to a human cDNA insert encoding TGF-β1 (kindly provided by Dr. R. Derynck). The autoradiograph depicts three mRNA bands (3.5, 2.4 and 1.9 kb) encoding porcine TGF-β1 in the heart and they were icreased in the E as compared to the C. Lower panel shows the 1.4 kb band of GAPDH detected in above myocardial RNA preparations.

atrial and ventricular extracts of different species [17,18,20]. Bernotat-Danielowski et al from our group tried to localize the bFGF antigen in the porcine ischemic myocardium using a monoclonal antibody, and were unable to see any labelling by immunohistochemical methods [53]. This may be explained by the low detection limit of immunostaining methods and presumably, bFGF is transcribed in the heart at a low level which may not contribute in the ischemia induced angiogenic processes. Recently Spier et al [94] have shown that freshly isolated adult rat heart myocytes contain bFGF, which increases several fold upon culturing cells for few days and these cells in culture express the fibroblast growth factor receptor (flg) gene.

Transforming growth factor-β1

Transforming growth factor-β1 (TGF-β1) is a 25 kDa homodimeric polypeptide differentiation factor largely found in platelets and most organs, including heart [23-24,55]. Although TGF-β1 is an inhibitor of endothelial cell proliferation, it has been found to be angiogenic when injected subcutaneously into newborn mice [56] or when applied locally in wound healing experiments [57]. The angiogenic response to TGF-β1 application is an indirect one, the primary response is the chemo-attraction for monocytes which then in turn stimulate angiogenesis [7,56]. TGF-β1 has been shown to contribute in myocardial protection during ischemic injury [58]. The physiological role of TGF-β1 in the heart remains to be well elucidated, however, its properties in vitro suggests that it might be an important molecule in various myocardial situations such as cardiac embryogenesis, hypertrophy, atherogenesis, healing of myocardial infarction and development of coronary collaterals [22,59,60].

We used RT-PCR for the detection of TGF-β1 in various myocardial RNA preparations by employing porcine specific TGF-β1 oligonucleotide primers [61]. A DNA product of 423 bp was amplified in cDNA preparations derived from normal and collateralized myocardium. The PCR product was verified by Southern hybridization as well as by reamplification of a smaller fragment using internal primers [62]. In a semi-quantitative approach, higher amplification of a TGF-β1 specific DNA fragment of 257 bp was observed after 15 cycles of RT-PCR in collateralized as compared to the normal myocardium [62)] This difference became more apparent when TGF-β1 expression was evaluated by Northen hybridization. We found enhanced expression of TGF-β1 mRNAs of 3.5, 2.4 (major) and 1.9 kb in the ischemic-collateralized myocardium in our porcine experimental model of progressive coronary artery occlusion (Figure 5). In another set of experiments, we used a porcine specific 257 bp DNA fragment amplified by RT-PCR in Northern hybridization and found a significantly increased mRNA (1.9kb) expression in the collateralized tissue as compared to the normally perfused tissue [32]. Employing in situ hybridization, we observed TGF-β1 specific mRNA transcripts predominantly in cardiac myocytes near fibrotic tissue and not in the area of inflammatory infiltrate (22).

We performed immunoblot analysis with a polyclonal anti TGF-β1 antibody which showed a specific band of 25 kD in myocardial protein extracts from normal and collateralized tissue [22]. By immunohistochemical methods, we observed TGF-β1 staining in the cardiac myocytes. Purkinje cells of the conduction system were consistently stained with TGF-β1 specific antibodies [32] indicating that TGF-β1 may influence the degree of differentiation in these cells. The cellular source of TGF-β1 in the heart is controversial. Thompson et al [23] found TGF-β1 mRNA and protein in the cardiac myocytes of the infacted tissue, whereas, Eghbali (24) could demonstrate mRNA expression of TGF-β1 only in the non-myocyte fraction of cardiac tissue. In contrast to the findings of Thompson et al [23], we could not find a significantly enhanced expression of TGF-β1 in the infarcted tissue [22]. By in situ hybridization technique, we found that cardiac myocytes predominantly express TGF-β1 mRNA and not the cells in damaged tissue or capillaries where only few silver grains were seen (22).

Other growth factors / cytokines in the heart

Insulin-like growth factors

The insulin-like growth factors (IGF) are subdivided into two groups: insulin-like growth factor I (IGF-I or somatomedin C) and insulin-like growth factor II (IGF-II). IGFs are single-chain peptid growth factors of approximately 7.5kD, which show a high homology to proinsulin and have in addition to the A-, B- and C -domain of proinsulin a

D-domain. IGF-I and IGF-II show 62% amino acid homolgy and are each the product of a single gene (reviewed in [63]). They occur in blood plasma, where they are bound to specific insulin-like growth factor binding proteins (IGFBP-1 to -6), are mainly produced by the liver, and are found in low concentrations in most body tissues, where they are locally produced as paracrine and autocrine growth factors. IGFs stimulate cellular proliferation and differentiation and are important factors in normal fetal and postnatal development [63]. Their mitogenic effects are mediated by specific receptors, the type 1 receptor, which has a tyrosine phosphorylation activity and is homologous to the insulin receptor, and the type 2 receptor, which has no similarity to the type 1 receptor and a greater affinity to IGF-II than to IGF-I [64]. IGF-I and -II are single gene products and their genes are localized on chromosome 12 (human) and on chromosome 11 (human) respectively. At least two mRNAs are encoded by the IGF-I gene, whereas expression of the IGF-II gene is tissue- and development-specific [63-65].

The insulin-like growth factors have multiple biological activities. IGF-I stimulates the growth of a variety of cultured cells including smooth muscle cells [66]. Endothelial cells after injury synthesize an increased amount of IGF-I [67]. IGF-II mRNA is increased in tumors of SMC [68] and it promotes proliferation and differentiation of myoblasts (66). In a recent paper [69] it is stated that " the IGFs are the only well-defined agents thus far shown to stimulate myogenesis". Lowe and co-workers [70] described that in the rat heart, expression of IGF-I inreases substantially during the first post-natal days indicating it´s importance during development. Furthermore, it was recently shown that in an in vivo model of cardiac growth using hypophysectomized rats which were treated with thyroid hormone (T3) the IGF-I gene expression is significantly increased. This indicates a autocrine role of cardiac IGF-I as a regulatory event in the T3 mediated growth effects [71].

In our model of microsphere induced ischemia IGF-I showed a weak, but constant expression of an mRNA of approximately 8.2 kb. An additional mRNA of about 1.0 kb was more weakly expressed. At least 5 different mRNAs were observed for IGF-II in the pig heart, the strongest signal appearing at approximately 2.8 kb and weaker signals at 1.7, 1.9, 4.8, and 6.0 kb (Figure 6). The expression of IGF-II mRNAs was not changed in microembolized pigs [72]. In situ hybridization studies using sense and antisense mRNA transcripts for IGF-II identified myocytes as the IGF-II producing cells (Kluge et al., unpublished) It is not clear why there is an expression of insulin-like growth factors in the pig heart, even in the region not affected by

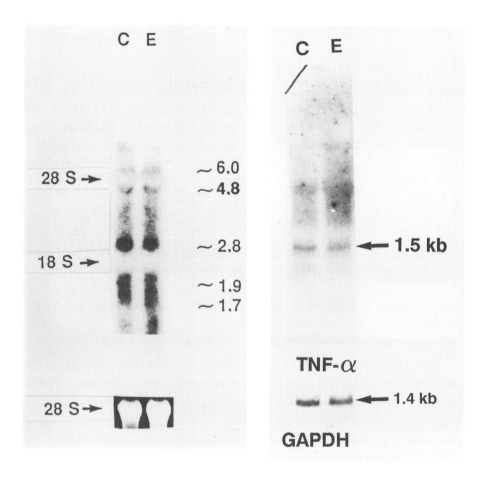

Figure 6 (left). Northern blot analysis of the IGF-II mRNA in the microembolized tissue. Total RNA from the microembolized (E) and control (C) myocardial tissue was used for the Northern hybridization with a radiolabelled human IGF-II cDNA probe (procurred from ATCC). Five different mRNA bands of 6, 4.8, 2.8, 1.9 and 1.7 kb were detected and they remain unchanged during microembolization. Lower panel shows the 28S rRNA band of above blot.

Figure 7 (right). Detection of TNF-α mRNA in the porcine myocardium. Using a human cDNA probe (purchased from ATCC) encoding TNF-α in Northern hybridization, a single band of 1.5 kb is visible in the porcine myocardium which is not affected by myocardial ischemia. The lower panel depicts the GAPDH mRNA band of 1.4 kb used as a reference.

ischemia. We think that the IGFs are trophic factors, necessary for the heart to maintain its normal function.

Tumor necrosis factor-α

Tumor necrosis factor-α (TNF-α) is a multipotent cytokine of 17 kD produced mainly by activated macrophages and has been implicated in several biologic processes including inflammation, immunoregulation, and angiogenesis (73). It acts directly on vascular endothelium to increase the adhesion of leukocytes during the inflammation [74]. TNF-α is similar in many ways to TGF-β: both polypeptides induce angiogenesis in vivo, promote tube formation in vitro, but inhibit endothelial cell proliferation in vitro indicating that TNF-α is an indirect angiogenic growth factor which may stimulate other cells to produce angiogenic factors [7,74]. Employing polymerase chain reaction (PCR) and Northern hybridization, we searched for mRNAs encoding TNF-α in the porcine normal and collateralized myocardium. Using porcine specific oligonucleotide primers, we amplified a DNA fragment of 483 bp encoding TNF-α from both normal and collateralized myocardium [32]. By Northern hybridization we detected TNF-α specific mRNA band of 1.5 kb in the porcine myocardium (Fig. 7) Slightly induced expression of TNF-α mRNA in the collateralized myocardium as compared to the normally perfused myocardium was observed in the ameroid constrictor model. Similar results were obtained for the TNF-α expression in the ischemic region of the microembolized pigs (Sharma et al unpublished). From these results it may be inferred that the TNF-α is transcribed in the adult heart at a detectable mRNA level and may play a role in the inflammatory processes caused by myocardial ischemia.

Interleukin-1

Interleukin-1 (IL-1) is a multifunctional cytokine, primarily involved in the regulation of inflammatory processes. It mediates most of the acute-phase response to infection including induction of fever, production and release of acute-phase proteins in hepatocytes and of prostaglandins and collagenase by fibroblasts and synovial cells [75]. Recent evidence indicates that IL-1 produced within tissues contributes to local inflammatory reactions [76]. Other biological activities of interleukin-1 include induction of growth of fibroblasts, bone resorption, ICAM-1 expression and growth and differentiation of B- and T-cells [77]. Two genes are expressed for IL-1: IL-1α and IL-1ß. Although these genes show only 20-30% amino acid homology they were shown to bind the same high-affinity receptor [78] and they may be derived from a common ancestral gene. IL-1 does not posses a typical hydrophobic signal sequence for secretion and may be processed extracellulary by limited proteolysis from a high molecular mass intracellular precursor of 33 kDa to an active form of 17 kDa [79,80].

IL-1 is produced mainly by macrophages/monocytes, T-cells, B-cells, fibroblasts, keratinocytes, astrocytes and endothelial cells [77] and has a wide range of target cells including T-cells, B-cells, fibroblasts and many others. Recent evidence indicates that there are direct actions of IL-1 on vascular smooth muscle cells. Trinkle and co-workers [81] showed that the content of contractile proteins of rat thoraric aorta was significantly affected by this cytokine, e.g. γ-actin isoforms were enhanced and the vascular smooth muscle specific α-isoactin was decreased. It also induces prostanoid-dependent hypotension in rabbits in vivo [82] and stimulates human smooth muscle cells to secrete interleukin-6 [83].

In our model of microsphere-induced ischemia the region of putative collateral growth is characterized by an increased number of macrophages/monocytes as a sign for regional inflammatory response and by endothelial cell proliferation. Because monocytes/macrophages are the richest source for IL-1 we investigated the expression of these genes in the ischemic porcine heart. Using northern blot hybridization, we found that IL-1α and IL-1ß were neither expressed in normal nor in ischemic porcine myocardium [72]. However, using RT-PCR we could detect a DNA fragment encoding IL-1β in the porcine heart. Han and co-workers [84] found unchanged IL-1ß mRNA expression in non-failing and failing human heart by PCR, whereas, IL-1α was not expressed. It may be inferred from these findings that IL-1α and IL-1ß are not involved in ischemia induced processes in porcine heart.

Interleukin-6

Interleukin-6 (IL-6), a secreted single chain protein of 28 kDa (184 amino acids), encoded on chromosomes 7 (human) and 5 (mouse), respectively, is another pluripotent cytokine. It is released from a variety of cell types including monocytes/macrophages, fibroblasts, T- and B-cells, keratinocytes, endothelial cells, astrocytes, mesangial cells, and bone marrow stroma cells (for review see: [77,85]). Recently, it was shown that IL-6 is also expressed by vascular smooth muscle cells in atherosclerotic lesions of genetically hyperlipidemic rabbits [86]. IL-6 has a wide variety of biological functions including induction of B-cell differentiation and acute-phase response [87-89]. Furthermore, it induces macrophage differentiation, hematopoietic stem cell growth, maturation of megakaryocytes, neural cell differentiation, mesangial cell growth, and myeloid leukemic cell differentiation [77]. Recently, S. Morimoto and collegues [90] showed that treatment of cultured rat vascular smooth muscle cells with recombinant IL-6 resulted in an increased c-myc mRNA level, followed by increase in DNA synthesis and cell number, indicating that IL-6 may play a role in the proliferation of these cells. It is also reported that human vascular smooth muscle cells after IL-1 stimulation or during proliferation not only express the IL-6 gene, but that IL-6 is a major secretory product of these cells [83]. Therefore it is conceivable to assume that this pleiotropic cytokine may have functions in the heart, especially when there is an accumulation of monocytes/macrophages in regions of local ischemia, followed by local inflammatory reactions. In fact, we found a low, but constant mRNA expression of IL-6 in porcine myocardium not only in the ischemic region of the heart, but also in the control region (Figure 8), where there are hardly any monocytes/macrophages [72]. In 1986 , T. Hirano et al. [87] reported that IL-6 was expressed in cardiac myxoma cells at much higher levels than in activated lymphocytes, and that the mRNA size was larger than 1.3 kb found in other tissues and cells. In our porcine model of microsphere-induced ischemia, the mRNA-size was 1.3 kb, which is in accordance with the results reported by Richards and Saklatvala [91] who cloned the porcine IL-6 cDNA, which has 83.2% homology to the human IL-6 cDNA, the probe which we have used in our studies. There is now evidence that in patients suffering from acute myocardial infarction IL-6 may affect the progression and the healing process of this illness, because IL-6 serum levels seem to be elevated compared to normal patients [92]. With all these results it appears that IL-6 may play a role in the heart. But it is unknown why this cytokine is expressed at low but constant levels in normal myocardium. It is possible that IL-6 is a trophic factor for the heart, necessary to maintain its normal function.

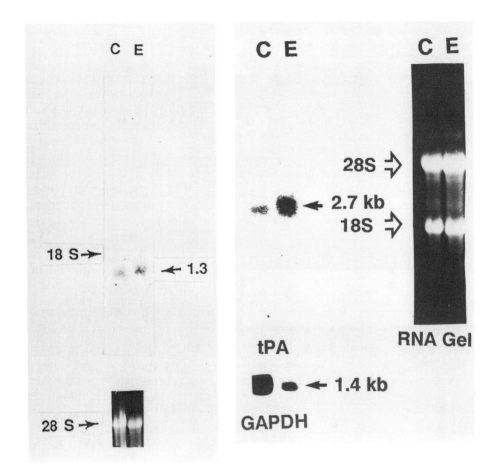

Figure 8 (left). Expression of IL-6 in the porcine myocardium Total RNA isolated from the microembolized (E) and normal (C) myocardial tissue was hybridized with a human cDNA probe encoding IL-6. A single mRNA species of 1.3 kb was detected in both tissues with slight induction in the E as compared to C. 28S rRNA band of above blot is shown in the lower panel.

Figure 9 (right). Expression of t-PA in the microembolized and normal myocardium. Similar amounts of total RNA from ischemic microembolized (E) and control (C) tissue was hybridized with a radiolabelled human t-PA cDNA probe (provided by Dr. S. Degen). The positions of 28S and 18S rRNA bands are marked on the ethidium bromide stained gel(right panel). One mRNA species of 2.7 kb encoding t-PA was detected in the swine myocardium which was significantly induced in the ischemic tissue as compared to the control. Filters were also hybridized with GAPDH for reference purposes.

Myocardial ischemia induces the expression of plasminogen activators and their inhibitor

We examined the expression pattern of plasminogen activator/plasmin system which plays a key role in the tissue remodelling by studying urokinase- and tissue- type plasminogen activators (uPA and tPA) and their physiological inhibitor, PAI-1 in the porcine myocardium subjected to the ischemic conditions by an ameroid constrictor or microspheres. Both uPA and tPA have been shown to be involved in fibrinolysis, extracellular matrix degradation and angiogenesis [95]. Over expression of PAI-1 in vivo impairs the fibrinolytic balance and correlates with thrombotic disorders [96]. In our both experimental models, we found that myocardial ischemia induces the expression of tPA and uPA in the porcine heart [97]. Significantly enhanced mRNA expression of tPA was seen in the myocardial tissues where infarction was noticed (Figure 9) and in such tissue the expression of glyceraldehyde 3-phosphate dehydrogenase (GAPDH) was drastically decreased (Figure 9). PAI-1 mRNAs of 3.5 kb (major) and 3.1 kb (minor) were also significantly induced in the microembolized pigs after 3 days of microspheres infusion (Figure 10). However, the magnitude of expression of plasminogen activators and their inhibitor varied from group to group depending on the degree of stenosis and myocardial necrosis [97]. Mohri et al [98] have shown the tissue distribution of tPA where they found immunoreactive tPA in the vascular endothelial cells mainly of veins. Intesity of uPA and PAI-1 staining was markedly increased in the extracellualr matrix around viable myocytes in the necrotic area of micrembolized pigs. The increased expression of PAs and PAI-1 in the ischemic myocardium suggest their role in the tissue degradation related to the coronary angiogenesis and/or infarct healing processes.

Conclusion

Our findings on the expression of a variety of growth factors in the porcine heart and their induction during myocardial ischemia indicated that the myocardial response to the coronary artery occlusion is mainly associated with the induction of a angiogenic cascade. This cascade does involve other regional myocardial changes including micronecrosis, inflammation and tissue repair. We have accumulated evidences that myocardial ischemia induced by an ameroid onstrictor or by coronary microembolization leads to the enhanced expression of different

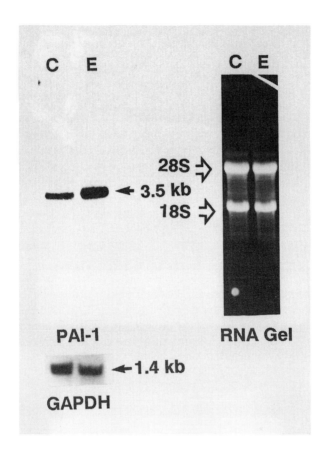

Figure 10. Northern blot analysis of PAI-1 expression in the microembolized and normal myocardium. 15 μg of total RNA from ischemic microembolized (E) and control (C) tissue was subjected to Northern hybridization with a radiolabeled human PAI-1 cDNA probe (provided by Dr. P. Andreasen). The positions of 28S and 18S rRNA bands are marked on the ethidium bromide stained gel (right panel). One major mRNA band of 3.5 kb encoding PAI-1 was detected in the swine myocardium which was significantly induced in the ischemic tissue as compared to the control. Lower panel shows the GAPDH mRNA band used as reference.

140

angiogenic growth factors like aFGF, VEGF, and TGF-β1 as well as proteases and their inhibitor in the porcine heart. Increased expression of these molecules in response to ischemia and micronecrosis clearly point to their important contribution in the myocardial angiogenic processes. Additionally, other growth factors and cytokines (bFGF, TNF-α, IGF-I and II, IL-1 and IL-6) are also expressed in the normal and ischemic myocardium, which are probably vital for the normal functioning of the heart or they have functions in the normal heart which are not yet known. The significant amount of aFGF and VEGF expression in the heart raises questions of further control mechanisms of these growth factors function.

Acknowledgements

We thank the physiology team of Drs. M. Mohri, S. Sack, R.J. Schott and M. Arras for the surgical work. We are grateful to Profs. W. Schaper and J. Schaper for critically reading the manuscript of this chapter and their continuous support. Technical assistance of Mrs. C. Ullmann, B. Münckel and E. Neubauer and photographic help of Mrs. A. Möbs is highly acknowledged.

References

1. Schaper W. The Collateral Circulation of the heart. Amsterdam, North Holland Publishing Co 1971.
2. Kass RW, Kotler MN, Yazdanfar S. Stimulation of coronary collateral growth: Current developments in angiogenesis and future clinical applications. Am Heart J 1992; 123: 486-496.
3. Görge G, Schmidt T, Ito BR, Pantely GA, Schaper W. Microvascular and collateral adaptation in swine hearts following progressive coronary artery stenosis. Basic Res Cardiol 1989; 84: 524-535.
4. Schaper W, Bernotat-Danielowski S, Nienaber C, Schaper J. In: Fozzard HA et al. editors. Collateral Circulation. The Heart and Cardiovascular System (Second edition) Raven Press, Ltd., New York, 1992; 1427-1463.
5. Schaper W, Jageneau A, Xhonneux R. Development of collateral circulation in the pig and the dog heart. Cardiologia 1967; 51: 321-335.
6. Folkman J, Shing Y. Angiogenesis. J Biol Chem 1992; 267: 10931-10934.

7. Klagsbrun M, D' Amore PA. Regulators of Angiogenesis. Ann Rev. Physiol 1991; 53: 217-239.
8. D' Amore PA, Thompson RW. Mechanism of angiogenesis. Ann Rev Physiol 1987; 49: 453-464.
9. Rifkin DB, Gross Jl, Moscatelli D, Jaffe E. Pathobiology of the endothelial cells Academic press. New York. 1982; pp 191-197.
10. Montesano R. Regulation of angiogenesis in vitro. Eur J Clin Invest. 1992; 22, 504-515.
11. Folkman J, Klagsbrun M. Angiogenic Factors. Science 1987; 235: 442-447.
12. Sharma HS, Kandolf R, Markert T, Schaper W. Localization of endothelial cell growth factor-a mRNA in the pig heart during collateralization. Circulation 1989; 80: II-453.
13. Sharma HS, Wünsch M, Schott RJ, Kandolf R, Schaper W. Angiogenic growth factors possibly involved in coronary collateral growth. J Mol Cell Cardiol (Supplement V) 1991; 23: S.18.
14. Sharma HS, Sassen L, Verdouw PD, Schaper W. Myocardial ischemia and reperfusion leads to the induced expression of a potent mitogen vascular endothelial growth factor. Eur Heart J 1992; 13: 249.
15. Schaper W, De Brabander M, Lewi P. DNA synthesis and mitosis in coronary collateral vessel of the dog. Circ Res 1971; 28: 671-67.9
16. Kumar S, Shahabuddin S, Haboubi N, West D, Arnold F, Carr T. Angiogenesis factor from human myocardial infarcts. Lancet 1983; 2: 364-368.
17. Quinckler W, Maasberg M, Bernotat-Danielowski S, Luthe N, Sharma HS, Schaper W. Isolation of heparin-binding growth factors from bovine, porcine and canine hearts. Eur J Biochem 1989; 181: 67-73.
18. Kardami E, Fandrich RR. Basic fibroblast growth in atria and ventricles of the vertebrate heart. J Cell Biol 1989; 109: 1865-1875.
19. Risau W, Ekblom P. Production of heparin-binding angiogenesis factor by the embryonic kideney. J Cell Biol 1986; 103: 1101-1107.
20. Casscells W, Spier E, Sasse J, Klagsburn M, Allen P, Lee M, Calvo B, Chiba M, Haggroth L, Folkman J, Epstein S. Isolation, characterization and localization of heparin-binding growth factors in the hearts. J Clin Inv 1990; 85: 433-441.
21. Sasaki H, Hoshi H, Hong Y, Suzuki T, Kato T, Sasaki H, Saito M, Youki H, Karube K, Kono S, Onodera M, Saito T, Aoyagi S. Purification of acidic fibroblast growth factor from bovine heart and its localization in the cardiac myocytes. J Biol Chem 1989; 264: 17606-17612.

22. Wünsch M, Sharma HS, Markert T, Bernotal- Danielowski S, Schott RJ, Kremer P, Bleese N, Schaper W. In situ localization of transforming growth factor-ß1 in the porcine heart: Enhanced expression after chronic coronary artery constriction. J Mol Cell Cardiol 1991; 23: 1051-1062.

23. Thompson NL, Basoberry F, Spier EH, Casscells W, Fevvans VJ, Flanders KC, Kondaiah P, Geiser AG, Sporn MB. TGF-ß1 in acute myocardial infarction in rats. Growth Factor 1988; 1: 91-99.

24. Eghbali M. Cellular origin and distribution of transforming growth factor ß in the normal rat myocardium. Cell Tissue Res 1989; 256: 553-558.

25. Sharma HS, Wünsch M, Schmidt M, Schott RJ, Kandolf R, Schaper W. In: eds. Steiner, Weisz, Angiogenesis, Key Principles-Science-Technology-Medicine, Langer, 1992; 255-260.

26. Schaper W, Goerge G, Winkler B, Schaper J. The collateral circulation of the heart. Prog Cardiovasc Dis 1988; 31: 57-77.

27. Litvak J, Siderides E, Vineberg AM. The experimental production of coronary artery insufficiency and occlusion. Am Heart J 1957; 53: 505-518.

28. Mohri M, Tomoike H, Noma M , Inone T, Hisana K, Nakamura M. Duration of ischemia is vital for collateral development. Circ Res 1988; 64: 287-296.

29. White FC, Roth DM, Bloor CM. Coronary collateral reserve during exercise induced ischemia in swine. Basic Res Cardiol 1989; 84: 42-54.

30. Chilian WM, Mass HJ, Williams SE, Layne SM, Smith ES, Schael KW. Microvascular occlusions promote coronary collateral growth. Am J Physiol 1990; 258: H1103-H1110.

31. Pasyk S, Schaper W, Schaper J, Pasyk K, Miskiewicz G, Steinscifer B. DNA synthesis in coronary collaterals after coronary artery occlusion in concious dog. Am J Physiol 1982; 242: H1031-H1037.

32. Sharma HS, Schaper W. The role of growth factors during development of a collateral circulation in the porcine heart. In: Schaper W, SchaperJ. editors, Collateral Circulation. Kluwer Academic Publishers, USA 1992; 123-147.

33. Mohri M, Zimmermann R, Bernotat-Danielowski S, Sack S, Schwarz ER, Araas M, Schaper J, Schaper W. Coronary microembolization increases frowth factor expression in the porcine hearts. Circulation 1991; 84 (Supplement II): II-395 .

34. Mohri M, Sack S, Schwarz ER, Arras M, Zimmermann R, Bernotat-Danielowski S, Schaper J, Schaper W. Selective coronary microembolization increses acidic fibroblast growth factor in the ischemic porcine myocardium. Circ Res 1992; (in press).

35. Wong DTW. Histone gene (H3) expression in chemically transformed oral keratinocytes. Exp Mol Path 1988; 49: 206-214.

36. Leung DW, Cachianes G, Kuang WJ, Goeddel DV, Ferrara N. Vascular endothelial growth factor is a secreted angiogenic mitogen. Science 1989; 246: 1306-1309.

37. Keck PJ, Hauser SD, Kvivi G, Sanzo K, Warren T, Feder J, Connolly DT. Vascular permeability factor, an endothelial cell mitogen related to PDGF. Science 1989; 246:1309-1312.

38. Ferrara N, Houck KA, Jakeman LB, Winer J, Leung DW. The vascular endothelial growth family of polypeptides. J Cell Biochem 1991; 47: 211-218.

39. Tischer E, Gospodawowicz D, Mitchall R, Silva M, Schilling J, Lau K, Crisp T, Fiddes JC, Abraham JA. Vascular endothelial growth factor: A new member of the platelet derived growth factor gene family. Biochem Biophys Res Comm 1989; 165: 1198-1206

40. Breier G, Albrecht U, Sterrer S, Risau W. Expression of vascular endothelial growth factor during embryonic angiogenesis and endothelial cell differentiation. Development 1992; 114: 521-532.

41. Phillips HS, Hains J, Leung DW, Ferrara N. Vascular endothelial growth factor is expressed in rat corpus luteum. Endocrinol 1990; 127: 965-967.

42. Sharma HS, Schaper W. Adult porcine heart is a rich source of the polypeptide mitogen vascular endothelial growth factor - Personal Communication.

43. Pepper MS, Ferrara N, Orci L, Montesano R. Vascular endothelial growth factor (VEGF) induces plasminogen activators and plasminogen activator inhibitor-1 in microvascular endothelial cells. Biochem Biophys Res Comm 1991; 181: 902-906.

44. Burgess WH, Maciag,T. The heparin binding fibroblast growth factor family proteins. Ann Rev Biochem 1989; 58: 575-606.

45. Gospodarowicz D, Ferrara N, Schweigerer L, Neufeld G.Structural characterization and biological fuctions of fibroblast growth factor. Endocrine Rev 1987; 8: 95-109.

46. Moscatelli D. High and low affinity binding sites of basic fibroblast growth factor on cultured cells: Absence of a role for low affinity binding in the stimulation of plasminogen activator by bovine capillary endothelial cells. J Cell Physiol 1987; 131: 123-130.

47. Vlodavsky L, Friendman R, Sullvan R, Sasse J, Klagsbrun M. Aortic endothelial cells synthesize basic fibroblast growth factor which remain cell associated and platelet derived growth factor like protein which is secreted. J Cell Physiol 1987; 131: 402-408.

48. Delli-Bovi P, Curatola AM, Kern FG, Greco A, Ittmann M, Basilico C. An oncogene isolated by transfection of Kaposi's sarcoma DNA encodes a growth factor that is member of the FGF family. Cell 1987; 50: 729-730.

49. Dickson C, Smith R, Brookes S, Peters G. Proviral insertions within the int-2 can generate multiple anomalous transcripts but leave the protein coding domain intact. J Virol 1990; 64: 784-793.

50. Schnürch H, Risau W. Differentiating and mature neurons express the acidic fibroblast growth factor gene during chick neural development. Development 1991; 111: 1143-1154.

51. Schmidt M, Sharma HS, Schaper W. Amplification and sequencing of a mRNA encoding acidic fibroblast growth factor from porcine heart. Biochem Biophys Res Comm 1991; 180: 853-859.

52. Schaper W. Development and role of coronary collaterals. Trends Cardiovas Med 1991; 1: 256-261.

53. Bernotat-Danielowski S, Schott R, Sharma H, Kremer P, Schaper W. Fibroblast growth factor (FGF), an endothelial mitogen, is localized in cardiomyocytes of the ischemic collaterlized pig heart. Circulation 1990; 82: III-37.7

54. Weiner HL, Swain J L. Acidic fibroblast growth mRNA expression by cardiac myocytes in culture and the protein is localized to the extra cellular matrix. Proc Natl Acad Sci USA 1989; 86: 2683-2687.

55. Sporn MB, Robert AB. In: Sporn MB, Roberts AB. editors. Peptide growth factors and their receptors I. Springer Verlag, New York 1990; 419-472,.

56. Roberts AB, Sporn MB, Assoian RK, Smith JM, Roche NS, Wakefield LM, Heine UI, Liotta LA, Falanga V, Kehvl JH, Fauci AS. TGF-ß: Rapid induction of fibrosis and angiogenesis in vivo and stimulation of collagen formation in vitro. Proc Natl Acad Sci USA 1986; 83: 4167-4171.

57. Mustoe TA, Pierce GF, Thopson A, Gramates P, Sporn MB, Deul TF. Accelerated healing of inscisional wounds in rats induced by TGF-ß1. Science 1987; 237: 1333-1335.

58. Lefer AM. Mechanism of the protective effects of transforming growth factor-ß in reperfusion injury. Biochem Pharmacol 1991; 42: 1323-1327.

59. Casscells W, Bazoberry F, Speir E, Thompson N, Flanders K, Kondaiah P, Ferrans VJ, Epstein SE, Sporn M. Transforming growth factor ß1 in the normal heart and in myocardial infarction. Annals New York Acad Sci 1990; 593: 148-160.

60. Schaper W, Sharma HS, Quinkler W, Markert T, Wünsch M, Schaper J. Molecular biologic concepts of coronary anastomoses. J Am Coll Cardiol 1990; 15: 513-518.

61. Derynck R, Rhee L. Sequence of the porcine TGF-ß1 precursor. Nucleic Acid Res 1987; 15: 3187.

62. Sharma HS, Wünsch M, Brand T, Verdouw PD, Schaper W. Molecular biology of the coronary vascular and myocardial responses to ischemia. J Cardiovasc Pharmacol 1992; 20: S23-S31.

63. Humbel RE. Insulin-like growth factors I and II. Eur J Biochem 1990; 190: 445-462.

64. Rechle MM, Nissley SP. The nature and regulation of the receptors for insulin-like growth factors. Ann Rev Physiol 1985; 47: 425-442.

65. Brown AL, Graham DE, Nissley SP, Hill DJ, Strain AJ, Rechler MM. Developmental regulation of insulin-like growth factor II mRNA in different rat tissues. J Biol Chem 1986; 261: 13144-13150.

66. Johnson SE, Allen RE. The effects of bFGF, IGF-I, and TGF-ß on RMo skeletal muscle cell proliferation and differentiation. Exp Cell Res 1990; 187: 50-254.

67. Cercek B, Fishbein MC, Forrester JS, Helfant RH, Fagin JA. Induction of vascular insulin-like growth factor-I mRNA after ballon denudation precedes neointimal proliferation. Circulation 1989; 80: II-453.

68. Heldin CH, Westermark B. Growth factors as transforming proteins. Eur J Biochem 1989; 184: 487-496.

69. Magri KA, Ewton DZ, Florini JR. The role of the IGFs in myogenic differentiation. In: Raizada MK, LeRoith D. Molecular Biology and physiology of insulin and insulin-like growth factors. Plenum Press, New York 1991; 57-76.

70. Lowe WL, Roberts CT, Lasky SR, LeRoith D. Differential expression of alternative 5' untranslated regions in mRNAs encoding rat insulin-like growth factor I. Proc Natl Acad Sci USA 1987; 84: 8946-8950.

71. Kupfer JM, Rubin SA. Differential regulation of insulin-like growth factor I by growth hormone and thyroid hormone in the heart of juvenile hypophysecto-mized rats. J. Mol. Cell Cardiol. 1992; 24: 631-639.

72. Zimmermann R, Kluge A, Mohri M, Sack S, Verdouw PD, Sharma HS, Schaper W. Expression of interleukins and growth factors in ischemic pig heart. J Mol Cell Cardiol 1992; 24 (Suppl. I): 233.

73. Beutler B, Cerami A. Cachetin and tumor necrosis factor as two sides of the same biological coin. Nature 1986; 320: 584-588.

74. Sherry B, Cerami A. Cachetin/tumor necrosis factor exerts endocrine, paracrine, and autocrine control of inflammatory responses. J Cell Biol 1988; 107: 1269-1277.

75. Lord PCW, Wilmoth LMG, Mizel SB, McCall CE. Expression of interleukin-1α and ß genes by human blood polymorphonuclear leukocytes. J Clin Invest 1991; 87: 1312-1321.

76. Dinarello CA. Biology of interleukin 1. FASEB J 1988; 2: 108-115

77. Akira S, Hirano T, Taga T, Kishimoto,T. Biology of multifunctional cytokines: IL 6 and related molecules (IL 1 and TNF). FASEB J 1990; 4: 2860-2867.

78. Kilian PL, Kaffka KL, Stern AS, Woehle D, Benjamin WR, Dechiara TM, Gubler U, Farrar JJ, Mizel SB, Lomedico PT. Interleukin-1α and interleukin-1ß bind to the same receptor on T cells. J Immunol 1986; 136: 4509-4514.

79. Whicher JT, Evans SW. Cytokines in disease. Clin Chem 1990; 36/7, 1269-1281.

80. Rubartelli A, Cozzolino F, Tali M, Sitia R. A novel secretory pathway for interleukin-1ß, a protein lacking a signal sequence. EMBO J 1990; 9: 1503-1510.

81. Trinkle LA, Beasley D, Moreland RS. Interleukin-1ß alters actin expression and inhibits contraction of rat thoracic aorta. Am J Phys 1992; 262: C828-833.

82. Okusawa S, Gelfand JA, Ikejima T, Connoly RJ, Dinarello CA. Interleukin 1 induces a shock-like state in rabbits. Synergism with tumor necrosis factor and the effect of cyclooxygenase inhibition. J Clin Invest 1988; 81: 1162-1172.

83. Loppnow H, Libby P. Proliferating interleukin 1 activated human vascular smooth muscle cells secrete copius interleukin 6. J Clin Invest 1990; 85: 731-738.

84. Han RO, Ray PE, Baughman KL, Feldman AM. Detection of interleukin and interleukin-receptor mRNA in human heart by polymerase chain reaction. Biochem Biophys Res Comm 1991; 181: 520-523.

85. Bendtzen K. Interleukin 1, interleukin 6 and tumor necrosis factor in infection, inflammation and immunity. Immunol Lett 1988; 19: 183-192.

86. Ikeda U, Ikeda M, Seino Y, Takahashi M, Kano S, Shimada K. Interleukin-6 gene transcripts are expressed in atherosclerotic lesions of genetically hyperlipidemic rabbits. Atherosclerosis 1992; 92: 213-218.

87. Hirano T, Yasukawa K, Harada H, Taga T, Watanabe Y, Matsuda T, Kashiwamura S, Nakajima K, Koyama K, Iwamatsu A, Tsunasawa S, Sakiyama F, Matsui, Takahara Y, Tanigushi T, Kishimoto T. Complementary DNA for a novel human interleukin (BSF-2) that induces B lymphocytes to produce immunoglobulin. Nature 1986; 324: 73-76.

88. Baumann H, Richards C, Gauldie J. Interaction between hepatocyte-stimulating factors, interleukin-1 and glucocorticoids for regulation of acute phase proteins in human hepatoma (Hep-G2) cells. J Immunol 1988; 139: 4122-4128.

89. Geiger T, Andus T, Klapproth J, Hirano T, Kishimoto T, Heinrich PC. Induction of acute phase-proteins by interleukin 6 in vivo. Eur J Immunol 1988; 18: 717-721.

90. Morimoto S, Nabata T, Koh E, Shiraishi T, Fukuo K, Imanaka S, Kitano S, Miyahita Y, Ogihara T. Interleukin-6 stimulates proliferation of cultured vascular smooth muscle cells independently of interleukin-1ß. J Cardiovascular Pharmacology 1991; 17 (Suppl. 2): S117-S118.

91. Richards CD, Saklatvala J. Molecular cloning and sequence of porcine interleukin 6 cDNA and expression of mRNA in synovial fibroblasts in vitro. Cytokine 1991; 3: 269-276.

92. Ikeda U, Ohkawa F, Seino Y, Yamamoto K, Hidaka Y, Kasahara T, Kawai T, Shimada K. Serum interleukin 6 levels become elevated in acute myocardial infarction. J Mol Cell Cardiol 1992; 24: 579-584.

93. Berse B, Brown LF, Van De water L, Dvorak HF, Senger DR. Vascular permeability factor (vascular endothelial growth factor) gene is expressed differentially in normal tissues, macrophages, and tumors. Mol Biol Cell 1992; 3: 211-220.

94. Speir E, Tanner V, Gonzalez AM, Farris J, Baird A, Casscells W. Acidic and basic fibroblast growth factors in the adult rat heart myocytes: Localization, regulation in culture, and effects on DNA synthesis. Circ Res 1992; 71: 251-259.

95. Schneiderman J, Loskutoff DJ. Plasmin activator inhibitor. Trends Cardiovas Med 1991; 1 (3): 99-102.

96. Vassalli J-D, Sappino A-P, Belin D. The plasminogen activator / plasmin system. J Clin Invest 1991; 88: 1067-1072.

97. Sharma HS, Mohri M, Sack S, Schaper W. Induction of plasminogen activator inhibitor-1 (PAI-1) expression during microembolization. J Mol Cell Cardiol 1992; 24: S.233.

98. Mohri M, Sack S, Zimmermann R, Arras M, Schaper J, Schaper W. Tissue- and urokinase- type plasminogen activator (tPA and uPA) and type-1 PA inhibitor after coronary microembolization in the pig heart. J Cell Mol Cardiol 1992; 24: (Supplement I) S.49.

9. The role of growth factors in angiogenesis

ROBERT J. SCHOTT and LINDA A. MORROW

Introduction

Although a role for growth factors in angiogenesis was first recognized in 1971 an explosion in growth factor identification and characterization has occurred over the last 5 years. Widespread use of recombinant DNA technology has led to the identification of new peptide growth factors (and in many cases their receptors) which are capable of stimulating angiogenesis. For example, the family of Heparin Binding Growth Factors (HBGF's), which includes Fibroblast Growth Factor (FGF), has had five new members identified since 1987, bringing the total in 1992 to seven. There are currently four receptors for the HBGF family which have been identified and partially characterized. Despite cloning and in vitro characterization of growth factors, their contribution to developmental, physiologic or pathologic angiogenesis remains largely speculative [1]. Growth factors are considered angiogenic on the basis of in vitro or biologic assays, but the in vivo activity of any particular growth factor appears to be contextual, i.e. modulated by the presence of other growth factors, as well as the extracellular milieu and participating cell types [2]. Angiogenesis is a complex process shaped by the interplay of stimulatory and inhibitory factors, the choreography of which is an important subject for angiogenesis research.

This section endeavors to provide background on those growth factors which by virtue of angiogenic (or antiangiogenic) properties have been implicated in developmental, physiologic or pathologic angiogenesis. It encompasses and supplements information presented in a recent review of this rapidly evolving area of investigation [3].

An overview of angiogenesis

New blood vessel growth has traditionally been studied in the context of other biologic processes, i.e. development, tumor growth, wound healing, and collateralization in the heart, among others. This is a convenient, although perhaps arbitrary basis for classifying angiogenesis, which unfolds in a morphologically uniform manner, modulated by an overlapping set of growth factors irrespective of the biologic setting.

Embryonic angiogenesis

The circulatory system arises from the mesoderm of the yolk sac, where undifferentiated mesenchymal cells condense to form angiogenic cell clusters. These angiogenic clusters differentiate to form both the blood vessels and the blood-forming elements [4]. Recent studies in amphibian embryos implicate growth factors with angiogenic potential (including members of the FGF and/or Transforming Growth Factor (TGF) family) as necessary for mesoderm induction in early embryogenesis [5]. These observations suggest that the growth factors shaping development in early embryogenesis are the same factors which stimulate post-developmental angiogenesis. The economy of biology which this represents is intuitively attractive but not yet proven.

Post-embryonic angiogenesis

The morphology of angiogenesis in fully differentiated tissue has been described in a variety of settings. There are uniform features which begin with disruption of basement membranes followed by digestion of the extracellular matrix; migration and proliferation of the capillary or venular endothelium, and then formation and closure of the nascent vascular tubes [6,7]. Pericytes migrate to the apex of the new capillary loop and may be important in turning off angiogenesis. TGF-ß has been implicated in turning off angiogenesis in this setting [8]. The capillary endothelial cell contains the necessary information for the development of new microvascular networks [7]. Neovascularization associated with diverse processes including ovulation, wound healing and tumorigenesis appears to unfold along similar pathways [6].

Angiogenesis in the heart

Angiogenesis in the adult heart has been described as either "non-sprouting" or "sprouting", based on the histologic appearance. In the former, there is expansion of preexisting channels with proliferation of smooth muscle and endothelium, whereas sprouting angiogenesis is marked by proliferation of capillary and venular endothelium, and invasion of tissue to form new capillary beds [9]. Both varieties have been associated with the same peptide growth factors although the physiology is not well understood [10]. Elucidating the physiology of new vascular growth has important clinical implications particularly in cardiology, where collateralization of chronically ischemic myocardium is a beneficial form of adaptation [11].

Other forms of cardiac angiogenesis include recanalization of thrombus and intraarterial angiogenesis, both of which are associated with atherosclerotic heart disease [12] (For review see Eisenstein [13]). Myocardial hypertrophy is also accompanied by growth of the coronary vasculature [14]. Protamine inhibition of collateralization in hypertrophy suggests that Heparin Binding Growth Factors (HBGF's, FGF's) are important [15], but otherwise little is known about growth factor participation in the angiogenesis associated with myocardial hypertrophy. The signaling pathways for the initiation, execution and termination of either sprouting or non-sprouting angiogenesis are the subject of speculation. The in-vitro models and bioassays for peptide growth factors pertain to sprouting angiogenesis, and the bulk of the molecular work has been done in this area [1]. However, because the same growth factors may participate in both types of angiogenesis, the distinction between the two is not maintained throughout the remainder of this chapter.

An overview of growth actors

The era of growth factors and their relationship to angiogenesis was opened in 1971 when Folkman et al. demonstrated that extracts from tumor cells were angiogenic when injected into the dorsal air sack cavity of rats. Named Tumor Angiogenesis Factor (TAF), these extracts (originally identified only as a fraction from a Sephadex column) were mitogenic for capillary endothelial cells [16]. TAF was later assigned to the FGF family [17].

Angiogenesis factors have been subsequently divided into two categories: peptide growth factors and low-molecular weight or secondary angiogenesis factors. Protein growth factors once painstakingly purified from biologic sources have, in the last decade, been identified and expressed based on the cDNA clones. Advances in molecular biology are largely responsible for the torrent of new data on peptide growth factors and pertinent techniques will be reviewed briefly.

Techniques for the evaluation of growth factors

The laborious work of protein purification and sequencing has been complemented (and in many instances supplanted) by recombinant DNA techniques in which the gene for a candidate growth factor (or receptor) is cloned. Cloning and sequencing of the cDNA for peptide growth factors allows for structural comparisons among peptides and for high level expression of the protein. Large quantities of easily obtained pure protein facilitate in vitro studies and bioassays. The nucleotide sequence from one peptide factor (or receptor) can be exploited using a variety of strategies to clone structurally related factors [18,19]. Thus, once one member of a growth factor superfamily or receptor is identified, additional factors are more easily cloned and the protein sequence determined prior to any understanding of the biologic significance of the molecule.

The polymerase chain reaction (PCR) has been used to detect the presence of growth factors in tissue [20], or to screen for structurally related clones [21]. Cross-linking of growth factor to cell surface proteins has been used to identify receptors [22]. Site directed mutagenesis, and other studies using chemical and enzymatic techniques to alter peptide structure, have permitted localization of the functional domains of both the growth factors and their receptors at the amino acid level [23]. Recently X-ray crystallography has been used to resolve the tertiary structure of TGF-ß [24].

Once a candidate growth factor has been isolated, the angiogenic activity is characterized in cultured cells and in bioassays, which include the chicken chorioallantoic membrane (CAM), corneal pocket, hamster cheek pouch, and disc assays. In vitro, cultured endothelial and other cell lines are incubated with growth factors, and observed for proliferation, differentiation or transformation. (For review, see Auerbach et al. [25]) More recently, angiogenesis factors have been assayed for their ability to stimulate vessel formation in 3-dimensional matrices, as well as in situ[26]. Growth factor purification on affinity chromatography columns was made possible after the serendipitous discovery that members of the FGF family bind heparin [17].

With the availability of growth factors in quantity, physiologic experiments have been made possible in which factors (e.g. FGF) are administered in large animal models to study the effects on the heart [27].

Using these and other experimental tools, investigators have gained considerable insight into the structure and activity of several peptide factors with angiogenic activity. Discussed next are those peptide growth factors which have angiogenic activity in vitro and or in bioassays.

The fibroblast growth factors (FGF's)

The first angiogenic growth factors to be identified and extensively characterized are members of the Fibroblast Growth Factor (FGF) family (or Heparin Binding Growth Factor, HBGF). Although FGF was named because it was first recognized as a mitogen for fibroblasts, FGF's are now known to be mitogens for a variety of cells, including vascular endothelium (reviewed by Gospodarowicz et al. [17,28]). The FGF family now includes acidic FGF and basic FGF, along with five additional members: HST [29], *int-2* [30], FGF-5 [31], FGF-6[18], and KGF (Kaposi's Sarcoma Oncogene)[32]. These last five have been identified based on structural and functional similarities to acidic and basic FGF (see below).

Acidic and basic FGF

Acidic FGF (aFGF) and basic FGF (bFGF) are 140 and 146 amino acid (15 to 17 kD) single chain peptides, respectively. aFGF and bFGF share a 53% homology at the amino acid level [33] and are likely divergent products of the same ancestral gene. The conservation of sequence across species further implies evolutionary conservation of gene product function. The lack of a hydrophobic leader sequence characteristic of secreted proteins for both the a and the b-FGF peptide suggests either an autocrine or paracrine mode of action for FGF. Chemical and site-directed mutagenesis studies of the FGF molecule have identified functional domains for heparin-binding and receptor-binding [23].

Several FGF receptors (FGFR) have been cloned and structurally characterized. Structural motifs include multiple immunoglobulin-like extracellular domains, a transmembrane domain, and an intracellular tyrosine kinase domain through which the signal is transduced to the nucleus [22]. Alternative splicing of the FGFR gene gives rise to different receptor isoforms with differing binding affinities for aFGF and bFGF [34]. Recently two additional members of this FGFR-tyrosine kinase family have been cloned. [19,35]. Distribution of FGFR-4 receptor appears limited to the lung, suggesting a mechanism for FGF tissue-specific activity [19]. A second class of low affinity heparin-like FGF receptors, found on the cell surface and in the ECM, has been found to be necessary for high affinity FGF-FGFR binding [36], and may explain heparin's ability to promote angiogenesis in many models [37].

bFGF is distributed widely, including vascular endothelium [38], vascular smooth muscle [39], cardiac myocytes [40,41], and in general, organs which are heavily vascularized. The distribution aFGF appears to be more limited than that of bFGF, and aFGF has not been reported in vascular endothelium [17]. However, aFGF mRNA has been detected in normal and collateralizing pig myocardium [20] by using the polymerase chain reaction, which can detect and amplify rare transcripts. bFGF produced in endothelial cells is sequestered in the extracellular matrix (ECM) and basement membranes [38,42] bound to heparin or heparan sulfate glycosaminoglycans [43,44]. ECM-bound inactive FGF's could be released with tissue injury in a paracrine model of angiogenic stimulation [44]. Others have proposed autocrine models of angiogenesis [45].

In embryogenesis, FGF-like factors and bFGF have the potential to stimulate mesodermal differentiation [46,47]. In tumorigenesis, it has been shown that bFGF, altered to included a signal peptide, induces malignant transformation when transfected into host cells [48]. A switch to export of bFGF has been implicated in tumor angiogenesis associated with the growth of fibrosarcomas in transgenic mice [49]. aFGF and bFGF stimulate mitogenesis in several cell types, including endothelial cells [17,50,51]. In cultured endothelial cells, FGF has been shown to stimulate several angiogenesis-related responses: cell migration [45] and invasion of a synthetic matrix where they form tubular structures resembling capillaries [50]. bFGF also stimulates release of plasminogen activator and collagenase which may digest the basement membrane preceding migration of endothelial cells [50,52,53]. Gelatin sponges releasing physiologic amounts of aFGF induce luxuriant neovessel formation when implanted into rats [26]. Heparin promotes angiogenesis in vitro [54] and collateralization in vivo [37], whereas the heparin antagonist protamine inhibits collateralization [15]. This is consistent with the observation that heparan proteoglycans are necessary for high affinity receptor binding by bFGF, and that heparin can reconstitute binding activity in mutant cells lacking native heparan proteoglycans [36].

In summary, bFGF has the capacity to stimulate most of the individual components of new capillary growth, including: 1) endothelial cell proliferation, 2) release of proteases which digest the basement membrane, 3) endothelial cell migration, and 4) organization of endothelial cells into tubules. Whether bFGF stimulates any or all of these functions during angiogenesis in vivo is not presently known. FGF is present throughout the heart and we know that heparin promotes myocardial angiogenesis. These observations provide strong circumstantial evidence for FGF participation in myocardial angiogenesis.

Transforming growth factor-ß (TGF-ß)

These peptides were isolated from neoplastic cells and named Transforming Growth Factors for their ability to transform non-neoplastic fibroblasts in culture. Two factors (subsequently found to be unrelated) were identified: TGF-α and TGF-ß [55]. While TGF-ß acts both to stimulate and inhibit growth depending on the setting, TGF-ß appears to inhibit angiogenic growth.

TGF-ß is a homodimeric 25 kD protein derived from a 112 amino acid monomer [56]. Five isoforms of TGF-ß have been recognized (TGF-ß 1-5), although only TGF-ß 1, 2, and 3 are recognized in mammals [57].

The receptors for TGF-ß include two high affinity receptors (I and II) which are known to be transmembrane proteins [58]. The TGF-ß type II receptor protein structure has been characterized and found to have a cytoplasmic serine-threonine kinase domain which may be the signaling mechanism [59]. A third, somewhat lower affinity receptor (previously designated III), has been identified as the proteoglycan betaglycan and has been recently characterized [60,61].

TGF-ß is widely distributed throughout normal tissue and tumors in a latent form [58,62]. Activation of latent TGF-ß to the active form is currently under investigation and has been found to require cell to cell contact, plasminogen activator, plasmin and binding to cell surface receptors [63,64]. In addition, TGF-ß receptors are equally widespread, suggesting that TGF-ß may have an important ongoing role in modulation of cell function [65]. Receptors I and II have differing affinities for the various isoforms of TGF-ß, while betaglycan has a similar affinity for all forms [66]. While receptors I and II are thought to be important in signal transduction, betaglycan may control the ability of TGF-ß to interact with the cell [60,61].

TGF-ß is pluripotent and its biologic function is, like most peptide growth factors, dependent upon other growth factors present, as well the stage of cellular differentiation. TGF-ß is mitogenic for osteoblasts and Schwann cells [58], morphogenic in the case of adult rabbit cardiac fibroblasts, which are induced to display phenotypic features of cardiac myocytes [67]; antiproliferative for epithelial cells [68], endothelial cells [69], T and B lymphocytes [70]; and chemotactic for fibroblasts and monocytes [70]. Functional differences in TGF-ß isoforms are currently being investigated; most of what follows pertains to TGF-ß1.

A role for TGF-ß in angiogenesis was suggested by experiments in which injection of TGF-ß into newborn mice induced granulation tissue with neovascularization and collagen production [71]. The angiogenic response may be mediated through the secretion of products from monocytes which are attracted to the injection site by TGF-ß.

Monocytes secrete the angiogenic factor TNF-α following stimulation by TGF-ß [72,73]. Subsequent studies suggest that TGF-ß1 stimulates production of plasminogen activator inhibitor [74,75] which retards dissolution of the extracellular matrix and new capillary formation [74]. bFGF and TGF-ß have opposing effects on the plasminogen activator activity of cultured endothelial cells. TGF-ß also inhibits the angiogenic effect of bFGF in cultured endothelial cells [53].

Two additional functions of TGF-ß that may be important in angiogenesis include stimulation of extracellular matrix formation. in addition to increasing the transcription of collagen and fibronectin in human, rat, mouse and chicken fibroblasts [58,71,76]. This function, like control of proteolysis, may have an important role in regulating the formation of new vessels. TGF-ß also functions to regulate endothelial cell growth and differentiation. Depending on culture conditions, TGF-ß may inhibit endothelial cell growth (in monolayer) or promote the formation of branching tubular-like structures [77].

At present TGF-ß is an important regulatory growth factor whose in vivo roles are currently known to include tissue inflammation and wound healing. Its in vivo role in angiogenesis is unclear at present, and may be mediated indirectly through other growth factors such as TNF-α.

The epithelial growth factor (EGF) family

Members of this family of peptides include EGF, isolated by Cohen in the early 1960's; and TGF-α, as well as two other members [78,79]. Membership in the EGF family is defined by several features including recognition of the EGF receptor (which has a cytoplasmic tyrosine kinase domain), mitogenicity in EGF-responsive cells, and common structural motifs [78]. EGF has a wide distribution, including the a granules of platelets. EGF stimulates endothelial cell migration and proliferation. Both TGF-α and EGF stimulate angiogenesis in bioassays, with TGF-α reported as more potent [80]. Although the physiologic role of EGF is not known, its distribution suggests participation in development, as well as epithelial regeneration [79].

The platelet derived growth factor (PDGF) family

PDGF

Presently not recognized as an angiogenic factor, PDGF is one of several peptides found in the alpha-granules of platelets, as well as in macrophages and endothelial cells. It is mitogenic for vascular smooth muscle and connective tissue, including fibroblasts [81], and has been recently shown to facilitate capillary formation in vitro [82]. PDGF exists as one of three dimeric combinations of A and B chains [83]. It is a chemoattractant for neutrophils and macrophages and may stimulate the cellular proliferation of atherosclerosis and wound repair. The precise physiologic role of PDGF is at present unknown [81].

VEGF

In 1989 Gospodarowicz et al. purified an endothelial cell-specific mitogen from cultured pituitary-derived folliculo stellate cells (FSdGF) [84]. (It has been labelled Vascular Permeability Factor (VPF), or Vascular Endothelial Growth Factor (VEGF), which is used in this chapter.) Within months the gene for VEGF was cloned and the sequence was published virtually simultaneously by several teams of investigators [21,85-88]. It is included in the PDGF family here because of the weak sequence homology with the PDGF-B chain (18% identity in human tumor cell-derived VEGF, with conservation of the 8 cysteine residues, and even greater homology with the transforming region of thePDGF-related oncogene v-sis) [87]. Unlike FGF, the VEGF peptide has a leader sequence, suggesting that it is secreted from cells. VEGF is angiogenic in the corneal pocket assay [86], and the mitogenic activity appears specific for endothelial cells and not vascular smooth muscle. Northern analysis and in-situ hybridization demonstrate VEGF expression in a variety of organs including the heart [9,89]. A VEGF receptor has been identified on cell surface of endothelial cells [90,91], and binding sites are present throughout adult rat endothelium, including the heart [92] The receptor for VEGF has recently been cloned [93]. Interestingly hypoxia has been shown to stimulate the expression of VEGF in ovarian granulosa cells [94]. Receptor binding of VEGF appears to be dependent on heparan proteoglycans [95], (a similar dependence of heparin like molecules has also been shown for bFGF [36]). As with other peptide growth factors, the biologic role of VEGF is uncertain, but several features of the molecule have led to intense scrutiny and speculation about the possible role of VEGF in angiogenesis. These features include the pattern of

158

VEGF expression, along with widespread endothelial distribution of binding sites, VEGF's angiogenic capacity in vivo, and structural features (i.e. it is secreted).

Other angiogenic peptides

Angiogenin

Angiogenin was the first angiogenic peptide to be purified from tumor cells [96]. The same lab sequenced the peptide [97] and then cloned the gene in 1985 [96]. It is a 14 kD homodimeric member of the pancreatic ribonuclease family and is not a member of previously described growth factors. It is angiogenic in the CAM and rabbit corneal assays [96]. Although the biologic function of angiogenin is unknown, the pattern of mRNA expression is not temporally related to maximal vascular growth in the developing rat [99]. Despite the presence of angiogenin receptors on endothelial cells [100], it is not an endothelial cell mitogen.

Angiotropin

Angiotropin is a 4.5 kD copper containing peptide growth factor purified from macrophages [101]. Angiotropin stimulates endothelial cell migration and tube formation in vitro, but is not mitogenic for endothelial cells [101]. It has not been cloned, and the tissue distribution and receptors for angiotropin have not been characterized.

Platelet derived endothelial cell growth factor (PD-ECGF)

In 1987 a 45 kD endothelial cell mitogen, distinct from PDGF, was purified from human platelets. (Two micrograms of pure protein were isolated from 900 liters of blood [102].) The protein was partially sequenced, and this information was used to synthesize oligonucleotide probes for the screening of a human placental cDNA library, where a clone containing the complete open reading frame for PD-ECGF was isolated. Like aFGF and bFGF, PD-ECGF does not have a leader peptide. PD-ECGF is distinct from other growth factors; is chemotactic for endothelial cells in culture and is angiogenic in the CAM assay [103]. PD-ECGF is produced by a variety of cells in culture, including human vascular smooth muscle cells [104]. The in vivo role of PD-ECGF is presently unknown.

TNF-α

TNF-alpha is a pluripotent peptide secreted by activated macrophages [105]. Hypoxia has been shown to stimulate the release of TNF-α from macrophages [106,107]. Because of anti-tumor activity TNF-α was initially suspected to have anti-angiogeneic activity. In vitro, TNF-α was indeed found to inhibit bFGF stimulated endothelial cell growth; however, in vivo bioassays revealed TNF-α to be a potent stimulator of angiogenesis, albeit of an inflammatory nature, with associated capillary leak [107].

Low molecular weight (non-peptide) angiogenesis factors

Several low molecular weight, non-peptide angiogenesis factors have been described. (For review see [108,109]). One role of secondary angiogenesis messengers may be to stimulate release of, or act as chemotactic stimuli for, the primary peptide growth factors. Hypothesized mechanisms include displacement or chemical release of peptide growth factors (e.g. bFGF) from the extracellular matrix [110,111]. Nicotinamide and other pyridine derivatives have indirect angiogenesis activity in-vitro [110,111]. The angiogenic activity of adenosine has been controversial [111,112].

Myocardial angiogenesis

Evidence for growth factor mediation of myocardial angiogenesis is incomplete, but it is possible to speculate on a cascade for neovascularization of the myocardium. Injury (e.g. myocardial infarction) may result in displacement of growth factors from sites within the basement membrane or ECM; or factors may be released from endothelial cells by unknown mechanisms, stimulating angiogenesis via autocrine or paracrine mechanisms. Two candidate growth factors implicated in myocardial angiogenesis are bFGF and VEGF. Non-peptide co-factors from the ECM such as Heparan proteoglycans may be exposed following injury and increase the affinity of bFGF or VEGF for its receptor. Alternatively, activated macrophages or platelets present at the site of injury may release other growth factors, which directly stimulate angiogenesis (i.e. angiotropin and TNF-α from macrophages, PD-ECGF from platelets) or indirectly act by stimulating

160

the release of other factors (i.e. TGF-ß and the release of TNF-α). Other growth factors (e.g. PDGF) may stimulate smooth muscle proliferation or influence the architecture of vasculature growth in ways that are presently not defined.

Most growth factors act by binding cell surface receptors, transducing a signal to the nucleus via a tyrosine kinase receptor mechanism. Transcription is stimulated, followed by endothelial cell division and directed migration of endothelial cells, perhaps along a gradient of secondary angiogenic stimuli. Once the nascent vessels are formed, ECM components are synthesized, and migration of pericytes may signal the completion of neovascularization.

Conclusion

The list of growth factors with angiogenic potential is growing, stimulated by advances in research techniques. It is not clear why so many factors with angiogenic potential exist, although Folkman suggests that redundancy underscores the essential nature of the angiogenic response [6]. Additionally, these factors or their close relatives have other biologic activities, including developmental morphogenesis, tumorigenesis, regeneration of injured tissue, and immunosignaling. Recent advances in the understanding of these factors include primary peptide sequence for all but one peptide growth factor included in this review, identification of cell surface receptors for many, and extensive characterization of biologic potential. What is yet to be defined is the orchestration of the various peptide growth factors in blood vessel growth.

References

1. Folkman J, Klagsbrun M. Angiogenic Factors. Science 1987; 235: 442-447.
2. Sporn M, Roberts A. Autocrine growth factors and cancer. Nature 1985; 313: 745-747.
3. Schott R, Morrow L. Growth Factors and Angiogenesis. Cardiovascular Research, in press.
4. Gilbert SF. Developmental Biology. (3rd ed.) Sunderland, MA: Sinauer Associates, 1991: 891.
5. de Pable F, Roth J. Endocrinization of the early embryo: an emerging role for hormones and hormone-like factors. Trend Biochem Sci 1990; 15: 339-342

6.   Folkman J, Klagsbrun M. A family of angiogenic peptides. Nature 1987; 329: 671-672.
7.   Folkman J, Haudenschild C. Angiogenesis in vitro. Nature 1980; 288: 551-556.
8.   Antonelli-Orlidge A, Smith S, D'Amore P. Influence of pericytes on capillary endothelial cell growth. Annu Rev Respir Dis 1989; 140: 1129-1131.
9.   Schaper W. Angiogenesis in the adult heart. Bas Res Cardiol 1991; 86(suppl 2): 51-56.
10. Schaper W, Sharma H, Quinkler W, Markert T, Wünsch M, Schaper J. Molecular biologic concepts of coronary anastomoses. J Am Coll Cardiol 1990; 15: 513-8.
11. Sasayama S, Fujita M.   Recent insights into coronary collateral circulation. Circulation 1992; 85: 1197-1204
12. Barger A, Beeuwkes R, Lainey L, Silverman K. Hypothesis: vasa vasorum and neovascularization of human coronary arteries. N Engl J Med 1984; 310: 175-177.
13. Eisenstein R. Angiogenesis in arteries: review. Pharmac Ther 1991; 49: 1-19.
14. Tomanek R. Response of the coronary vasculature to myocardial hypertrophy. J Am Coll Cardiol 1990; 15: 528-533.
15. Flanagan M, Fujii A, Colan S, Flanagan R, Lock J. Myocardial angiogenesis and coronary perfusion in left ventricular pressure-overload hypertrophyin the young lamb. Circ Res 1991; 68: 1458-1470.
16. Folkman J, Merler E, Abernathy C, Williams G. Isolation of a tumor factor responsible for angiogenesis. J Exp Med 1971; 133: 275-288.
17. Gospodarowicz D, Ferrara N, Schweigerer L, Neufeld G. Structural characterization and biologic functions of fibroblast growth factor. Endocrine Rev 1987; 8: 95-114.
18. Marics I, Adelaide J, Raybaud F, et al. Characterization of the HST-related FGF.6 gene, a new member of the fibroblast growth factor gene family. Oncogene 1989; 4: 335-340.
19. Holtrich U, Bräuninger A, Strebhardt K, Rübsamen-Waigmann H. Two additional protein-tryosine kinases expressed in human lung: fourth member of the fibroblast growth factor receptor family and an intracellular protein-tyrosine kinase. Proc Natl Acad Sci USA 1991; 88: 10411-10415.
20. Schmidt M, Sharma HS, Schott, RJ, Schaper, W. Amplification and sequencing of mRNA encoding acidic fibroblast growth factor aFGF from porcine heart. Biochem Biophys Res Comm 1991; 180: 853-859.

21. Conn G, Bayne M, Soderman D, et al. Amino acid and cDNA sequences of a vascular endothelial cell mitogen that is homologous to platelet-derived growth factor. Proc Natl Acad Sci USA 1990; 87: 2628-2632.

22. Lee P, Johnson D, Cousens L, Fried V, Williams L. Purification and complementary DNA cloning of a receptor for basic fibroblast growth factor. Science 1989; 245: 57-60.

23. Burgess W, Shaheen A, Ravera M, Jaye M, Donohue P, Winkles J. Possible dissociation of the heparin-binding and mitogenic activities of Heparin-binding (Acidic Fibroblast) Growth Factor-1 from its receptor-binding activities by site-directed mutagenesis of a single lysine residue. J Cell Biol 1990; 111: 2129-2138.

24. Daopin S, Piez K, Ogawa Y, Davies D. Crystal structure Transforming Growth Factor-ß2: an unusual fold for the superfamily. Science 1992; 257: 369-373

25. Auerbach R, Auerbach W, Polakowski I. Assays for angiogenesis: a review. Pharmac Ther 1991; 51: 1-11.

26. Thompson J, Anderson K, DiPietro J, et al. Site-directed neovessel formation in vivo. Science 1988; 241: 1349-1352.

27. Banai S, Jaklitsch MT, Casscells W, Shou M, Shrivastav S, Correa R, Epstein SE, Unger EF. Effects of acidic fibroblast growth factor on normal and ischemic myocardium. Circ Research 1991; 69(1): 76-85.

28. Gospodarowicz D, Neufeld G, Schweigerer L. Fibroblast growth factor. Mol Cell Endocrinol 1986; 46: 187-204.

29. Yoshida T, Miyagawa K, Odagiri H, et al. Genomic sequence of hst, a transforming gene encoding a protein homologous to fibroblast growth factors and the int-2-encoded protein. Proc Natl Acad Sci USA 1987; 84: 7305-7309.

30. Moore R, Casey G, Brookes S, Dixon M, Peters G, Dickson C. Sequence, topography and protein coding potential of mouse int-2: a putative oncogene activated by mouse mammary tumour virus. EMBO 1986; 5: 919-924.

31. Zhan X, Bates B, Hu X, Goldfarb M. The human FGF-5 oncogene encodes a novel protein related to fibroblast growth factors. Mol Cell Biol 1988; 8: 3487-3495.

32. Delli Bovi P, Curatola A, Kern F, Greco A, Ittmann M, Basilico C. An oncogene isolated by transfection of Kaposi's sarcoma DNA encodes a growth factor that is a member of the FGF family. Cell 1987; 50: 729-737.

33. Esch F, Baird A, Ling N, et al. Primary structure of bovine pituitary basic fibroblast growth factor (FGF) and comparison with the amino-terminal sequence of bovine brain acidic FGF. Proc Natl Acad Sci USA 1985; 82: 6507-6511.

34. Johnson D, Lee P, Lu J, Williams L. Diverse forms of a receptor for acidic and basic fibroblast growth factors. Mol Cell Biol 1990; 10: 4728-4736.

35. Keegan K, Johnson D, Williams L, Hayman M. Isolation of an additional member of the fibroblast growth factor receptor family, FGFR-3. Proc Natl Acad Sci USA 1991; 88: 1095-1099.

36. Yayon A, Klagsbrun M, Esko J, Leder P, Ornitz D. Cell surface, heparin-like molecules are required for binding of basic fibroblast growth factor to its high affinity receptor. Cell 1991; 64: 841-848.

37. Unger E, Sheffield C, Epstein SE. Creation of an anastomoses betweenan extracardiac artery and the coronary circulation. Circulation. 1990; 82: 1449-1466.

38. Vlodavsky I, Folkman J, Sullivan R, et al. Endothelial cell-derived basic fibroblast growth factor: synthesis and deposition into subendothelial extracellular matrix. Proc Natl Acad Sci USA 1987; 84: 2292-2296.

39. Winkles J, Friesel R, Burgess W, et al. Human vascular smooth muscle cell both express and respond to heparin-binding growth factor I (endothelial cell growth factor). Proc Natl Acad Sci USA 1987; 84: 7124-7128.

40. Quinkler W, Maasberg M, Bernotat-Danielowski S, Lüthe N, Sharma H, Schaper W. Isolation of heparin binding growth factors from bovine, porcine, and canine hearts. Eur J Biochem 1989; 181: 67-73.

41. Casscells W, Speir E, Sasse J, et al. Isolation, characterization, and localization of heparin-binding growth factors in the heart. J Clin Invest 1990; 85: 433-441.

42. Folkman J, Klagsbrun M, Sasse J, Wadzinski M, Ingber D, Vlodavsky I. A heparin-binding angiogenic protein - basic fibroblast growth factor - is stored within basement membrane. Am J Pathol 1988; 130: 393-400.

43. Baird A, Ling N. Fibroblast growth factors are present in the extracellular matrix produced by endothelial cells in vitro: implications for a role of heparinase-like enzymes in the neovascular response. Biochem Biophy Res Comm 1987; 142: 428-435.

44. Ruoslahti E, Yamaguchi Y. Proteoglycans as modulators of growth factor activities. Cell 1991; 64: 867-869.

45. Mignatti P, Morimoto T, Rifkin D. Basic fibroblast growth factor released by single, isolated cells stimulates their migration in an autocrine manner. Proc Natl Acad Sci USA 1991; 88: 11007-11011.

46. Slack J, Darlington B, Heath J, Godsave S. Mesoderm induction in early Xenopus embryos by heparin-binding growth factors. Nature 1987; 326: 197-200.

47. Kimelman D, Kirschner M. Synergistic induction of mesoderm by FGF and TGF-ß and the identification of an mRNA coding for FGF in the early Xenopus embryo. Cell 1987; 51: 869-877.

48. Rogelj S, Weinberg R, Fanning P, Klagsbrun M. Basic fibroblast growth factor fused to a signal peptide transforms cells. Nature 1988; 331: 173-175.

49. Kandel J, Bossy-Wetzel E, Radvanyi F, Klagsbrun M, Folkman J, Hanahan D. Neovascularization is associated with a switch to the export of bFGF in the multistep development of fibrosarcoma. Cell 1991; 66: 1095-1104.

50. Montesano R, Vassalli J-D, Baird A, Guillemin R, Orci L. Basic fibroblast growth factor induces angiogenesis *in vitro*. Proc Natl Acad Sci USA 1986; 83: 7297-7301.

51. Thomas K, Rios-Candelore M, Gimenez-Gallego, et al. Pure brain-derived acidic fibroblast growth factor is a potent angiogenic vascular endothelial cell mitogen with sequence homology to interleukin 1. Proc Natl Acad Sci USA 1985; 82: 6409-6413.

52. Gross J, Moscatelli D, Rifkin D. Increased capillary endothelial cell protease activity in response to angiogenic stimuli *in vitro*. Proc Natl Acad Sci USA 1983; 80: 2623-2627.

53. Saksela O, Moscatelli D, Rifkin D. The opposing effects of basic fibroblast growth factor and transforming growth factor beta on the regulation of plasminogen activator activity in capillary endothelial cells. J Cell Biol 1987; 105: 957-963.

54. Folkman J, Weisz P, Joullié M, Li W, Ewing W. Control of angiogenesis with synthetic heparin substitutes. Science 1989; 243: 1490-1493.

55. Anzano M, Roberts A, Smith J, Sporn M, DeLarco J. Sarcoma growth factor from conditioned medium of virally transformed cells is composed of both type alpha and type beta transforming growth factors. Proc Natl Acad Sci USA 1983; 80: 6264-6268.

56. Derynck R, Jarrett J, Chen E, et al. Human transforming growth factor-ß complementary DNA sequence and expression in normal and transformed cells. Nature 1985; 316: 701-705.

57. Roberts A, Kim S, Noma T, et al. Multiple forms of TGF-beta: distinct promoters and differential expression. Ciba Found Symp 1991; 157: 7-15.

58. Sporn M, Roberts A, Wakefield L, de Crombrugghe B. Some recent advances in the chemistry and biology of transforming growth factor-beta. J Cell Biol 1987; 105: 1039-1045.

59. Lin HY, Wang XF, Ng-Eaton E, Weinberg RA, Lodish HF. Expression cloning of the TGF-beta type II receptor, a functional transmembrane serine/threonine kinase. Cell 1992;68:775-785.

60. López-Cassillas F, Cheifetz S, Doody J, Andres J, Lane W, Massagué J. Structure and expression of the membrane proteoglycan betaglycan, a component of the TGF-ß receptor system. Cell 1991; 67: 785-795.

61. Wang X-F, Lin H, Ng-Eaton E, Downward J, Lodish H, Weinberg R. Expression cloning and characterization of the TGF-ß type III receptor. Cell 1991; 67: 797-805.

62. Miyazono K, Heldin C. Latent forms of TGF-beta: molecular structure and mechanisms of activation. Ciba Found Symp 1991; 157: 81-89.

63. Dennis PA, Rifkin DB. Cellular activation of latent transforming growth factor beta requires binding to the cation-independent mannose beta-phosphate/insulin-like growth factor type II receptor. Proc Natl Acad Sci USA 1991; 88: 580-584.

64. Gaffen JD. Interaction between the cell surface and the extracellular matrix. Br J Rheum 1992; 31: 74-76.

65. Wakefield L, Smith D, Masui T, Harris C, Sporn M. Distribution and modulation of the cellular receptor for transforming growth factor-beta. J Cell Biol 1987; 105: 965-975.

66. Boyd F, Cheifetz S, Andres J, Laiho M, Massagué J. Transforming growth factor-beta receptors and binding proteoglycans. J Cell Sci(suppl) 1990; 13: 131-138.

67. Eghbali M, Tomek R, Woods C, Bhambi B. Cardiac fibroblasts are predisposed to convert into myocyte phenotype: specific effect of transforming growth factor ß. Proc Natl Acad Sci USA 1991; 88: 795-799.

68. Lynch S, Colvin R, Antoniades H. Growth factors in wound healing. J Clin Invest 1989; 84: 640-646.

69. Heimark R, Twardzik D, Schwartz S. Inhibition of endothelial regeneration by type-beta transforming growth factor from platelets. Science 1986; 233: 1078-1080.

70. Kehrl J. Transforming growth factor-beta: an important mediator of immunoregulation. Int J Cell Cloning 1991; 9: 438-50.

71. Roberts A, Sporn M, Assoian R, et al. Transforming growth factor type ß: rapid induction of fibrosis and angiogenesis *in vivo* and stimulation of collagen formation *in vitro*. Proc Natl Acad Sci USA 1986; 83: 4167-4171.

72. Wiseman D, Polverini P, Kamp D, Leibovich S. Transforming growth factor-beta (TGFß) is chemotactic for human monocytes and induces their expression of angiogenic activity. Biochem Biophys Res Comm 1988; 157: 793-800.

73. McCartney F, Mizel D, Wong H, Wahl L, Wahl S. TGF-beta regulates production of growth factors and TGF-beta by human peripheral blood monocytes. Growth Factors 1990;4:27-35.

74. Pepper M, Belin D, Montesano R, Orci L, Vassalli J-D. Transforming growth factor-beta 1 modulates basic fibroblast growth factor-induced proteolytic and angiogenic properties of endothelial cells in vitro. J Cell Biol 1990; 111: 743-755.

75. Rifkin D, Moscatelli D, Bizik J, et al. Growth factor control of extracellular proteolysis. Cell Differ Dev 1990; 323: 313-318.

76. Ignotz R, Massagué J. Transforming growth factor-ß stimulates the expression of fibronectin and collagen and their incorporation into the extracellular matrix. J Biol Chem 1986; 261: 4337-4345.

77. Madri J, Pratt B, Tucker A. Phenotypic modulation of endothelial cells by transforming growth factor-beta depends upon the composition and organization of the extracellular matrix. J Cell Biol 1988; 10: 1375-1384.

78. Carpenter G, Cohen S. Epidermal growth factor. J Biol Chem 1990; 265: 7709-7712.

79. Carpenter G, Wahl M. The epidermal growth factor family. In: Sporn MB Roberts A, ed. Peptide Growth Factors and Their Receptors I. 1 ed. Berlin: Springer-Verlag, 1990: 69-171. vol 95

80. Schreiber A, Winkler M, Derynck R. Transforming growth factor-a: a more potent angiogenic mediator than epidermal growth factor. Science 1986; 232: 1250-1252.

81. Ross R. The pathogenesis of atherosclerosis - an update. N Engl J Med 1986; 314: 488-500.

82. Sato N, Nariuchi H, Tsuruoka N, et al. Actions of TNF and IFN-γ on angiogenesis in vitro. J Invest Dermatol 1990; 95: 85S-89S.

83. Heldin C-H, Westermark B. Platelet-derived growth factor: three isoforms and two receptor types. Trends Genet 1989; 5: 108-111.

84. Gospodarowicz D, Abraham J, Schilling J. Isolation and characterization of a vascular endothelial cell mitogen produced by pituitary-derived folliculo stellate cells. Proc Natl Acad Sci USA 1989; 86: 7311-7315.

85. Tischer E, Gospodarowicz D, Mitchell R, et al. Vascular endothelial growth factor: an new member of the platelet-derived growth factor gene family. Biochem Biophys Res Comm 1989; 165: 1198-1206.

86. Leung D, Cachianes G, Kuang W-J, Goeddel D, Ferrara N. Vascular endothelial growth factor is a secreted angiogenic mitogen. Science 1989; 246: 1306-1309.

87. Keck P, Hauser S, Krivi G, et al. Vascular permeability factor, an endothelial cell mitogen related to PDGF. Science 1989; 246: 1309-1312.

88. Conn G, Soderman D, Schaeffer M-T, Wile M, Hatcher V, Thomas K. Purification of a glycoprotein vascular endothelial cell mitogen from a rat glioma-derived cell line. Proc Natl Acad Sci USA 1990; 87: 1323-1327.

89. Berse B, Brown L, Sioussat T, Senger D, Dvorak H. Vascular permeability factor (vascular endothelial growth factor) expression in normal tissues and in tumors. J Cell Biol 1991; 115(3 Part 2): 2443, abstract.

90. Connolly D, Heuvelman DM, Nelson R et al. Tumor vascular permeability factor stimulates endothelial cell growth and angiogenesis. J Clin Invest 1989; 84: 1470-1478.

91. Vaisman N, Gospodarowicz D, Neufeld G. Characterization of the receptors for vascular endothelial growth factor. J Biol Chem 1990; 265: 19461-19466.

92. Jakeman LB, Winer J, Bennett GL, Altar CA, Ferrara. Binding sites for Vascular Endothelial Growth Factor are localized on endothelial cells in adult rat tissues. J Clin Invest 1992; 89: 244-53

93. De Vries C, Escobedo JA, Ueno H, Houck K, Ferrara N, Williams LT. The *fms*-like tyrosine kinase, a receptor for vascular endothelial growth factor. Science 1992; 255: 989-991

94. Koos R, Olson C. Hypoxia stimulates expression of the gene for vascular endothelial growth factor (VEGF), a putative angiogenic factor, by granulosa cells of the ovarian follicle, a site of angiogenesis. J Cell Biol 1991; 115(3 Part 2): 2444.

95. Gitay-Goren H, Soker S, Vlodavsky I, Neufeld G. The binding of Vascular Endothelial Growth Factor to its receptors is dependent on cell surface-associated heparin-like molecules. J Biol Chem. 1992; 267(9): 6093-6098.

96. Fett J, Strydom D, Lobb R, et al. Isolation and characterization of angiogenin, an angiogenic protein from human carcinoma cells. Biochem 1985; 24: 5480-5486.

97. Strydom D, Fett J, Lobb R, et al. Amino acid sequence of human tumor derived angiogenin. Biochem 1985; 24: 5486-5494.

98. Kurachi K, Davie E, Strydom D, Riordan J, Vallee B. Sequence of the cDNA and gene for angiogenin, a human angiogenesis factor. Biochem 1985; 24: 5494-5499.

99. Weiner H, Weiner L, Swain J. Tissue distribution and developmental expression of the messenger RNA encoding angiogenin. Science 1987; 237: 280-282.

100. Hu G-F, Chang S-I, Riordan J, Vallee B. An angiogenin-binding protein from endothelial cells. Proc Natl Acad Sci USA 1991; 88: 2227-2231.

101. Höckel M, Sasse J, Wissler J. Purified monocyte-derived angiogenic substance (angiotropin) stimulates migration, phenotypic changes, and "tube formation" but not proliferation of capillary endothelial cells in vitro. J Cell Physiol 1987; 133: 1-13.

102. Miyazono K, Okabe T, Urabe A, Takaku F, Heldin C-H. Purification and properties of an endothelial cell growth factor from human platelets. J Biol Chem 1987; 262: 4098-4103.

103. Ishikawa F, Miyazono K, Hellman U, et al. Identification of angiogenic activity and the cloning and expression of platelet-derived endothelial cell growth factor. Nature 1989; 338: 557-562.

104. Usuki K, Heldin N-E, Miyazono K, et al. Production of platelet-derived endothelial cell growth factor by normal and transformed human cells in culture. Proc Natl Acad Sci USA 1989; 86: 7427-7431.

105. Fràter-Schröder M, Risau W, Hallmann R, Gautschi P, Böhlen P. Tumor necrosis factor type a, a potent inhibitor of endothelial cell growth *in vitro*, is angiogenic *in vivo*. Proc Natl Acad Sci USA 1987; 84: 5277-5281.

106. Knighton D, Hunt T, Scheuenstuhl H, Halliday B. Oxygen tension regulates the expression of angiogenesis factor by macrophages. Science 1983; 221: 1283-1285.

107. Leibovich S, Polverini P, Shepard H, Wiseman D, Shively V, Nuseir N. Macrophage-induced angiogenesis is mediated by tumor necrosis factor-alpha. Nature 1987; 329: 630-632.

108. Klagsbrun M, D'Amore P. Regulators of angiogenesis. Annu Rev Physiol 1991; 53: 217-239.

109. Odedra R, Weiss J. Low molecular weight angiogenesis factors. Pharmac Ther 1991; 49: 111-124.

110. Kull F, Brent K, Parikh I, Cuatrecasas P. Chemical identification of a tumor-derived angiogenic factor. Science 1987; 236: 843-845.

111. Morris P, Ellis M, Swain J. Angiogenic potency of nucleotide metabolites: potential role in ischemia-induced vascular growth. J Mol Cell Cardiol 1989; 21: 351-358.

112. Dusseau J, Hutchins P, Malbasa D. Stimulation of angiogenesis by adenosine on the chick chorioallantoic membrane. Circ Res 1986; 59:163-170.

10. Atherosclerosis and platelet derived growth factors

GORDON A.A. FERNS and CLAIRE RUTHERFORD

Introduction

Coronary heart disease (CHD) accounts for more than 160,000 deaths per year in England and Wales [1], and is the major cause of mortality of men under 65 years of age in the Western world. The economic impact of CHD is correspondingly profound, with estimated costs for treating the condition in England and Wales alone exceeding £400 million per annum [2]. Our understanding of the cellular events that lead to atherosclerosis have improved substantially over recent years due to the availability of cell-specific monoclonal antibodies for immunocytochemical analysis [3]; the cloning of the genes for several growth factors and cytokines, which have permitted studies of gene expression; and the development of carefully devised animal models. The latter in particular have provided a means of studying the sequence of events that lead to the atherosclerotic plaque formation.

Atherogenesis: the cellular pathology

Atheroma is by far the most common cause of arteriosclerosis. The fully established atheromatous plaque generally consists of an accumulation of cells and lipid, both cellular and extracellular, within the arterial tunica intima. The biochemical and cellular composition of the plaque is variable, depending on its anatomical site, the predisposing risk factors (Table 1) and the age and sex of the individual.

Table 1. Risk Factors for Coronary Heart Disease

Hypercholesterolaemia
Hypertriglyceridaemia
Hypo-alpha-lipoproteinaemia
Cigarette smoking
Genetic Factors (Family History)
Raised plasma levels of clotting factors
Hypertension
Impaired glucose tolerance; Diabetes Mellitus
Obesity

Fatty-streaks

Fatty-streaks are the earliest and most common lesions of atherosclerosis. They may be found throughout the arterial tree and are frequently found in children [4]. They are essentially superficial accumulations of macrophages, macrophage-derived foam-cells and lymphocytes (Figure 1a and 1b) [5,6,7]. Medial smooth muscle cells enter the lesion at a later stage and may subsequently develop into smooth muscle-derived foam cells. In some cases they elaborate large quantities of extracellular matrix components, leading to the development of a proteoglycan-rich 'gelatinous' lesion.

The fibrous plaque

The fibrous plaque is the lesion that is most frequently associated with clinical sequelae. It usually consists of a 'cap' region, composed primarily of vascular smooth muscle cells and connective tissue, which overlies a cellular lipid-rich 'core', containing macrophages, lymphocytes and foam-cells. As the lesion matures, the core may become necrotic and patches of calcification may also develop within it. The base of the lesion contains a smooth muscle rich region that is delimited by the internal elastic lamina.

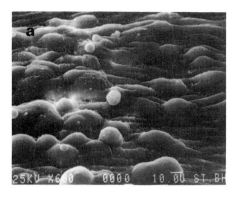 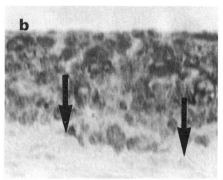

Figure 1. The fatty-streak. a) shows a scanning electron micrograph of the thoracic aorta of a rabbit fed a 2% cholesterol diet for one month. The endothelial surface is deformed by the presence of numerous underlying macrophage-derived foam-cells. bar=10 microns. b) shows a cross-section through a fatty-streak in the thoracic aorta of the same animal, immunostained with RAM-11, a macrophage-specific monoclonal antibody, showing DAB-positive, superficially located foam-cells. The internal elastic laminar is indicated by an arrow.

The complicated plaque

The stability of the fibrous plaque is in major part dependent on its cellular composition. Lesions that are rich in macrophages are prone to complications including cracking, fissuring, ulceration, haemorrhage, acute rupture and thrombosis, that finally lead to overt clinical disease [8]. The reason for this is thought to relate to the release of proteases, such as collagenase and elastase, from activated leukocytes within the plaque, which weaken the vessel wall.

The cellular participants in atherogenesis

The major cellular players in atherogenesis include: mononuclear cells (monocytes and lymphocytes), vascular smooth muscle cells, endothelial cells and platelets (Figure 2). The primary event in this process, according to the 'Response to Injury Hypothesis' [9], is the development of a dysfunctional vascular endothelium. One of a number of precipitating causes may lead to endothelial dysfunction, including;

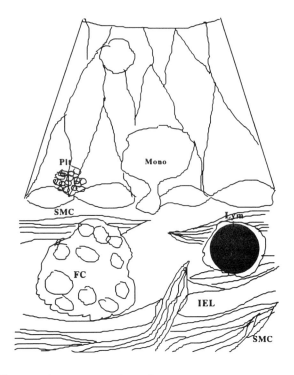

Figure 2. A diagramatic representation of the early atherosclerotic lesion, showing the major cellular participants. Plt=platelets; Mono=monocyte; FC=foam-cell; IEL=internal elastic lamina; SMC=smooth muscle cell.

hyperlipidaemia, particularly raised levels of plasma LDL; viral infection; mechanical injury (following balloon angioplasty); cigarette smoking [10]; and circulating endothelial cell toxins. Normal endothelial cells produce factors such as endothelium derived relaxing factor (EDRF) and prostacyclin (PGI_2) [11] which inhibit platelet aggregation and mononuclear cell adhesion. The production of these substances, or their bioactivity, is perturbed by endothelial injury, so that increased leukocyte adhesion is often one of the first manifestations of endothelial dysfunctionality observed in animal models of atherosclerosis. The adherent leukocytes subsequently enter the sub-endothelium by passing between the endothelial cell junctions. Here, monocytes differentiate into macrophages, and are subsequently converted into foam-cells by their incorporation of lipid. LDL accumulates within the intima by a process of trans-endothelial transport. The LDL then undergoes modification to a form that allows it to bind to scavenger receptors on macrophages and is subsequently taken up by these cells. This process not only results in foam-cell formation, but also leads to enhanced expression and release of cytokines and growth factors from the activated macrophage. Among these are; platelet derived growth factor (PDGF), transforming growth factors (TGF) α and ß, interleukin-1 (IL-1), macrophage colony stimulating factor-1 (M-CSF-1), basic fibroblast growth factor (bFGF) and tumour necrosis factor α (TNF α) [12]. The process is self-perpetuating, and the lesion expands by the continued recruitment of circulating monocytes. Medial smooth muscle cells are also attracted into the lesion by macrophage-derived and LDL-derived chemoattractants. Once within the intima these cells may proliferate rapidly. Indeed, the 'Monoclonal Hypothesis' of [13] suggests that the final population of intimal smooth muscle cells is derived from a very few precursor cells that proliferate in an almost neoplastic manner. These smooth muscle cells may also change from a contractile to synthetic phenotype, and are then a principle source of connective tissue within the plaque. These latter events contribute to the formation of a fibrous cap. At some anatomical sites (e.g. opposite flow-dividers), the accumulation of intimal cells is so great that it causes the overlying endothelium to become grossly deformed. In some cases this results in endothelial cell retraction, in other cases complete denudation ensues. In both instances the thrombogenic subendothelial matrix is exposed leading to the deposition of adherent platelet microaggregates. Platelets contain several growth factors that may contribute to atherosclerotic lesion progression [14,15,16,17] (Table 2),

Table 2. Platelet Associated Mitogens and Chemotactic Factors

Growth Factor/ Cytokine	SMC mitogen		SMC chemoattractant
PDGF	+++		+++
IGF-I	+		-
TGFß	+/-	*	-
Interleukin-1	+	*	-
Epidermal Growth Factor	++		-

* The response to TGFß is biphasic, the response to IL-1 is indirect and mediated by an autocrine network involving PDGF-AA

and sites that are predisposed to platelet adherence appear to be prone to rapid development of atherosclerotic lesions. T lymphocytes of both helper (CD4) and suppressor (CD8) phenotypes are a minor, but potentially important cellular constituent of the atherosclerotic plaque [5,6]. They are present during all stages of plaque development, from the fatty-streak to the advanced fibro-fatty lesion. There is also histological evidence supporting the view that at least some of these cells are in an activated state [18]. Precisely how these cells may contribute to atherogenesis is unknown, but it is possible that the environment within the plaque leads to the formation of neo-antigens that are perceived as foreign by the immune system, and that this leads to an auto-immune response. This notion is supported by recent studies which have identified circulating antibodies directed against epitopes on modified LDL in patients with atherosclerosis [19]. Activated T-cells also elaborate gamma-interferon, a cytokine that enhances MHC class II molecule expression on smooth muscle cells [20], and which would improve the potential for antigen presentation by smooth muscle cells and hence exacerbate the immune response.

Atherosclerosis: the biochemical events

Lipoproteins and oxygen related free radicals

Hypercholesterolaemia has been shown to be an important coronary risk factor by epidemiological and intervention studies and by experiments using animal models. Leukocyte margination and adhesion may be increased within days of starting a high cholesterol diet [7], and in man hyperlipidaemia is associated with increased leukocyte-endothelial cell binding [21]. This interaction is mediated by pairs of membrane associated cell adhesion molecules (CAMs), one of each pair being located on the monocyte, the other on the endothelial cell. The expression of endothelial cell CAMs can be induced in culture by atherogenic levels of LDL, minimally modified LDL or cell-modified LDL [22,23]. Monocytes, endothelial cells, smooth muscle cells and lymphocytes are all capable of modifying LDL [24,25]. The precise mechanism for this has not been established, but it may involve either enzymatic (lipoxygenase), or non-enzymatic (free-radical) processes. There is considerable evidence supporting the view that LDL is modified *in vivo*. LDL isolated from the arterial wall of animals with atherosclerosis has almost identical properties as oxidized LDL [26]; epitopes identified on modified LDL are also expressed in atherosclerotic lesions [19,27]; and anti-oxidants such as probucol have proven to be highly efficacious in ameliorating atherosclerosis in cholesterol-fed animals [28]. Modified LDL also has several biological properties that would tend to enhance lesion development [24]. It is cytotoxic, and its local generation by intimal macrophages may lead to the dysfunction of overlying endothelium. It causes altered endothelial cell expression of growth factors, such as PDGF [29], and other intracellular growth factors (bFGF and IGF-I) may be released following endothelial cell death. The transformation of monocytes into lipid-laden macrophages may also be associated with the release of growth factors, including PDGF [30]. These factors may act synergistically to promote intimal cell proliferation. Oxidized LDL is a monocyte and smooth muscle cell chemoattractant [31,32,33] and hence it would tend to increase the cellularity of the intima. It has also been reported to be cytostatic [31], so that cells that enter the intima are retained here. Oxidized LDL also appears to antagonize the biological effects of EDRF [34].

Syndromes of accelerated atherosclerosis

There are certain clinical states associated with very rapidly developing atherosclerosis. Among these are the autosomal co-dominant disorder Familial Hypercholesterolaemia (FH), and paradoxically, three strategies used to treat coronary atherosclerosis. In each case accelerated atherosclerosis is probably related to gross endothelial cell injury.

Familial hypercholesterolaemia

Genetic defects of the LDL receptor lead to the condition FH. Patients with FH have elevated levels of total and LDL cholesterol and a very high risk of premature atherosclerosis. Without treatment the clinical outcome is almost invariably premature death, often before the age of thirty. The Watanabe Heritable Hyperlipidaemic (WHHL) rabbit is an animal model equivalent of this condition. Arterial lesions that develop in WHHL rabbits are very similar in composition and structure to those associated with cholesterol feeding [7] and it has provided a useful insight into the disease process.

Percutaneous transluminal coronary angioplasty

Coronary angioplasty has been used clinically for more than a decade to treat single and multiple vessel coronary artery disease. Although it is a relatively safe and simple procedure, re-occlusion is a common late complication. The re-stenotic lesion is frequently vascular smooth muscle cell-rich. Although the agents responsible for the accumulation of intimal smooth muscle cells are largely unknown, several factors are either released from injured vascular smooth muscle cells or liberated from platelets. Platelet degranulation, and leukocyte adhesion at the sites of de-endothelialization, are an inevitable consequence of balloon inflation. Several studies employing animal models illustrate this fact (see Figure 3a and 3b), and have permitted a detailed analysis of the cell kinetics of neo-intimal lesion development. These studies have established that medial smooth muscle cell migration, and their subsequent proliferation are key events in neo-intima formation [35]. If animals are additionally cholesterol-fed, foam-cell rich lesions may quickly form (Figure 3c), providing a model which closely mirrors clinical disease.

Coronary artery by-pass grafting

Vein grafts become arterialized, developing a thickened neo-intima within days of implantation. Atherosclerotic lesions usually then evolve over a period of several months. In venous grafts, the lesions are characteristically superficial, uniform, concentric and usually contain a high proportion of foam-cells. Arterial grafts are less prone to atherosclerosis over the short term. Golden et al [36] have reported that neo-intimal cells from vascular grafts, express PDGF-A chain message and PDGF protein at higher levels than cells of a normal artery, and they suggest that this may in part account for intimal cell accumulation.

Transplantation atherosclerosis

Atherosclerosis may develop rapidly following cardiac transplantation, particularly at the sites of vascular anastomosis. As is the case with by-pass grafts, these lesions tend to be concentric. It is likely that surgical manipulation results in endothelial dysfunction acutely, and that immune mechanisms are involved in chronic injury. It is possible that drugs such as Cyclosporine A, used to prevent rejection, also have deleterious effects on endothelial function [36], hence their is a fine balance between maintaining optimum immunosuppression and causing drug-induced endothelial injury.

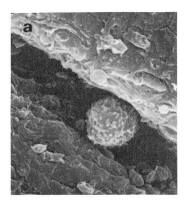
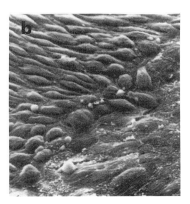
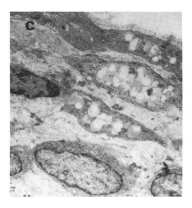

Figure 3. Electron micrographs showing: a) an adherent, activated leukocyte on the surface of a balloon catheterized rabbit carotid artery; numerous adherent, flattened platelets are also apparent; b) the junction between denuded and re-endothelialized regions of a rabbit common carotid artery, one month after surgery; the exposed smooth muscle cells are less thrombogenic at this time, forming what has been termed a 'pseudoendothelium'; and c) a ballooned carotid artery of a rabbit that received a 2% cholesterol diet, showing several intimal smooth muscle cell-derived foam-cells.

The role of growth factors in atherogenesis

Cell proliferation and migration are characteristic features of atherosclerosis. These processes are probably brought about by the synergistic interplay of several growth factors and cytokines. Following arterial injury it is likely that some of these at least, are platelet derived. In the absence of overt endothelial injury and platelet degranulation, growth factors are probably released by cells of the vessel wall. These may then act in an autocrine or paracrine manner. PDGF is a potent mitogen and chemoattractant, and is probably among the factors that are involved in atherogenesis.

Table 3. Human Vascular Cells Expressing PDGF or its Receptor

Cell Type	PDGF	PDGF-receptor
Endothelial cell	A and B	ß?
Smooth muscle cell	A	α and ß
Activated Monocyte	A and B	?
Lymphocyte	-	?
Platelet/Megakaryocyte	A* and B	-

* The composition of platelet PDGF is species dependent.
? Some authors have reported that PDGF is a monocyte chemoattractant [38], and that natural killer cells (large granular lymphocytes) have PDGF receptors [39]. Some authors have also reported that PDGF is an endothelium dependent vaso-relaxant in rat aorta [40].

Platelet derived growth factor

Ross et al [15] predicted the existence of a platelet derived growth factor on the basis of its ability to stimulate the growth of smooth muscle cells in culture. It was later isolated and purified as a cationic protein with a molecular weight of 28 to 35 KDa. The active molecule is dimeric, consisting of one of three combinations of two homologous polypeptide chains, termed PDGF-A and -B, linked by disulphide bonds. These are encoded by separate genes, that in man, have been localized to different chromosomes [41,42]. The gene for the B-chain is highly homologous to the proto-oncogene v-sis [43]). Recent studies have established that platelets are not the only cellular source of PDGF (reviewed by Raines et al. [44]), which is also synthesized by several other cell types [45,46,47] (Table 3). However the distribution of PDGF isoforms that is elaborated by a particular cell is lineage- and species-dependent. For example, human platelets contain PDGF-AA, -AB and -BB, whereas porcine platelets only contain PDGF-BB [48].

Table 4. The Biological Effects of PDGF

Mitogen and competence factor.
Directed cell migration.
Endothelium dependent relaxation.
Vasoconstriction.
Phosphorylation of intracellular proteins mediated by the tyrosine kinase activity of the PDGF receptor.
LDL receptor upregulation.
Nuclear proto-oncogene expression (c-myc, c-fos).
Early gene response (JE, KC, c-jun).
Intracellular alkalinization via sodium-hydrogen antiport.
Increased intracellular free calcium.
Activation of phospholipase C and A2.
Diacylglycerol, inositol triphosphate and arachidonic acid release.
Activation of protein kinase C.
Cytoskeletal re-arrangement.

PDGF receptor

The genes for the PDGF receptors are members of the split tyrosine kinase family [49]. The functional receptor is dimeric, being composed of combinations of α- and ß-subunits [50]. Although these subunits are homologous, they have a particular binding specificity for the PDGF polypeptide chains. The α-subunit can bind either A-or B-chain, whereas the ß-subunit can only bind the B-chain. The consequence of this is that PDGF-BB can interact productively with all three possible combinations of the PDGF receptor (α-α, α-ß and ßß), whereas PDGF-AA can only bind to a homodimeric α-α PDGF receptor. It is thought that receptor dimerization may be ligand-induced, whereby a dimeric PDGF molecule brings two 'floating' receptor subunits into apposition within the plasma membrane [51]. Cross-chain phosphorylation is thought to be one of the first steps in signal transduction. In this process each receptor subunit's intracellular domain acts as a substrate for the tyrosine kinase activity of the other. The fact that the PDGF receptor alpha- and ß- subunits may be differentially expressed during certain disease processes [52], permits the cells expressing them to vary in their responses to the PDGF isoforms to which they are exposed.

Putative role of PDGF in atherogenesis

From its biological properties listed in Table 4, it is clear that PDGF
may contribute to the atherogenic process at a number of stages. Several
strands of evidence suggest that this may indeed be the case. Some of
these are discussed below.

Expression of PDGF by the cells of the atherosclerotic plaque and the injured artery wall

Barrett and Benditt [53]) have reported that PDGF-B chain (v-sis)
expression is increased in atherosclerotic arteries, whereas PDGF-A
chain expression is unaffected, and is relatively low in normal and
diseased vessels. They also found that c-fms expression (a marker for
the presence of macrophages) was elevated in diseased arteries, and that
there was a good correlation between the expression of c-fms and
PDGF-B, suggesting that macrophages are the major source of
PDGF-BB. Ross et al [30] have recently investigated the expression of
PDGF-B chain in experimentally induced lesions of the cholesterol-fed
monkey, and also in advanced human lesions. PDGF-BB was identified
using a chain-specific monoclonal antibody, and was found to be
expressed primarily by macrophages, during all stages of lesion
development. PDGF was not present in all the macrophages in a lesion
simultaneously, and it is likely that PDGF is only expressed by
macrophages/ foam-cells during particular phases of their development.
Ross and his colleagues [30] also found that c-fms and IL-1 expression
were upregulated in atherosclerotic blood vessels, reinforcing the
hypothesis that activated macrophages were the source of PDGF. Using
in-situ hybridization, Wilcox and his colleagues [54], could find no
evidence for increased PDGF gene expression in atherosclerotic lesions.
However they did find that endothelial cells and 'mesenchymal' cells of
unidentified lineage did express both PDGF-A and -B chains. They also
found that the PDGF receptor ß-subunit was expressed by many of the
cells in the plaque. The discrepancies in these studies may be accounted
for in part by the type of pathological material examined. This was
different in each case, and as has already been eluded to, gene
expression would be expected to vary with stage of plaque
development.
    Following balloon catheter injury, there is a rapid modulation of
growth factor and growth factor receptor gene expression, within the
arterial wall. Among the early events in this process is an upregulation
of PDGF-A chain and reduction of PDGF receptor ß-subunit expression

[55]. There follows a gradual increase in the latter, particularly by cells of the neo-intima [55].

Effects of thrombocytopaenia on neo-intima development

The importance of platelets in intimal cell accumulation is apparent from studies using thrombocytopaenic animals. Moore et al [56], Friedman et al ([57] and Fingerle et al [58], all found that the intimal response to balloon catheter injury is diminished in thrombocytopaenia. The findings in the latter study indicated that the factors contained within platelets, exert their effects predominantly as smooth muscle cell chemoattractants, rather than as mitogens. Separate studies have suggested that PDGF may be the major platelet associated chemotactic factor [59]. Hence in the balloon injury model, PDGF may play a vital role.

Effects of PDGF antagonists in animal models of intimal hyperplasia

The importance of PDGF in neo-intima development has recently been tested more directly. A PDGF antagonist, Trapidil was found to inhibit arterial re-stenosis following balloon injury in the rabbit iliac artery [60]. These data are not conclusive because Trapidil's specificity as an antagonist of PDGF alone, is uncertain. However recent work by Ferns et al [59] and Jawien et al [61] have provided further evidence for the importance of PDGF in the arterial response to injury. Ferns et al [59] used a PDGF-specific polyclonal antibody to neutralize the effects of PDGF in the balloon catheterized athymic nude (nu/nu) rat. The size of the neo-intima was significantly reduced in the anti-PDGF treated animals, although cell proliferation (measured as thymidine uptake) was unaffected. Jawien et al [61] administered PDGF-BB to rats at different intervals after balloon injury. They found that PDGF treatment increased neo-intimal size without affecting cell proliferation during the first two weeks after injury. After the fourth week, they observed a small increase in thymidine index in the PDGF treated animals, indicating that smooth muscle cell-PDGF receptor expression may be enhanced at this time. Both studies suggest that PDGF's major activity is as a smooth muscle cell chemotactic factor. This also appears to be the case when endothelium is removed without significant medial cell injury, using a filament loop [62] (see Figure 4).

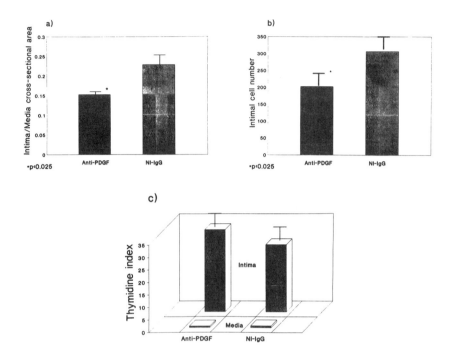

Figure 4. The effects of administering a neutralizing anti-PDGF or non-immune goat IgG to nude rats for eight days after 'gentle' (nylon filament loop) de-endothelialization on: a) intima: media cross-sectional area, b) intimal cellularity, and c) intimal and medial proliferation (measured as thymidine uptake) (from the data of Ferns et al [62]). Although neo-intimal cellularity was reduced by anti-PDGF IgG treatment, this appeared to be due to an effect on cell migration rather than proliferation.

Conclusions

It is clear that although PDGF plays a role in atherogenesis, other factors are also involved. Some of these will be discussed in subsequent chapters. It also seems likely that the importance of PDGF will be dependent on the aetiology of the atherosclerotic lesion; whether it is induced by mechanical injury, dyslipoproteinaemia or immune mechanisms. A clearer understanding of these processes is necessary before effective intervention strategies can be devised.

Acknowledgements

The authors are grateful to Ono Pharmaceutical Company Ltd, Japan, The British Heart Foundation, and the University of London Central Research Fund, for financial support.

References

1. Wells N. Coronary heart disease. The need for action. Paper 80. Office of Health Economics, London 1987.
2. Elkan W. Coronary heart disease: Economic aspects of prevention. Lipid Review 1988; 2: 41-46.
3. Tsukada T et al. Immunocytochemical analysis of cellular components in atherosclerotic lesions. Arteriosclerosis 1986; 6: 601-613.
4. Stary HC. Evolution of atherosclerotic plaques in the coronary arteries of young adults. Arteriosclerosis 1983; 3: 471a.
5. Masuda J, Ross R. Atherogenesis during low-level hypercholesterolaemia in the non-human primate. II. Fatty-streak conversion to fibrous plaque. Arteriosclerosis 1990; 10: 178-187.
6. Masuda J, Ross R. Atherogenesis during low-level hypercholesterolaemia in the non-human primate. I. Fatty-streak formation. Arteriosclerosis 1990; 10: 164-177.
7. Rosenfeld ME et al. Fatty streak initiation in Watanabe Heritable Hyperlipemic and comparably hypercholesterolemic fat-fed rabbits. Arteriosclerosis 1987; 7: 9-23.
8. Richardson PD et al. Influence of plaque configuration and stress distribution on fissuring of coronary atherosclerotic plaques. Lancet 1989; ii: 941-944.
9. Ross R. The pathogenesis of atherosclerosis: an update. N Engl J Med 1986; 314: 488-500.
10. Woolf N, Wilson-Holt N. Cigarette smoking and atherosclerosis. In: Greenhaugh RM ed. Smoking and arterial disease. Pitman Medical 1981; pp 46-59.
11. Vane JR et al. Regulatory functions of the vascular endothelium. N Engl J Med 1990; 323: 27-36.
12. Nathan CF. Secretory products of macrophages. J Clin Invest 1987; 79: 319-326.
13. Benditt EP, Benditt JM. Evidence for a monoclonal origin of human atherosclerotic plaques. Proc Natl Acad Sci, USA 1973; 70: 1753-1756.

14. Assoian RK et al. Transforming growth factor ß in human platelets. identification of a major storage site, purification and characterisation. J Biol Chem 1983; 258: 7155-7160.
15. Ross R et al. A platelet-dependent serum factor that stimulates the proliferation of arterial smooth muscle cells. Proc Natl Acad Sci, USA 1974; 71: 1207-1210.
16. Oka Y, Orth DN. Human plasma epidermal growth factor/ ß-urogastrone is associated with blood platelets. J Clin Invest 1983; 72: 249-259.
17. Hawrylowicz CM et al. Platelet-derived IL-1 induces human endothelial adhesion molecule expression and cytokine production. J Exp Med 1991; 174: 785-790.
18. Hansson GK et al. Detection of activated T lymphocytes in the human atherosclerotic plaque. Am J Path 1989; 135: 169-175.
19. Palinski W et al. Low density lipoprotein undergoes oxidative modification in vivo. Proc Natl Acad Sci, USA 1989; 86: 1372-1376.
20. Hansson GK et al. Gamma interferon regulates vascular smooth muscle proliferation and Ia antigen expression in vivo and in vitro. Circ Res 1988; 63: 712-719.
21. Losche W et al. Functional behaviour of mononuclear cells from patients with hypercholesterolaemia. Thromb Res 1992; 65: 337-342.
22. Berliner JA et al. Minimally modified low density lipoprotein stimulates monocytes endothelial interactions. J Clin Invest 1990; 85: 1260-1266.
23. Frostegard J et al. Biologically modified LDL increases adhesive properties of endothelial cells. Atherosclerosis 1991; 90: 119-126.
24. Steinberg D et al. Beyond cholesterol. Modifications of low density lipoprotein that increase its atherogenicity. N Engl J Med 1989; 320: 915-924.
25. Lamb DJ et al. The oxidative modification of low density lipoprotein by human lymphocytes. Atherosclerosis 1992; 92: 187-192.
26. Rosenfeld ME et al. Macrophage-derived foam cells freshly isolated from rabbit atherosclerotic lesions degrade modified lipoproteins, promote oxidation of low density lipoproteins and contain oxidation specific lipid-protein adducts. J Clin Invest 1991; 87: 90-99.
27. Haberland ME et al. Malondialdehyde-altered proteins occur in atheroma of Watanabe Hyperlipidemic rabbits. Science 1988; 241: 215-218.
28. Kita T et al. Probucol prevents the progression of atherosclerosis in Watanabe Heritable Hyperlipidemic rabbits, an animal model of Familial Hypercholesterolemia. Proc Natl Acad Sci, USA 1987; 84: 5928-5931.
29. Fox PL, DiCorletto PE. Modified low density lipoproteins suppress production of a platelet-derived growth factor-like protein by cultured endothelial cells. Proc Natl Acad Sci, USA 1986; 83: 4774-4778.

30. Ross R et al. Localization of PDGF-B protein in macrophages in all phases of atherogenesis. Science 1990; 248: 1009-1012.

31. Quinn MT et al. Oxidatively modified LDL: Potential role in recruitment and retention of monocyte/ macrophage during atherogenesis. Proc Natl Acad Sci, USA 1987; 84: 2995-2999.

32. Quinn MT et al. Lysophosphatidyl choline: A chemotactic factor for human monocytes and its potential role in atherogenesis. Proc Natl Acad Sci, USA. 1988: 85; 2805-2809.

33. Autio I et al. Oxidized low density lipoprotein is chemotactic for arterial smooth muscle cells in culture. FEBS 1990; 277: 247-249.

34. Chin JH et al. Inactivation of endothelial derived relaxing factor by oxidized lipoproteins. J Clin Invest 1992; 89: 10-18.

35. Clowes AW et al. Mechanisms of stenosis after arterial injury. Lab Invest 1983; 49: 208-215.

36. Golden MA et al. Platelet-derived growth factor activity and mRNA expression in healing vascular grafts in baboons. Association in vivo of platelet-derived growth factor mRNA and protein with cellular proliferation. J Clin Invest 1991; 87: 406-414.

37. Ferns GAA et al. Vascular effects of cyclosporine A in vivo and in vitro. Am J Path 1990; 137: 403-414.

38. Deuel T et al. Chemotaxis of monocytes and neutrophils to platelet-derived growth factor. J Clin Invest 1982; 69: 1046-1049.

39. Gersuk G et al. Inhibition of human natural killer cell activity by platelet-derived growth factor. J Immunol 1988; 141: 4031-4038.

40. Cunningham LD et al. Platelet derived growth factor receptors on macrovascular endothelial cells mediate relaxation via nitric oxide in rat aorta. J Clin Invest 1992; 89: 878-882.

41. Betsholtz C et al. The human platelet-derived growth factor A-chain; cDNA sequence, chromosomal localization and expression in tumour cell lines. Nature 1986; 323: 226-232.

42. Dalla-Farera R et al. Chromosomal localization of the human homolog (c-sis) of the simian sarcoma virus onc gene. Science 1982; 218: 686-688.

43. Doolittle RF et al. Simian sarcoma virus onc gene, v-sis, is derived from the gene (genes) encoding a platelet-derived growth factor. Science 1983; 221: 275-277.

44. Raines EW et al. Platelet-derived growth factor. In: Sporn MB, Roberts A. editors. Handbook of Experimental Pharmacology, Vol 95/I. Peptide Growth Factors and Their Receptors. Springer-Verlag, Berlin 1990: 174-262.

45. Sjolund M et al. Arterial smooth muscle cells express platelet derived growth factor (PDGF) A chain mRNA, secrete a PDGF-like mitogen, and bind exogenous PDGF in a phenotype- and growth state-dependent manner. J Cell Biol 1988; 106: 403-413.

46. Collins T et al. Cultured human endothelial cells express platelet-derived growth factor B chain: cDNA cloning and structural analysis. Nature 1985; 316: 748-750.

47. Shimokado K et al. A significant part of macrophage-derived growth factor consists of at least two forms of PDGF. Cell 1985; 43: 277-286.

48. Bowen-Pope DF et al. Sera and conditioned media contain different isoforms of platelet derived growth factor (PDGF) which bind to different classes of PDGF receptor. J Biol Chem 1989; 264: 2502-2508.

49. Yarden Y et al. Structure of the receptor for platelet derived growth factor helps define a family of closely related growth factor receptors. Nature 1986; 323: 226-232.

50. Seifert RA et. Two different subunits associate to create isoform specific platelet-derived growth factor receptors. J Biol Chem 1989; 264:8771-8778.

51. Bishayee S et al. Ligand-induced dimerization of the PDGF receptor. J Biol Chem 1989; 264: 11699-11705.

52. Gronwald RGK et al. Differential regulation of expression of two platelet-derived growth factor receptor sub-units by transforming growth factor ß. J Biol Chem 1989; 264: 8120-8125.

53. Barrett TB, Benditt EP. Platelet-derived growth factor gene expression in human atherosclerotic plaques and normal artery wall. Proc Natl Acad Sci, USA 1988; 85: 2810-2814.

54. Wilcox JN et al. Platelet derived growth factor mRNA detection in human atherosclerotic plaques by in situ hybridization. J Clin Invest 1988;82: 1134-1143.

55. Majesky MW et al. PDGF ligand and receptor gene expression during repair of arterial injury. J Cell Biol 1989; 111: 2149-2158.

56. Moore S et al. Inhibition of injury induced thromboatherosclerotic lesions by anti-platelet serum in rabbits. Thromb Haemostasis 1976; 35: 70-81.

57. Friedman RJ et al. The effect of thrombocytopaenia on experimental arteriosclerotic lesion formation in rabbits: smooth muscle cell proliferation and re-endothelialization. J Clin Invest 1977; 60: 1191-1201.

58. Fingerle J et al. Role of platelets in smooth muscle cell proliferation and migration after vascular injury in rat carotid artery. Proc Natl Acad Sci, USA 1989; 86: 8412-8416.

59. Ferns GAA et al. Anti-PDGF IgG inhibits the arterial response to balloon injury. Science 1991; 253: 1129-1132.

60. Liu MW et al. Trapidil in preventing restenosis after balloon angioplasty in the atherosclerotic rabbit. Circulation 1990; 81: 1089-1093.

61. Jawien A et al. Platelet-derived growth factor promotes smooth muscle migration and intimal thickening in a rat model of balloon angioplasty. J Clin Invest 1991; 89: 507-511.

62. Ferns GAA et al. Arterial response to gentle de-endothelialization is modulated by anti-PDGF IgG in the nude (nu/ nu) rat carotid. Clin Sci 1992; in press.

11. Effects of TGF-ß on vascular smooth muscle cell growth

PETER L. WEISSBERG, D.J. GRAINGER and JAMES C. METCALFE

Introduction

In the normal adult artery the majority of the vascular smooth muscle cells (VSMCs) are confined to the media of the vessel. These VSMCs undergo little if any growth and express smooth muscle-specific contractile proteins which enable them to maintain vascular tone. However, abnormal VSMC growth occurs in a number of vascular disease processes. In hypertension the artery wall becomes thickened as a result of growth (probably hypertrophy) of contractile VSMCs within the media. The increased wall to lumen ratio results in an elevated vascular resistance which maintains the hypertension. By contrast, in obliterative vascular conditions such as atherosclerosis VSMCs migrate into the intima and proliferate. The intimal VSMCs differ from medial VSMCs in that they contain few contractile filaments and many synthetic organelles which allow them to synthesise and secrete extracellular matrix proteins which contribute to the bulk of the lesion.

At present the factors responsible for inducing VSMC hypertrophy or hyperplasia *in vivo* are poorly understood but a large number of naturally occuring polypeptides have been identified which will enhance VSMC migration and/or growth *in vitro*. These include recognised growth factors such as platelet-derived growth factor (PDGF), epidermal growth factor (EGF), basic fibroblast growth factor (bFGF), endothelium-derived growth factor (EDGF) and insulin-like growth factor 1 (IGF-1) and vasoactive peptides such as angiotensin II (AII), endothelin, serotonin, noradrenalin and vasopressin. Many of these mitogens are synthesised or secreted at the sites of vascular injury or inflammation and are likely, therefore, to play a role in promoting VSMC growth *in vivo*. However, their growth promoting influences are opposed by factors which modulate the extent and nature of the growth response. A potential candidate for this role is transforming growth factor beta (TGFß), a cytokine which is also expressed at sites of vascular injury and which may act to modify the proliferative response to vascular injury and the hypertrophic response in hypertension.

Transforming growth factor ß

The transforming growth factors beta are members of a family of growth regulators which have diverse effects on many different cell types (reviewed in ref 47). TGFß-1 is the best characterised member of the family and most of the studies on the effects of TGFß on VSMC growth have been carried out using TGFß-1. Generally TGFß has been found to promote proliferation of anchorage-independent cells and inhibit proliferation of anchorage-dependent cells. It is thought to play a major role in wound healing where it upregulates expression of extracellular matrix proteins and down regulates expression of matrix degrading enzymes. (reviewed in refs 1 & 2).

TGFß is released by platelets [3], macrophages [4] and VSMCs [5] at the sites of vascular injury and high levels of both mRNA and protein have been demonstrated in proliferative vascular lesions suggesting an important role for TGFß [5,6]. However, TGFß is synthesised and released as an inactive propeptide [7], therefore its presence does not necessarily imply biological activity. The latent propeptide must be cleaved to form the active peptide by proteases such as plasmin before it can exert any biological effect [7]. Since VSMCs and endothelial cells at the site of vascular injury can synthesise and release tissue-type plasminogen activator (tPA) [8], a local mechanism exists for activation of secreted TGFß. Furthermore, the level of tPA activity will depend on the expression of plasminogen activator inhibitor-1 (PAI-1) which is also synthesised in the vessel wall [9] and possibly as a result of increased local concentrations of TGFß [10]. Thus a potential self-regulating loop for the activation of TGFß exists in the vessel wall.

Proteolytic activation of the propeptide is not the only local mechanism involved in determining the biological activity of TGFß. It has been shown that TGFß binds with high affinity to alpha 2 macroglobulin thereby rendering it unable to bind to cell surface receptors. However, the association between TGFß and alpha 2 macroglobulin can be reversed by polyanionic glycosaminoglycans such as heparin [12]. Since these are also normally present in the vessel wall where they are synthesised by both VSMCs and endothelial cells, this provides another potential local regulatory influence. In addition, the response to active TGFß may depend on the phenotypic state of the VSMCs and this, in turn, may be influenced by their extracellular environment, as discussed below. Therefore, because the biological effects of TGFß can be regulated at so many different levels, the demonstration of its presence in vascular lesions provides insufficient information to determine its function.

Effects of TGFß on VSMC proliferation in vitro

TGFß appears to exert different effects according to the culture conditions used and not all the reports on the effects of TGFb on VSMC proliferation agree. In one of the earliest reports Assoian and Sporn [3] found that TGFß inhibited proliferation of mitogen-stimulated subconfluent monolayers of bovine aortic VSMCs but enhanced the effects of mitogens on VSMCs grown in soft agar. Consistent with this, Ouchi et al.[13] reported that TGFß can inhibit EGF-induced DNA synthesis in monolayers of rat aortic VSMCs. However, a more complex effect was reported by Majack who found that TGFß inhibited proliferation of sparsely plated rat VSMCs but enhanced proliferation of densely plated cells [14]. He postulated that this effect of TFGß on densely plated cultures might be responsible for their characteristic "hills and valleys' pattern at confluence.

In studies on neonatal human VSMCs in culture, Battegay et al.[15] found that TFGß had a bimodal effect on proliferation with a small stimulatory effect at low concentrations (<0.1ng/ml) and inhibition at high concentrations regardless of cell density. They suggested that this was because low concentrations of TGFß induced expression of PDGF A isoform which acted as an autocrine or paracrine growth factor, whilst high concentrations of TGFß inhibited expression of the PDGF a receptor required to bind PDGF AA. They argued that the effects of TGFß demonstrated by Majack [14] could be explained on the basis of the concentration of TGFß available per cell, the concentration per cell being high at low cell density and low at high cell density. They also postulated that limited diffusion of TGFß through agar might result in low concentrations reaching suspended cells thereby explaining the stimulatory effect of TGFß under these conditions [3]. A similar bimodal effect of TGFß on porcine arotic VSMCs was reported by Hwang et al [16] who also showed that high concentrations of TGFß (10ng/ml) inhibited PDGF-induced DNA synthesis. By contrast however, Janat and Liau [14] found that TGFß did not induce expression of PDGF A mRNA in rabbit aortic VSMCs yet it enhanced PDGF-induced mitogenesis . However, the effects of TGFß were not consistent in all VSMC strains tested, suggesting some heterogeneity of response.

These diverse reports on the effects of TGFß on VSMC proliferation cannot easily be reconciled. Some of the differences may be species dependent since VSMCs from rat, rabbit, pig and man exibit a number of differences in culture. Another important consideration is potential heterogeneity of VSMCs both within a population derived from a single vessel and between those derived from vessels of different ages. Recent studies from our own and other laboratories [18-24] have provided strong evidence for heterogeneity of VSMCs within a single vessel. Furthermore, there is substantial evidence showing that neonatal VSMCs behave differently form adult cells. In particular, we have found that TGFß has a marked effect on the morphology and growth characteristics of clones of VSMCs grown from neonatal rats (see below). Thus the results of experiments on the effects of TGFß on VSMC proliferation *in vitro* must be interpreted with caution. Nevertheless, despite these caveats, there does appear to be a consensus of opinion that concentrations of TGFß greater than 0.1ng/ml inhibit VSMC proliferation in a cencentration dependent manner [25-27].

Effect of TGFß on VSMC cell cycle

The mechanism by which TGFß inhibits VSMC proliferation appears to depend on the mitogen used to stimulate the cells. Morisaki et al.[26] demonstrated that TGFß delayed expression of the *c-myc* proto-oncogene and inhibited DNA synthesis in PDGF-stimulated rabbit aortic VSMCs, clearly demonstrating an effect on the G1 phase of the cell cycle. However, this effect was much greater in cells stimulated with single mitogens than in cells stimulated with serum. Consistent with these findings, we have found that TGFß inhibits DNA synthesis in rat aortic VSMCs stimulated with either PDGF or EGF. However, in serum-stimulated cells we have found that TGFß has little effect on DNA synthesis. Instead it exerts an antiproliferative effect by prolonging the G2 phase of the cell cycle such that all the cells complete the cell cycle, but at a slower rate (Grainger et al, unpublished observations). These findings confirmed similar observations made by Bjorkerud [27] on human VSMCs and Owens et al.[25] on normotensive rat VSMCs. Thus, depending on the culture conditions, TGFß can either prevent (G1 effect) or slow (G2 effect) proliferation .

Heparin, which is known to release TGFß from its binding

proteins [12], also inhibits VSMC proliferation *in vitro* [28-30]. McCaffrey et al.[12]showed that heparin increased the concentration of free TGFß by preventing its association with alpha 2 macroglobulin and found that the short term antiproliferative effects of heparin required the presence of active TGFß. More recently they have shown that fucoidan, a polyanionic substance which is structurally distinct from heparin and which has little anticoagulant activity, binds to TGFß more avidly than heparin and is a more potent antiproliferative agent than heparin on VSMCs *in vitro* and following balloon injury in the rat carotid [32]. In recent experiments we have found that heparin inhibits proliferation of serum-stimulated rat VSMCs by extending the G2 phase of the cell cycle [32] and that this effect can be abolished by a neutralizing antibody to TGFß [19]. Thus it appears that heparin may exert a substantial part of its antiproliferative effect on VSMCs *in vitro* and possibly *in vivo* via release of TGFß.

Effect of TGFß on VSMC phenotype and extracellular matrix formation.

TGFß has been shown to be involved in the differentiation of a number of different cell types including adipocytes, myocytes and chondrocytes [33]. When VSMCs are dispersed in cell culture they lose contractile proteins and modulate to a 'synthetic' phenotype as they proliferate [34-36]. Since the majority of VSMCs in atheromatous plaques appear to be in a synthetic phenotype [37] it has been suggested that a change form a contractile to a synthetic phenotype is necessary for VSMC proliferation. However, we [38] and others [39] have shown that loss of smooth muscle-specific proteins occurs spontaneously in cell culture in the absence of mitogens where no proliferation occurs. This indicates that the phentoypic change is due not to mitogenic stimulation but to removal of the cells from their extracellular matrix. The matrix contains large quantities of collagen and glycosaminoglycans which could maintain the VSMCs in their contractile state. Consistent with this hypothesis it has been shown that VSMCs plated onto a collagen matrix [40]or into medium containing heparin remain in the contractile phenotype even in the presence of serum [39]. Furthermore, we have shown that, as for the effect of heparin on cell proliferation, its effect on VSMC phenotype can be abolished by neutralizing antibodies to TGFß [19]. However, TGFß does not exert its antiproliferative effect via inhibition of phenotypic modulation since it is equally effective at slowing proliferation of passaged VSMCs which have lost their capacity to re-express substantial quantities of smooth muscle-specific contractile proteins. Thus TGFß is capable of maintaining VSMCs in the contractile phenotype and inhibiting their proliferation by independent effects. Furthermore, since VSMCs in primary cultures treated with heparin or TGFß remain in the contractile phenotype yet proliferate [19,32], albeit at a slower rate than in the absence of TGFß, this demonstrates that the change from a contractile to a synthetic phenotypic is not obligatory for proliferation. These findings are consistent with those of Bjorkerud who showed that TGFß inhibited proliferation of human VSMCs in culture and promoted expression of a smooth muscle actin in cells which continued to proliferate with a prolonged cell cycle time [27].

The effect of TGFß on cells which have modulated to a synthetic phenotype in culture may be different from the effect on contractile VSMCs. A number of groups have shown that cultured VSMCs synthesise and secrete large quantities of extracellular matrix proteins including sulphated glycoproteins [41,42] collagen [43] and thrombospondin [17,44,45]. Thrombospondin is a high molecular weight protein which is also stored in a granules of platelets and is synthesised by a number of connective tissue cells. Its function is to bind cell surfaces to matrix macromolecules and it has been suggested that its synthesis and deposition are essential for VSMC proliferation. Majak et al [45] showed that TGFß induces an increase in thrombospondin mRNA in VSMCs and that this effect was density dependent, delayed compared with PDGF A mRNA expression and was blocked by cycloheximide. This suggested that TGFß induced thrombospondin production via PDGF AA. By contrast, Janat and Liau demonstrated that TGFß and PDGF induced thrombospondin expression in rabbit VSMCs by independent mechanisms which could act synergistically [17]. In addition, TGFß induces increased synthesis of fibronectin in a number of cell types [1] and fibronectin has been shown to enhance the phenotypic modulation from contractile to synthetic in cell culture [40]. Thus the available evidence suggests that although TGFß serves to maintain VSMCs in their contractile phenotype, it enhances production of extracellular matrix proteins which favour maintenance of the synthetic phenotype in cells which have been allowed to modulate. Furthermore, TGFß also increases expression of a number of protease inhibitors including PAI-1, collagenase inhibitors and tissue inhibitor of metalloproteinase which favour the accumulation of extracellular matrix proteins [1].

Effects of TGFß on proliferation of VSMC clones

The conventional view of the participation of VSMCs in proliferative vascular lesions assumes a homogeneous population of contractile

VSMCs which modulate to a synthetic phenotype on migrating into the intima and proliferating. However, there is increasing evidence in favour of heterogeneity of VSMCs [18-24]. By cloning VSMCs from neonatal and adult rat aortae we have identified three types of VSMC which may represent phenotypes in a VSMC lineage (Grainger et al, submitted). One group consists of small cells which grow with a cobblestone morphology and proliferate in the absence of added mitogens, suggesting the production of an autocrine growth factor. In many ways these cells resemble VSMCs grown by others from neonatal rat aortae. The second group consists of intermediate size, spindle-shaped cells which grow in a characteristic 'hills and valleys' pattern and are reminiscent of the predominant cell morphology in standard cultures of adult aortic VSMCs. These cells will not grow in the absence of added mitogens. The third group consists of large, often multinucleate cells with limited proliferative capacity. All three types could be isolated from both neonatal and adult rat aortae. However, aortae from young rats yielded high proportions of the small cell clones whilst aortae from older rats yielded fewer small cell clones and higher proportions of intermediate and large cell clones.

These findings are consistent with two related hypotheses; firstly, that small neonatal-like cells exist in the adult vessel wall and may proliferate preferentially in the context of vascular injury and secondly, that these cells mature to the larger cell types with increasing age. The latter hypothesis necessarily implies an ability for small cells to change to intermediate and large cells. Consistent with this we have found that if small cells, whose morphological and growth charactistics are stable over many passages in culture, are treated with exogenous TGFß they rapidly become larger, spindle-shaped cells with all the characteristics of intermediate size cells. Furthermore, if these cells are plated at low cell density, a proportion of them will convert to large, polyploid, non-proliferating cells.

Thus there are at least two distinct ways in which TGFß may influence VSMC phenotype *in vitro* and possibly, therefore, *in vivo*. Firstly, it maintains expression of VSMC-specific contractile proteins in 'differentiated' adult VSMCs. Secondly, it is capable of causing 'maturation' of small, cobblestone VSMCs to intermediate size, spindle-shaped cells. However, it should be stressed that these are two entirely distinct effects since the 'maturation' process is not associated with upregulation of contractile proteins.

From the above account it is clear that the effects of TGFß on VSMCs are varied and complex and influenced by a number of factors which might prevail in the intact vessel wall. Prediction of the role of TGFß in vascular disease *in vivo* is therefore problematic.

Nevertheless, there are sufficient experimental data to permit hypotheses to be formulated on its role in both hypertension and obliterative vascular disease.

Role of TGFß in hypertension

In hypertension there is increased thickness of the vessel media with a consequent decrease in maximum lumen diameter leading to increased vascular resistance. This is due to growth of VSMCs within the media (reviewed in ref 46). At present the nature of the VSMC growth in hypertension is unclear. In large conductance vessels, such as the aorta, it is thought to be due predominantly to VSMC hypertrophy (enlargement without proliferation). This notion is supported by an increased incidence of polyploid cells within the aortic media in hypertensive animals [47,48]. However, in resistance vessels such as the mesenteric arteries, VSMC proliferation may contribute [49]. It was once thought that the VSMC growth in hypertension was a consequence of elevated blood pressure. However, more recently attention has focused on the possibility that the increased vascular tone which characterises hypertension and the coincident VSMC hypertrophy and/or hyperplasia may be caused independently by a common stimulus. In this context a number of investigators have found that, under certain circumstance, the vasoconstrictor peptide AII might be mitogenic for VSMCs [50-53].

When VSMCs from normotensive rats are stimulated with AII in the absence of other mitogens there is upregulation of the protooncogenes *c-myc, c-fos* and *c-jun*, increased expression of PDGF A mRNA and increased protein synthesis, yet there is no DNA synthesis [54,55]. However, when VSMCs are stimulated with AII they also synthesise TGFß [56-58]. Therefore, any mitogenic effect of AII might be inhibited by TGFß and the net effect of AII stimulation would be arrest in G1 and hypertrophy without proliferation [25]. In support of this, Dzau's group has shown firstly, that conditioned medium from VSMCs which have been stimulated by AII contains PDGF A peptide and secondly, that AII stimulation of VSMCs leads to DNA synthesis and proliferation in the presence of a neutralizing antibody to TGFß [55]. More recent experiments using antisense oligonucleotides to TGFß have confirmed the role of TGFß in inhibiting a proliferative response to AII [59]. Furthermore, they postulate that AII can induce activation of secreted TGFß by stimulating expression of tPA by the VSMCs [55].

Whilst the above model provides a plausible explanation for VSMC hypertrophy it does not account for the increased incidence of polyploidy in hypertension. However, as discussed above, the effects of TGFß on the cell cycle of VSMCs depends on the conditions involved; inhibition in G1 when stimulated by single mitogens such as PDGF or prolongation of G2 when stimulated with serum. Owens et al [25] showed that when serum-stimulated rat VSMCs in culture were treated with TGFß, their rate of proliferation was slowed and the cells increased in size and protein content. Furthermore, chronic treatment with TGFß resulted in an accumulation of cells in the G2 phase of the cell cycle and subsequent removal of TGFß resulted in an increased number of polyploid cells. Since the VSMCs involved in hypertension remain within the media of the vessel and are surrounded by an heparin-containing extracellular matrix, any TGFß produced should be freely available and should serve to maintain the cells in their contractile state. Thus the known effects of TGFß could explain both VSMC hypertrophy and polyploidy in hypertension. However, these effects do not explain the hyperplasia which may occur in some hypertensive vessels.

Recent experiments on VSMCs from spontaneously hypertensive rats (SHR) have provided another potential role for TGFß in hypertension. SHR-VSMCs proliferate more rapidly than VSMCs from normotensive strains in vitro. [60-63] Hamet et al [64] demonstrated that SHR-VSMCs increased DNA synthesis in response to TGFß when plated at high density, but not at low density. No such effect was seen in cells from normotensive Wistar-Kyoto (WKY) rats. Stouffer and Owens [65] showed that AII induced DNA synthesis in high density cultures of SHR-derived VSMCs. However DNA synthesis was delayed compared with that induced by growth factors such as EGF, bFGF or PDGF suggesting the induction of an intermediate mitogen. The mitogenic effect of AII was abolished by an antibody to TGFß. Curiously however, they failed to detect any direct effect of TGFß on SHR-derived VSMC growth when added alone to the medium, indicating that additional autocrine factors were required for the AII-mediated proliferative response. Taken with the results from studies on normotensive rats cited above, these data suggest that the cellular response to AII and possibly TGFß may be genetically determined and may therefore be involved in the vascular changes in some forms of hypertension. However, the relevence of these findings to human hypertension remain to be established.

The role of TGFß in atherosclersotic vascular disease

In obliterative vascular diseases such as atherosclerosis, VSMCs migrate from the media and proliferate in the intima where they secrete extracellular matrix proteins and form a lipid-rich plaque which encroaches on the vascular lumen. A similar but more rapid process occurs in response to intimal damage following therapeutic angioplasty leading to restenosis in a high proportion of cases [66]. Inappropriate intimal VSMC proliferation also occurs in vascular bypass grafts and the arteries of transplanted organs leading ultimately to graft occlusion and organ failure respectively [67]. By contrast with hypertension, where the VSMCs remain in the media of the vessel and remain in a contractile phenotype, in atherosclerosis and the response to intimal injury the VSMCs involved in the lesion are in the intima and generally conform to the synthetic phenotype.

One explanation for these findings is that that medial VSMCs migrate into the intima in response to injury or endothelial dysfunction and in so doing change from a contractile cell with limited synthetic capacity to a cell with limited contractile capacity which is geared to synthesise and secrete matrix proteins and proliferate. Having done so it might be anticipated that the effects of TGFß would be twofold; firstly to constrain or prevent the proliferative response to circulating or locally produced mitogens and secondly to induce synthesis and secretion of extracellular matrix proteins. Thus the predicted effect of TGFß would be to reduce the cellularity and increase the matrix component of a plaque.

An alternative hypothesis proposes firstly, that VSMCs in the intima share characteristics with neonatal VSMCs and secondly, that they are derived from a population of neonatal-like VSMCs in the vessel wall whose characteristics allow them to migrate and proliferate preferentially following vascular injury [68,69]. This hypothesis implies heterogeneity of the VSMCs in the vessel wall and is entirely compatible with the observations of Benditt and Benditt who showed that the VSMCs in many atheromatous plaques are monoclonal [70]. Walker et al.[71] showed that cultured VSMCs from intimal lesions following balloon-induced intimal injury in the rat carotid artery had a cobblestone morphology and secreted PDGF-like activity into the medium. These cells were similar to those grown previously from the normal media of neonatal rats [72]. By contrast, VSMCs grown from the healthy media of the undamaged carotid artery grew with the characteristic 'hills and valleys' morphology and produced little PDGF-like activity. It follows that the intimal phenotype was either induced or selected in response to injury. However, the fact that medial VSMCs did not adopt a similar phenotype when induced to proliferate *in vitro* suggests that the intimal-phenotype cells in the lesion may have been selected from a distinct cell population. Consistent with this,

Dartsch et al. [24] showed that VSMCs derived from human restenosing lesions proliferate more rapidly in culture and have a different morphology from cultured VSMCs derived from the normal media or primary athreomatous plaques.

Taken together with our recent findings on VSMC clones, described above, these studies provide compelling evidence for VSMC hererogeneity *in vitro*. Furthermore, they support, but do not confirm the hypothesis that a subpopulation of small, neonatal-like cells may proliferate preferentially following vascular injury. If such cells exist in the adult vessel wall, albeit at low frequency, then it should be possible to define culture conditions which favour their growth. In this context it is interesting to note that by culturing VSMCs from the adult rat aorta in plasma-derived serum, Schwartz et al.[73] obtained VSMCs which grew with a cobblestone morphology and which clearly did not require PDGF to sustain growth. However, until specific cell markers become available to identify such cells within the vessel wall *in vivo* the hypothesis remains unproven. Nevertherless, a model for the response to intimal injury which incorporates these findings can be proposed in which small, neonatal-like cells migrate preferentially into the intima in response to intimal damage and proliferate in response to circulating or local mitogens and proliferation is sustained by the production of an autocrine growth factor(s). If such cells are then exposed to active TGFß they would change into intermediate spindle-shaped cells which no longer produce an autocrine growth factor and are therefore less prone to proliferate. With the passage of time a proportion of these cells would modulate further to the non-proliferative large cells. This model does not exclude the possibility that some intermediate cells from the media may also migrate into the intima, change phenotype and, under the influence of TGFß, lay down extracellular matrix.

What is the role for TGFß in vivo?

Recent experiments involving balloon-induced intimal injury in animals have provided unequivocal evidence for increased TGFß mRNA and protein expression within the developing neointimal lesion [5]. More importantly, Nikol et al. [6] have demonstrated that TGFß is produced by VSMCs within human vascular lesions and is particularly highly expressed in restenosing lesions. From the above account it can clearly be seen that the presence of TGFß does not necessarily imply biological activity. Nevertheless, The correlation between TGFß expression and neointima formation has led to speculation that TGFß is acting to promote rather than inhibit VSMC proliferation. This notion appears to be supported by the demonstration by Majeski et al. [5] that an infusion of recombinant TGFß into rats two weeks after endothelial injury increases DNA synthesis in neointimal VSMCs. However, this simply confirms that pharmacological doses of TGFß can be mitogenic for VSMCs and the authors themselves caution against interpreting these results as indicating a growth-promoting role for locally produced TGFß within the vessel wall. It is equally possible that in such highly active lesions TGFß is constraining VSMC proliferation since the response of the VSMCs will be determined by their phenotypic state, local mitogens and the extracellular environment.

Summary

Further careful studies are needed in appropriate models to define the role of TGFß in vascular disease . It is to be hoped that novel techniques such as those for introducing new genes or antisense oligonucleotides into the vessel wall [74-80] may provide the tools to establish whether pharmacological manipulation of TGFß expression or activity is likely to be of benefit in the treatment of human vascular disease.

Acknowledgements

PLW is a British Heart Foundation (BHF) Senior Research Fellow. The BHF Vascular Smooth Muscle Cell Group is supported by BHF Group and Project Grants to JCM and PLW. DJG is a Wellcome Prize Student.

References

1. Massague J. The transforming growth factor-ß family. Annu Rev Biol 1990; 6: 597-41.
2. Sporn MB, Roberts AB. Transforming growth factor-ß: Recent progress and new challenges. J Cell Biol 1992; 119: 1017-21.
3. Assoian RK, Sporn MB. Type beta transforming growth factor in human platelets: release during platelet degranulation and action on vascular smooth muscle cells. J Cell Biol 1986; 102: 1217-23.

4.   Assoian RK, Fleurdelys BE, Stevenson HC, Miller PJ, Madtes DK, Raines EW, Ross R, Sporn MB. Expression and secretion of type beta transforming growth factor by activated human macrophages. Proc Natl Acad Sci USA. 1987; 84: 6020-4.

5.   Majesky MW, Lindner V, Twardzik DR, Schwartz SM. Production of transforming growth factor beta-1 during repair of arterial injury. J Clin Invest 1991; 88: 904-10.

6.   Nikol S, Isner JM, Pickering G, Kearney M, Leclerc G, Weir L. Expression of transforming growth factor-ß1 is increasing in human vascular restenosis lesions. J Clin Invest 1992; 90: 1582-92.

7.   Lyons RM, Gentry LE, Purchino AF, Moses HL. Mechanism of activation of latent recombinant transforming growth factor ß1 by plasmin. J Cell Biol 1990; 110: 1361-7.

8.   Clowes AW, Clowes MM, Au YP, Reidy MA, Belin D. Smooth muscle cells express urokinase during mitogenesis and tissue-type plasminogen activator during migration in injured rat carotid artery. Circ Res 1990; 67: 61-7.

9.   Schneiderman J, Sawdy M, Loskutoff D. Chronic dexamethasone treatment modulates the response of the PAI-1 gene to lipopolysaccharide in rats. Thromb Haem 1991; 65: 652-7.

10. Reilly CF, McFall RC. Platelet-derived growth factor and transforming growth factor-ß regulate plasminogen activator inhibitor-1 synthesis in vascular smooth muscle cells. J Biol Chem 1991, 266: 9419-27.

11. O'Connor-McCourt MD, Wakefield LM. Latent transforming growth factor-S in serum. A specific complex with a2-macroglobulin. J Biol Chem 1987; 262: 14090-99.

12. McCaffrey TA, Falcone DJ, Brayton CF, Agarwal LA, Welt FG, Weksler BB. Transforming growth factor-beta activity is potentiated by heparin via dissociation of the transforming growth factor-beta/alpha 2-macroglobulin inactive complex. J Cell Biol 1989; 109: 441-8.

13. Ouchi Y, Hirosumi J, Watanabe M, Hattori A, Nakamura T, Orimo H. Inhibitory effect of transforming growth factor-beta on epidermal growth factor-induced proliferation of cultured rat aortic smooth muscle cells. Biochem Biophys Res Comm 1988; 157: 301-7.

14. Majack RA. Beta-type transforming growth factor specifies organizational behaviour in vascular smooth muscle cultures. J Cell Biol 1987;105:465-71.

15. Battegay EJ, Raines EW, Siefert RA, Bowen-Pope DF, Ross R. TGF-ß induces bimodal proliferation of connective tissue cells via complex control of an autocrine PDGF loop. Cell 1990; 63: 515-24.

16. Hwang DL, Latus LJ, Lev-Ran A. Effects of platelet-contained growth factors (PDGF, EGF, IGF-1, and TGF-ß) on DNA synthesis in porcine aortic smooth muscle cells in culture. Exp Cell Res 1992; 200: 358-60.

17. Janat MF, Liau G. Transforming growth factor ß1 is a powerful modulator of platelet-derived growth factor action in vascular smooth muscle cells. J Cell Physiol 1992; 150: 232-42.
18. Grainger DJ, Metcalfe JC, Weissberg PL. Primary confluent vascular smooth muscle cells (VSMCs) are inhomogeneous with respect to smooth muscle specific myosin heavy chain (SM-MHC) content. Clin Sci 1991; 81: 25p.
19. Weissberg PL, Grainger DJ, Shanahan CM, Metcalfe JC. Approaches to the development of selective inhibitors of vascular smooth muscle cell proliferation. Cardiovas Res: in press.
20. Dilberto PA, Gordon G, Herman B. Regional and mechanistic differences in platelet-derived growth factor isoform-induced alterations in cytosolic free calcium in porcine vascular smooth muscle cells. J Biol Chem 1991; 266: 12612-7.
21. Babaev VR, Bobryshev YV, Stenina OV, Tararak EM, Gabbiani G. Heterogeneity of smooth muscle cells in atheromatous plaques of human aorta. Am J Physiol 1990; 136: 1031-42.
22. Orekhov AN, Krushinsky AV, Andreva ER, Repin VS, Smirnov VN. Adult human aortic cells in primary culture: heterogeneity in shape. Heart Vessels 1986; 2: 193-201.
23. Dartsch P, Weiss HD, Betz E. Human vascular smooth muscle cells in culture: growth characteristics and protein pattern by use of serum-free media supplements. Eur J Cell Biol 1990; 51: 285-94.
24. Dartsch PC, Voisard R, Bauriedel G, Hofling B, Betz E. Growth characteristics and cytoskeletal organization of cultured smooth muscle cells from human primary stenosing and restenosing lesions. Arteriosclerosis 1990; 10: 62-75.
25. Owens GK, Geisterfer AA, Yang YW, Komoriya A. Transforming growth factor-beta-induced growth inhibition and cellular hypertrophy in cultured vascular smooth muscle cells. J Cell Biol 1988; 107: 771-80.
26. Morisaki N, Kawano M, Koyama N, Koshikawa T, Umemiya K, Saito Y, Yoshida S. Effects of transforming growth factor-ß on growth of aortic smooth muscle cells. Atherosclerosis 1991; 88: 227-34.
27. Bjorkerud S. Effects of transforming growth factor-ß1 on human arterial smooth muscle cells in vitro. Arteriosclerosis and Thrombosis 1991; 11: 892-902.
28. Castellot JJ, Beeler DL, Rosenberg RD, Karnovsky MJ. Structural determinants of the capacity of heparin to inhibit the proliferation of vascular smooth muscle cells. J Cell Physiol 1984; 120: 315-20.
29. Reilly CF, Kindy MS, Brown KE, Rosenberg RD, Sonenshein GE. Heparin prevents vascular smooth muscle cell progression through the G1 phase of the cell cycle. J Biol Chem 1989; 264: 6990-5.

30. Reilly CF, Fritze LMS, Rosenberg RD. Antiproliferative effects of heparin on vascular smooth muscle cells are reversed by epidermal growth factor. J Cell Physiol 1987; 131: 149-57.

31. McCaffrey TA, Falcone DJ, Borth W, Brayton CF, Weksler BB. Fucoidan is a non-anticoagulant inhibitor of intimal hyperplasia. Biochem Biophys Res Comm 1992; 184: 773-81.

32. Grainger DJ, Witchell C, Shachar-Hill Y, Weissberg PL, Metcalfe JC. Heparin partially inhibits proliferation of vascular smooth muscle cells (VSMCS) by extending the G2 phase of the cell cycle. Clin Sci 1991; 81: 22p.

33. Massague J. The TGF-ß family of growth and differentiation facotrs. Cell 1987; 49: 437-8.

34. Chamley-Campbell JH, Campbell GR, Ross R. Phenotype-dependent response of cultured aortic smooth muscle cells to serum mitogens. J Cell Biol 1981; 89: 379-83.

35. Thyberg J, Palmberg L, Nilsson J, Ksaizek T, Sjolund M. Phenotype modulation in primary cultures of arterial smooth muscle cells. On the role of platelet-derived growth factor. Differentiation 1983; 25: 156-63.

36. Chamley-Campbell J, Campbell GR, Ross R. The smooth muscle cell in culture. Physiol Rev 1979; 59: 1-61.

37. Mosse PRL, Campbell GR, Wang ZL, Campbell JH. Smooth muscle phenotypic expression in human carotid arteries. I. Comparison of cells from diffuse intimal thickenings adjacent to atheromatous plaques with those of the media. Lab Invest 1985; 53: 556-62.

38. Grainger D, Hesketh R, Metcalfe JC, Weissberg PL. First entry into M phase causes a large accumulation of non-muscle myosin in rat vascular smooth muscle cells. Biochem J 1991; 277: 145-51.

39. Chamley-Campbell JH, Campbell GR. What controls smooth muscle phenotype? Atherosclerosis 1981; 40: 347-57.

40. Hedin U, Bottger BA, Forsberg E, Johansson S,Thyberg J. Diverse effects of fibronectin and laminin on phenotypic properties of cultured arterial smooth muscle cells. J Cell Biol 1988; 107: 307-319.

41. Schonherr E, Jarvelainen HT, Sandell LJ, Wight TN. Effects of platelet-derived growth factor and transforming growth factor-ß 1 on the synthesis of large versican-like chondroitin sulfate proteoglycan by arterial smooth muscle cells. J Biol Chem 1991; 266: 17640-7.

42. Chen JK, Hoshi H, McKeehan WL. Stimulation of human arterial smooth muscle cell chondroitin sulfate proteoglycan synthesis by transforming growth factor-beta. In Vitro Cell Dev Biol 1991; 27: 6-12.

43. Schlumberger W, Thie M, Rauterberg J, Robenek H. Collagen synthesis in cultured aortic smooth muscle cells. Modulation by collagen lattice culture transforming growth factor-beta 1, and epidermal growth factor. Arterioscler Thromb 1991; 11: 1660-6.

44. Kobayashi S, Yamamoto T. The molecular biologic study of the expression of thrombospondin in vascular smooth muscle cells and mesangial cells. J Diabet Complications 1991; 5: 121-3.

45. Majack RA, Goodman LV, Dixit VM. Cell surface thrombospondin is functionally essential for vascular smooth muscle cell proliferation. J Cell Biol 1988; 106: 415-22.

46. Owens GK. Control of hypertrophic versus hyperplastic growth of vascular smooth muscle cells. Am J Physiol 1989; 257: H1755-H1765.

47. Owens G, Rabinovitch P, Schwartz S. Smooth muscle cell hypertrophy versus hyperplasia in hypertension. Proc Natl Acad Sci 1981; 78: 7759-63.

48. Owens G, Schwartz S. Vascular smooth muscle cell hypertrophy and hyperploidy in Goldblatt hypertensive rat. Cir Res 1983; 53: 491-501.

49. Mulvany M, Baandrup U, Gundersen H. Evidence for hyperplasia in mesenteric resistance vessels of spontaneously hypertensive rats using a three-dimensional disector. Circ Res 1985; 57: 749-800.

50. Dzau V J, Gibbons GH, Pratt RE, Molecular mechanisms of vascular renin-angiotensin system in myointimal hyperplasia. Hypertension 1991; 18[suppl II]: II-100-II-105.

51. Dzau V, Gibbons GH. Autocrine-paracrine mechanisms of vascular myocytes in systemic hypertension. Am J Cardiol 1987; 60: 99I-103I.

52. Geisterfer AAT, Peach MJ, Owens GK. Angiotensin II induces hypertrophy, not hyperplasia, of cultured rat aortic smooth muscle cells. Circ Res 1988; 62: 749-56.

53 Stouffer G, Owens GK. Angiotensin II-induced mitogenesis of spontaneously hypertensive rat-derived cultured smooth muscle cells is dependent on autocrine production of transforming growth factor-ß. Circ Res 1992; 70: 820-8.

54. Naftilan AJ, Pratt RE, Dzau VJ. Induction of platelet-derived growth factor A chain and c-myc gene expressions by angiotensin II in cultured rat vascular smooth muscle cells. J Clin Invest 1989; 83: 1419-24.

55. Gibbons GH, Pratt RE, Dzau VJ. Vascular smooth muscle cell hypertrophy vs hyperplasia. J Clin Invest 1992; 90: 456-61.

56. Hahn AWA, Resink TJ, Bernhardt J, Ferracin F, Buhler F. Stimulation of autocrine platelet-derived growth factor AA-homodimer and transforming growth factor ß in vascular smooth muscle cells. Biochem Biophys Res Comm 1991; 178: 1451-8.

57. Scott-Burden T, Resink TJ, Hahn AW, Buhler FR. Induction of thrombospondin expression in vascular smooth muscle cells by angiotensin II. J Cardiovas Pharmacol 1990; 16 (suppl 7): S17-20.

58. Powell JS, Rouge M Muller RK, Baumgartner HR. Cilazapril suppresses myointimal proliferation after vascular injury: effects on growth factor induction in vascular smooth muscle cells. Basic Res Cardiol 1991; (86 suppl 1): 65-74.

59. Itoh H, Pratt RE, Dzau VJ. Antisense oligonucleotides complementary to PDGF mRNA attenuate angiotensin II-induced hypertrophy. Hypertension 1990; 16: 325.

60. Yamori Y, Igawa T, Kanabe T, Kihara M, Nara Y, Horie R. Mechanisms of structural vascular changes in genetic hypertension: analysis on cultured vascular smooth muscle cells from spontaneously hypertensive rats. Clin Sci 1981; 61: 121S-123S.

61. Hamet P, Hadrava V, Kruppa U, Tremblay J. Vascular smooth muscle cell hyperresponsiveness to growth factors in hypertension. J Hypertens 1988; 6 (suppl 4): S36-S39.

62. Scott-Burden T, Resink TJ, Baur U, Burgin M, Buhler FR. Epidermal growth factor responsiveness in smooth muscle cells from hypertensive and normotensive rats. Hypertension 1989; 13: 295-304.

63. Hadrava V, Tremblay J, Hamet P. Abnormalities in growth characteristics of aortic smooth muscle cells in spontaneously hypertensive rats. Hypertension 1989; 13: 589-97.

64. Hamet P, Hadrava V, Kruppa U, Tremblay J. Transfoming growth factor ß1 expression and effect in aortic smooth muscle cells from hypertensive rats. Hypertension 1991; 17: 896-901.

65. Stouffer GA, Owens GK. Angiotensin II-induced mitogenesis of spontaneously hypertensive rat-derived cultured smooth muscle cells is dependent on autocrine production of transforming growth factor-ß. Circ Res 1992; 70: 820-8.

66. McBride W, Lange RA, Hillis LD. Restenosis after successful coronary angioplasty. Pathophysiology and prevention. N Engl J Med 1988; 318: 1734-7.

67. Barnhart GR, Pascoe EA, Mills AS, Szentpetery S, Eich DM, Mohanakumar T, Hastillo A, Thompson JA, Hess ML, Lower RR. Accelerated coronary arteriosclerosis in cardiac transplant recipients. Transplantation Rev 1987; 1: 31-46.

68. Majesky MW, Schwartz SM. Smooth muscle diversity in arterial wound repair. Toxicol Pathol 1990; 18: 554-9.

69. Schwartz SM, Campbell GR, Campbell JH. Replication of smooth msucle cells in vascular disease. Circ Res 1986; 58: 427-44.

70. Benditt EP, Benditt JM. Evidence for a monoclonal origin of human atherosclerotic plaques. Proc Natl Acad Sci USA 1973; 70: 1753-6.

71. Walker LN, Bowen-Pope DF, Ross R, Reidy MA. Production of platelet-derived growth factor-like molecules by cultured arterial smooth muscle cells accompanies proliferation after arterial injury. Proc Natl Acad Sci USA 1986; 83: 7311-15.

72. Seifert RA, Schwartz SM, Bowen-Pope DF. Developmentally regulated production of platelet-derived growth factor-like molecules. Nature 1984; 311: 669-71.

73. Schwartz SM, Foy L, Bowen-Pope DF, Ross R. Derivation and properties of platelet-derived growth factor-independent rat smooth muscle cells. Am J Pathol 1990; 136: 1417-28.

74. Nabel EG, Plautz G, Nabel GJ. Site-specific gene expression *in vivo* by direct gene transfer into the arterial wall. Science 1990; 249: 1285-8.

75. Nabel EG, Plautz G, Nabel GJ. Gene transfer into vascular cells. JACC 1991; 17: 189B-94B.

76. Nabel EG, Plautz G, Boyce FM, Stanley JC, Nabel GJ. Recombinant gene expression *in vivo* within endothelial cells of the arterial wall. Science 1989; 244: 1342-4.

77. Lim CS, Chapman GD, Gammon TS, Muhlstein JB, Bauman RP, Stack RS, Swain JL. *In vivo* gene transfer into canine coronary artery and peripheral arteries. Circulation 1991; 83: 2007-11.

78. Chapman GD, Lim CS, Gammon RS, Culp SC, Desper JS, Bauman RP, Swain JL, Stack RS. Gene transfer into coronary arteries of intact animals with a percutaneous balloon catheter. Circ Res 1992; 71: 27-33.

79. Flugelman MY, Jakitsch MT, Newman KD, Casscells W, Bratthauer MT, Dichek DA. Low level *in vivo* gene transfer into the arterial wall through a perforated balloon catheter. Circulation 1992; 85: 1110-7.

80. Simons M, Edelman ER, DeKeyser J-L, Langre R, Rosenberg RD. Antisense *c-myb* oligonucleotides inhibit intimal arterial smooth muscle cell accumulation *in vivo*. Nature 1992; 359: 67-70.

12. Some aspects of growth signal transduction in vascular smooth muscle cells

ANDREW C. NEWBY and NICHOLAS P. J. BRINDLE

INTRODUCTION

Proliferation of vascular smooth muscle cells (VSMC) is a characteristic feature of repair following vascular injury and adaptation to increased intraluminal pressure such as occurs in arteriovenous fistulas and in pulmonary hypertension. The intimal smooth muscle accumulation in atherosclerosis, restenosis after angioplasty and in vein grafts is arguably a consequence of these same repair and haemodynamic adaptation mechanisms [1]. Intimal VSMC proliferation becomes of pathological significance when it causes an obstruction of normal flow and can then lead to heart failure (especially if in the pulmonary circulation), angina pectoris (if in the coronary circulation), cerebral ischaemia or peripheral organ ischaemia. These circulatory diseases together represent the most prevalent causes of morbidity and mortality in the developed world [2] and there is therefore an intense clinical and basic research effort aimed at improving therapy, one target for which is the design of clinically useful inhibitors of VSMC proliferation. Frustratingly, despite some 50 or so recent clinical trials of agents that have been shown to be effective in tissue culture or animal models, none of these has been of consistent benefit in preventing angioplasty restenosis in man [3], which indicates the need for more potent and selective agents. One promising approach to achieving such inhibitors is to intervene in the intracellular signalling pathways that mediate proliferation. Such a strategy rationally depends on knowledge of the signalling pathways themselves and the extent to which these are tissue-specific for VSMC. In this article, we will attempt to overview the relative limited information regarding these pathways in VSMC, relying where necessary on analogies with other cell types.

Growth factor signal transduction pathways

Table 1. Some growth factors for VSMC

Growth factor	Receptor tyrosine Kinase	Induces PI turnover	Induces PDGFAA
Platelet derived growth factor (PDGF)	+	+	+
Basic fibroblast growth factor (bFGF)	+	+	+
Epidermal growth Factor (EGF	+	+	?
Insulin-like gowth factor-1 (IGF-1)	+	+/-	?
5-hydroxytryptamine (serotonin)	-	+	?
Endothelin-1 (ET-1)	-	+	+
Angiotensin II (ang II)	-	+	+
Interleukin-1 (IL-1)	-	-	+
Transforming growth Factor ß (TGF-ß)	-	-	+

Table 1 contains a list of some of the agents that have been shown to be mitogenic for VSMC. These agents can be immediately subdivided into those that appear to have a direct mitogenic effect such as platelet-derived growth factor (PDGF), basic fibroblast growth factor (bFGF), epidermal growth factor (EGF) and insulin-like growth factor-1 (IGF-1). A distinct group, for which the mitogenic effect is likely to be indirect, includes the cytokines interleukin-1 (IL-1) and transforming growth factor ß (TGF-ß) that induce the formation of the direct mitogen, PDGFAA [4, 5, 6]. An intermediate situation relates to agents, including serotonin endothelin-1 (ET-1) and angiotensin II (ang II) may have both direct and indirect mitogenic actions. These agents can be shown to be weak mitogens on their own but to potentiate the effect of PDGF [7, 8, 9, 10, 11]. However, ET-1 and ang II also induce the formation of PDGF and TGFß, which might stimulate proliferation indirectly [11, 12]. The agents in Table 1 can also be subdivided according to the known properties of their receptors. Interestingly, direct mitogens have in common an intrinsic tyrosine kinase activity activity, while those with indirect actions definitely do not. Because receptors with tyrosine kinase activity can potentially activate the gamma isoform of inositol-specific phospholipase C (PIC), they may also mobilize Ca^{2+} and activate protein kinase C (PKC). However, those purely Ca^{2+}-mobilizing hormones such as serotonin, ang II and ET-1 that do not have tyrosine kinase activity fall into the category of agents that may have either direct or indirect mitogenic actions. Based on the above arguements a simple working hypothesis can be formulated:

1. Mitogenic stimulation requires the activation of membrane receptor tyrosine kinase activity, although activation of non tyrosine kinase cytokine receptors may induce production of mitogens and lead to indirect stimulation of proliferation.
2. Activation of PIC can contribute directly and/or indirectly to the mitogenic response.

Each of these hypotheses will now be considered in detail.

Early responses to membrane receptor tyrosine kinase activation

PDGF, bFGF, EGF and the IGF-1, all act through receptors which have intrinsic tyrosine kinase activity that is stimulated by growth factor binding. The structural and functional characteristics of this group of receptors has been well reviewed [13, 14]. In summary, all consist of an extracellular ligand binding domain, a transmembrane region and an intracellular portion which contains the tyrosine kinase domain (see

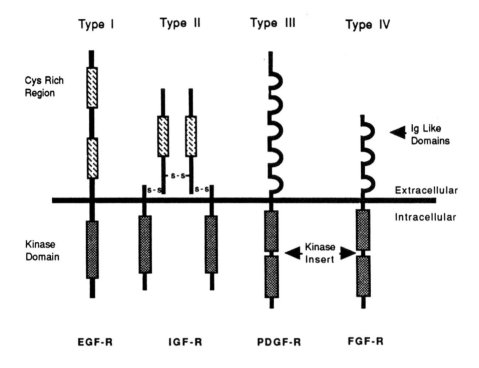

Figure 1. A schematic diagram of growth factor receptor structure.

Figure 1). The IGF-1 receptors are tetrameric structures consisting 2 pairs of identical subunits joined by disulphide bonds. The receptors for the other growth factors are monomers, but growth factor binding induces dimerization. Activated receptor kinases phosphorylate other proteins on tyrosine residues and also phosphorylate themselves, usually at multiple sites.

The importance of the ligand induced kinase activition in growth signal transduction has been established by several studies showing that mutant receptors deficient in kinase activity, while still able to bind agonist, fail to stimulate proliferation [15, 16, 17]. Furthermore, inhibitors of tyrosine kinase activity, such as genistein, negate the mitogenic actions of growth factors in cells, including VSMC [18, 19].

In elucidating how kinase activation leads to mitogenesis, it is important to identify the substrates for these tyrosine kinases and much effort has been devoted over the past 10 years to just this, using model systems ranging from from mouse fibroblasts to Drosophila eye cells. There is, however, little direct information in VSMC. One common feature of tyrosine kinase substrates that has emerged is that they contain sequences of amino acids known as SH2 domains; regions of about 100 amino acids homologous to part of the viral src oncoprotein [20]. SH2 domains mediate binding of proteins to phosphotyrosine residues, thus permitting substrates to bind to autophosphorylated growth factor receptors [20]. This brings the protein into close association with the receptor kinase and permit sphosphorylation to occur. It is likely that the different autophosphorylation sites on receptors interact with different SH2 containing substrates. In VSMC, PDGF stimulates tyrosine phosphorylation of at least six proteins, however, with the exception of the PGDF receptor, the identity of these substrates is not known [21, 22].

A kinase cascade has been implicated transducing the receptor-kinase activation from cell surface to nucleus; immediate substrates for the recetor tyrosine kinase being themselves kinases or phosphatases. These secondary kinases or phosphatases, which may act specifically on tyrosine, threonine or serine residues, activate substrates that may again be kinases or phosphatases. Eventually this sequence culminates in phosphorylation of an effector protein, such as a transcription factor that modulates expression of specific genes. To date, kinases that have been shown to be activated in response to growth factors include ribosomal S6 kinase (pp90rsk), mitogen activated protein kinases (MAPK) and Raf-1 [23, 24, 25]. At the effector end of the model, it has been shown that pp90rsk or MAPK can phosphorylate transcription factors c-fos, c-myc and c-jun as well as p62TCF, and modulate their activities [26, 27, 28, 29]. Thus several potential components have been identified that can be organised into a kinase cascade (see Figure 2). Initially, stimulation of the receptor kinase is believed to activate the oncoprotein p21ras [30]. p21ras is not a kinase but its activation has recently been shown to be associated with serine phosphorylation and resulting stimulation of the kinase Raf-1 [31]. Raf-1 can act, via an intermediate combined threonine and tyrosine kinase, to cause phosphorylation of MAPK [32]. Thus stimulated, MAPK can act on transcription factors directly or via phosphorylation of pp90rsk [33]. Other agonists, such as those utilizing PKC, may also interact to synergise or modulate the final response through components

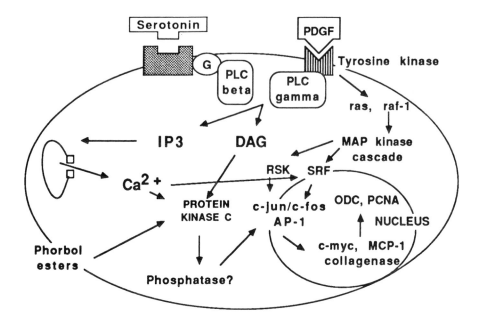

Figure 2. Pathways of mitogenic signal transduction.

of this kinase cascade (see Figure 2). For example, there is some evidence that PKC can increase ras activity [34]. The cascade outlined is therefore likely to be only part of a more complex network of pathways, and further interactions with other signalling systems will undoubtably be revealed.

Indeed, in addition to a kinase cascade, activated growth factor receptors have also been shown to interact with proteins involved in phosphoinositide (PI) metabolism and to have direct effects on possible transcription factors. The hydrolysis of plasma membrane phosphatidylinositol(4,5)bisphosphate (PIP$_2$) to generate the dual second messengers phosphoinositol(1,4,5)trisphosphate (IP$_3$) and diacylglycerol is catalysed by a family of phosphoinositide specific phospholipase C enzymes (PICs). As extensively reviewed [35, 36], one isoform, PIC-g contains two SH2 domains and hence is subject to tyrosine phosphorylation. Treatment of cells with PDGF or EGF results in a strong association of PIC-g with the growth factor receptor and an increase in tyrosine phosphate content, which correlates with increased PI hydrolysis. In addition, PIC-g also contains a src homology region 3 (SH3). This domain is seen in other tyrosine kinase substrates and is thought to mediate association of the protein with elements of the cytoskeleton [20]. Such an interaction with the cytoskeleton may permit PIC-g to act on phospholipids in the cell membrane. Tyrosine phosphorylation of the purified enzyme does not appear to affect activity [35], although it is enhanced in crude preparations [37]. This suggests that the stimulatory effect observed in cells may be by an indirect mechanism, possibly involving interaction with the cytoskeleton, as described above. The significance for mitogenesis of the growth factor-mediated activation of PIC-g and hence PI hydrolysis, has been brought into question by the following experiments. Mutation of a single specific tyrosine residue in the FGF receptor blocks its ability to interact with and phosphorylate PIC-g and abolishes stimulation of PI hydrolysis [38, 39], but has no effect on mitogenesis.

Another substrate for receptor tyrosine kinases is the Type I phosphatidylinositol kinase (PI3K), which is a heterodimeric protein with subunits of 110 and 85 kDa [40, 41]. The 85 kDa subunit contains both SH2 and SH3 domains and has been shown to associate with and be phosphorylated by activated PDGF and EGF receptors [42]. Association of PI3K with the activated PDGF receptor occurs at the kinase insert region of the receptor (see Fig. 1) [43, 44]. Deletion of this region eliminates PDGF stimulated PI3K association and mitogenesis but not PI hydrolysis, consistent with the idea that PI3K activation is essential for PDGF induced mitogenesis. However, it is also possible that in removing the insert domain the receptor is prevented from interacting with other essential mediators. It is likely that the physiological substrate of PI3K is PIP_2 [45, 46] because PDGF has been shown to increase phophoinositol(3,4,5)trisphosphate synthesis in mouse fibroblasts and rat VSMC. The product of PI3K does not lie on the classic IP_3 pathway and the function of inositol(1,3,4,5)tetrakisphosphate is not at present known, although it may itself be a novel intracellular messenger.

Another way in which receptor tyrosine kinases could transduce the growth factor signal is suggested in recent data on the proto-oncogene c-vav. This gene has homologies with known transcription factors and also has one SH2 and two SH3 domains [47] . When expressed in fibroblasts c-vav undergoes tyrosine phosphorylation in response to PDGF and EGF [48, 49]. Although c-vav expression has been reported only in haematopoietic cells, these observations raise the possibility that activated receptor kinases may directly act on proteins that could translocate to the nucleus and influence transcription.

As indicated above, the information on tyrosine kinase signalling pathways has been derived from a wide range of cell systems. In seeking to understand transduction of growth factor signals in VSMC, it will clearly be important to determine just what parts of these signalling systems operate and whether cell specific transduction cascades exist.

Early responses to PI turnover

The transduction pathways induced by growth factors are summarized schematically in Figure 2. One intial event is the hydrolysis of plasma membrane PIP_2 to generate the dual second messengers IP_3 and diacylglycerol [50]. The phosphoinositide specific phospholipase C (PIC) enzymes responsible belong to a family of at least 4 subtypes, of which the b and g isoforms are clearly associated with intracellular signalling. As detailed above, the g isoform is coupled to activation of tyrosine kinase receptors. The b isoform [35, 36] is activated in a rather different manner by a family of receptors, which includes those for serotonin, ET-1, and ang II, that contain 7 membrane-spanning domains [51]. These receptors lack intrinsic kinase activity but share the ability to activate members of the large family of guanyl-nucleotide binding transducing proteins (G-proteins) [52], members of which in turn can activate second messenger systems including PIC, adenylate cyclase and various ion channels. There is good evidence both from studies in intact cells and isolated membranes that G-proteins are essential mediators in the activation of PIC by this group of agents [36]. Once formed, IP_3 mediates the release of Ca^{2+} from endoplasmic reticulum stores [50]. Diacylglycerol activates one or more members of the PKC family of enzymes, in a process which involves translocation of the enzyme to the cytoplasmic face of the plasma membrane [53]. There are at least 8 isoenzymes of PKC [54], and VSMC cells appear to co-express more than one isoform [55]. It is assumed that the tissue specific expression of PKC isoforms has functional significance mediated by a difference in substrate specificity, although a clear picture of the roles of the individual isoforms has yet to emerge. All isoforms of the enzyme can be activated by synthetic diacylglycerols and their analogues, the tumour-promoting phorbol esters. These agents are mitogenic for cell including VSMC, which implies that activation of PKC alone may be a sufficient stimulus for proliferation [56, 57]. This conclusion is complicated, however, by the fact that phorbol esters elicit only a partial growth response in VSMC and may actually inhibit the response to an optimal mitogenic mixture, such as serum [55]. This may in part be mediated by down-regulation of the a isoform of PKC in response to prolonged activation [55], although other mechanisms are probably involved. Moreover, because G-protein linked mediators are poor mitogens on their own, but promote the action of other mitogens such as PDGF (see above), the primary role of PKC in VSMC may be to synergise with the tyrosine kinase pathway at the intracellular level. As discussed above, a mitogenic response can be obtained to FGF through a mutant receptor incapable of coupling to PIC-g. However, activation of another isoform of PIC by an endogenous G-protein linked mediator or basal activity of PKC may have been sufficient to sustain proliferation in these experiments. Consistent with this, inhibitors of protein kinase C, such as H7 and staurosporine are potent inhibitors of VSMC proliferation [58, 59]. These agents probably inhibit all PKC isoforms, but also inhibit cAMP and Ca^{2+}/calmodulin-dependent protein kinases [60]. This poor selectivity for PKC relative to these other kinases prompted us [61] to investigate the effect on VSMC proliferation of staurosporine derivatives with 100-fold greater specificity for PKC [60]. As shown in Table 2, 10 μM of the staurosporine derivatives, Ro 31-8220 or Ro 31-7549, profoundly inhibited the proliferative response of rabbit aortic VSMC to serum, PDGF plus serotonin or phorbol dibutyrate, without exerting a significant effect on viability measured by ATP concentration. In more detailed analysis (JW Assender, M Evans, AC Newby, unpublished observations), only minor differences in dose-response relationships were found for inhibition of the three mitogens, which is consistent with a common mechanism of action at the level of PKC. If so, this data implies that some activity of PKC is essential for a mitogenic response to agents that activate membrane tyrosine kinases.

Little work has been done in VSMC concerning the downstream events modulated by PKC activation, although this is partially understood in fibroblasts and some other cells. Two transcription activating factors that are present already in quiescent cells, namely serum response factor (SRF) and the oncogene c-jun, have been most strongly implicated in the initial events [62, 63]. These proteins are structurally unrelated and bind to distinct consensus sequences in the

Table 2. Effect of Ro 31-8220 and Ro 31-7549 on rabbit aortic VSMC proliferation and viability

Conditions	5% serum	20ng/ml PDGF+ 10 μM serotonin	0.1μM phorbol dibutyrate
	Thymidine incorporation (% control)		
10 μM Ro 31-8220	0.5±0.2*	9±4*	5±1*
10 μM Ro 31-7549	0.9±0.3*	8±3*	1.2±0.5*
	ATP concentration (% control)		
10 μM Ro 31-8220	110±20	120±10	110±10
10 μM Ro 31-7549	70±20	70±20	110±20

First passage rabbit aortic VSMC were rendered quiescent for 72 h in the absence of serum and then growth was reinitiated with the various mitogens shown. This led to a 65±14 (n=7), 4.7±0.9 (n=4) or 3.9±0.9 (n=4) fold stimulation of thymidine incorporation (1 μCi/ml) over the next 24 h in the presence of 5% FCS, 20 ng/ml of PDGFBB + 10μM serotonin or 0.1 μM phorbol dibutyrate, respectively. Values of thymidine incorporation and ATP concentration (by luminometry) were compared to those in the absence of PKC inhibitors. * p <0.001 vs control.

promotor region of a large group of so-called primary response genes that may number in total as many as 200 [63]. Both SRF and c-jun are phosphoproteins, which suggests that they may be regulated by phosphorylation/dephosphorylation. However, neither of these proteins appears to be directly activated by PKC [62]. Bacterially-expressed SRF is efficiently phosphorylated by casein kinase II on sites identical to those phosphorylated in intact cells and this promotes its interaction with DNA. Ca^{2+} elevation itself has been shown to stimulate c-fos expression fibroblasts [57], so the involvement of a calmodulin activated enzyme such as casein kinase II may be physiologically significant. Treatment of cells with phorbol ester actually decreases the phosphorylation of c-jun and this is believed to important for transcriptional activation [62]. The purified protein is a good substrate for glycogen synthase kinase 3, although this may not be the physiologically relevant kinase responsible for base-line phosphorylation of c-jun [62].

The SRF is 67kDa protein that binds alone to a consensus DNA sequence (for example in the c-fos gene) known as the serum response element (SRE); the binding of SRF may be enhanced also by a 62 kDa protein, p62TCF [63]. In contrast c-jun binds as a dimer to a distinct sequence, known as the TPA responsive element (TRE). For historical reasons, transcriptional activators at this site are often refered to as "activator protein-1" or AP-1 [62]. This nomenclature is unfortunate because a number of different proteins can express AP-1 activity, including the c-jun homodimer and dimers of the closely related proteins JunB and JunD. Interestingly, however, heterodimers of c-jun with c-fos (or members of this family, FosB Fra1, Fra2) have higher AP-1 activity than homodimers of the Jun family. Because c-fos is one of the most rapidly induced genes in response to growth factors, replacement c-jun dimers with c-fos/c-jun heterodimers could be one of the key events in triggering the primary response [62]. Members of the Fos family do not form homodimers and therefore do not show AP-1 activity on their own.

Among the earliest described primary response genes were the matrix-degrading metalloproteinases, collagenase and stromelysin [63]. We recently showed that metalloproteinase activity is essential for proliferation and emigration responses of VSMC in explants of rabbit aorta [64]. Seen in this light, collagenase induction is a rational part of the genetic response to growth factors. Induction of growth factor production and expression of growth factor receptors may also be a physiologically-important means of prolonging a growth response to a factor produced acutely, for example in response to injury [65]. Increasing the expression of monocyte chemotactic peptide -1 (the human equivalent of the rat early response gene JE) also appears most rational in the context of injury. Results discussed above suggest that activation of PIC-g is not rquired for a mitogenic response in cells adapted to tissue culture. It is possible nevertheless, that PIC-g and resulting PKC activation contributes to increased expression of genes, such as those for metalloproteinases, that are required for an optimal growth response in a tissue.

Are there unique features of the growth factor response in VSMC?

Recent success has been reported in inhibiting VSMC proliferation using antisense oligonucleotides to 2 ubiquitous cell cycle dependent proteins c-myb [66] and the 'proliferating cell nuclear antigen' (PCNA) [67]. In the former case [66], the oligonucleotides were applied to the external surface of vessels in live rats. The local application of antisense oligonucleotides or localized transfection [68] may therefore allow the targetting of any ubiquitous cell-cycle related protein for selective therapy. If a systemic therapy is to be developed, however, it should be directed ideally to a tranduction pathway specific for VSMC.

VSMC are kown to mount a typical primary response to growth factor stimulation [69, 70, 71] and vessel wall injury [72, 73], although many of the details of the proteins involved have not been documented. It is possible that cell-type specific utilization of transcriptional activators might suggest routes for selective inhibitory intervention but this remains to be demonstrated. A more obvious difference between VSMC and its close embryological relative, the fibroblast emerges when considering the interaction between the PKC pathways and another mediator, cAMP. Elevation of cAMP concentration appears to be a co-activator of proliferation in fibroblasts [56] but an inhibitor in VSMC [74]. Some primary response genes (for example c-fos) contain a cAMP response element (CRE) consensus sequence in their promotor region that interacts with the CRE binding protein, CREB [62, 63]. Activation of CREB is believed to underlie the growth response of fibroblasts to cAMP elevation and requires, in addition, an active cAMP-dependent protein kinase [62]. The different end-response to cAMP i.e. inhibition of proliferation of VSMC might be mediated upstream, downstream or at the level of early-response genes. For example, cAMP inhibits Ca^{2+} mobilization in a small number of tissues, including platelets [75] and contractile VSMC [76] and may therefore cocommitantly reduce PKC activation. However, we have recently observed that agonist stimulated Ca^{2+} elevation in cultured rabbit VSMC is not inhibited by cAMP [77], despite evidence for inhibition in aortic tissue [76]. This implies that the sensitivity of PIC to cAMP may be altered during modulation of VSMC into their proliferative phenotype. The effect of cAMP elevation on induction of early response genes does not appear to have been studied in VSMC. In preliminary studies [78], we found that a cAMP analogue only slowly reduced elevated c-myc expression in logarythmically growing rat aortic VSMC, concommittant with growth arrest, which argues against a direct action at the level of the c-myc promotor. In contrast, the effect of interferon g preceeded growth arrest. Timed additions of cAMP elevating agents to VSMC revealed that inhibition could be provoked as long as 12 hours after adding mitogens [79, 80, 81], which argues strongly for an effect of cAMP downstream of the early-immediate response. Data showing that cAMP is equally effective independent of the nature of mitogenic stimulation also argues for an effect on a late common pathway. The mechanism of cAMP inhibition of proliferation is therefore worthy of further study because it appears unique for VSMC amongst the vascular cells.

Acknowledgements

The authors work is supported by grants from the British Heart Foundation and the Heart Research Fund for Wales

References

1. Ip JH, Fuster V, Badimon L, Badimon J, Taubman MB, Chesebro JH. Syndromes of accelerated atherosclerosis: role of vascular injury and smooth muscle cell proliferation. J Am Coll Cardiol 1990; 15: 1667-1687.
2. Feinlieb M. Changing trends in atherosclerosis. In: Shepherd J, Morgan HG, Packard CJ, Brownlie SM editors Atherosclerosis: Developments, complications and treatment. Amsterdam: Elsevier Science Publishers, 1987: 53-64.
3. Califf RM, Fortin DF, Frid DJ, et al. Restenosis after coronary angioplasty: an overview. J Am Coll Cardiol 1991; 17 (Suppl B): 2B-13B.
4. Raines EW, Dower SK, Ross R. Interleukin-1 mitogenic activity for fibroblasts and smooth muscle cells is due to PDGF-AA. Science 1989; 243: 393-396.
5. Battegay E, Raines EW, Seifert RA, Bowen-Pope DF, Ross R. TGF-ß induces bimodal proliferation of connective tissue cells via complex control of an autocrine PDGF loop. Cell 1990; 63: 515-524.
6. Majack RA, Majesky MW, Goodman LV. Role of PDGF-A Expression in the Control of Vascular Smooth Muscle Cell Growth by Transforming Growth Factor-Beta. J Cell Biol 1990; 111(1): 239-247.

7. Araki S-I, Kawahara Y, Fukuzaki H, Takai Y. Serotonin plays a major role in serum-induced phospholipase C-mediated hydrolysis of phosphoinositides and DNA synthesis in vascular smooth muscle cells. Atherosclerosis 1990; 83: 29-34.

8. Hirata Y, Takagi Y, Fukuda Y, Marumo F. Endothelin is a potent mitogen for rat vascular smooth muscle cells. Atherosclerosis 1989; 78: 225-228.

9. Nakaki T, Nakayama M, Yamamoto S, Kato R. Endothelin-mediated stimulation of DNA synthesis in vascular smooth muscle cells. Biochem Biophys Res Comm 1989; 158(3): 880-883.

10. Weissberg PL, Witchell C, Davenport AP, Hesketh TR, Metcalfe JC. The Endothelin Peptides ET-1, ET-2, ET-3 and sarafotoxin S6b are Co-Mitogenic with Platelet-Derived Growth Factor for Vascular Smooth Muscle Cells. Atherosclerosis 1990; 85: 257-262.

11. Dzau VJ, Gibbons GH, Pratt RE. Molecular mechanisms of vascular renin-angiotensin system in myointimal hyperplasia. Hypertension 1991; 18(Suppl 2): II-100-II-105.

12. Hahn AWA, Resink TJ, Bernhardt J, Ferracin F, Bühler FR. Stimulation of autocrine platelet-derived growth factor AA-homodimer and transforming growth factorß in vascular smooth muscle cells. Biochem Biophys Res Commun 1991; 178: 1451-1458.

13. Ullrich A, Schlessinger J. Signal transduction by receptors with tyrosine kinase activity. Cell 1990; 61: 203-212.

14. Cadena DL, Gill GN. Receptor tyrosine kinases. FASEB J 1992; 6: 2332-2337.

15. Chen WS, Lazar CS, Poenie M, Tsien RY, Gill GN, Rosenfeld MG. Requirement for intrinsic protein tyrosine kinase in the immediate and late actions of the EGF receptor. Nature 1987; 328: 820-823.

16. Honegger AM, Szapary D, Schmidt A, et al. A mutant epidermal growth factor receptor with defective protein tyrosine kinase is unable to stimulate proto-oncogene expression and DNA synthesis. Mol Cell Biol 1987; 7: 4568-4571.

17. Williams LT. Signal transduction by the platelet-derived growth factor receptor. Science 1989; 243: 1564-1570.

18. Clegg KB, Sambhi MP. Inhibition of epidermal growth factor-mediated DNA synthesis by a specific tyrosine kinase inhibitor in vascular smooth muscle cells of the spontaneously hypertensive rat. J Hypertens 1989; 7: S144-S145.

19. Bilder GE, Krawiec JA, McVety K, et al. Tyrphostins inhibit PDGF-induced DNA synthesis and associated early events in smooth muscle cells. Am J Physiol 1991; 260: C721-C730.

20. Koch CA, Anderson D, Moran MF, Ellis C, Pawson T. SH2 and SH3 domains: elements that control interactions of cytoplasmic signaling proteins. Science 1991; 252: 668-674.

21. Tsuda T, Kawahara Y, Shii K, Koide M, Ishida Y, Yokoyama M. Vasoconstrictor-induced protein-tyrosine phosphorylation in cultured vascular smooth muscle cells. FEBS Letts 1991; 285: 44-48.

22. Koide M, Kawahara Y, Tsuda T, Ishida Y, Shii K, Yokoyama M. Stimulation of protein-tyrosine phosphorylation by endothelin-1 in cultured vascular smooth muscle cells. Atherosclerosis 1992; 92: 1-7.

23. Pelech SL, Sanghera JS. Mitogen-activated protein kinases: versatile transducers for cell signaling. TIBS 1992; 17: 233-238.

24. Rapp U. Role of Raf-1 serine/threonine protein kinase in growth factor signal transduction. Oncogene 1991; 6: 495-500.

25. Erikson RL. Structure, expression and regulation of protein kinases involved in the phosphorylation of ribosomal protein S6. J Biol Chem 1991; 266: 6007-6010.

26. Chen R-H, Chung J, Blenis J. Regulation of $pp90^{rsk}$ phosphorylation and S6 phosphotransferase activity in Swiss 3T3 cells by growth factor-, phorbol ester-, and cyclic AMP-mediated signal transduction. Mol Cell Biol 1991; 11: 1861-1867.

27. Alvarez E, Northwood IC, Gonzalez FA, et al. Pro-Leu-Ser/Thr-Pro is a consensus primary sequence for substrate protein phosphorylation. J Biol Chem 1991; 266: 15277-15285.

28. Pulverer BJ, Kyriakis JM, Avruch A, Nikolakaki E, Woodgett JR. Phosphorylation of c-*jun* mediated by MAP kinases. Nature 1991; 353: 670-674.

29. Gille H, Sharrocks AD, Shaw PE. Phosphorylation of transcription factor $p62^{TCF}$ by MAP kinase stimulates ternary complex formation at c-*fos* promoter. Nature 1992; 358: 414-417.

30. Downward J. Regulatory mechanisms for ras proteins. Bioessays 1992; 14: 177-184.

31. Williams NG, Roberts TM, Li P. Both $p21^{ras}$ and $pp60^{v-src}$ are required, but neither alone is sufficient, to activate the Raf-1 kinase. Proc Natl Acad Sci USA 1992; 89: 2922-2926.

32. Dent P, Haser W, Haystead TAJ, Vincent LA, Roberts TM, Sturgill TW. Activation of mitogen-activated protein kinase kinase by v-Raf in NIH 3T3 cells and *in vitro*. Science 1992; 257: 1404-1407.

33. Sturgill TW, Ray LB, Erikson E, Maller JL. Insulin-stimulated MAP-2 kinase phosphorylates and activates ribosomal protein S6 kinase II. Nature 1988; 334: 715-718.

34. Downward J, Graves JD, Warne GH, Rayter S, Cantrell DA. Stimulation of p21 ras upon T-cell activation. Nature 1990; 346: 719-723.

35. Rhee SG. Inositol-specific phospholipase C: interaction with the gamma1 isoform with tyrosine kinase. Trends in Biochem Sci 1991; 16: 297-301.

36. Meldrum E, Parker PJ, Carozzi A. The PtdIns-PLC superfamily and signal transduction. Biochim Biophys Acta 1991; 1092: 49-71.

37. Nishibe S, Wahl MI, Hernandez-Sotomayor SMT, Tonks NK, Rhee SG, Carpenter G. Increase of the catalytic activity of phospholipase C-g1 by tyrosine phosphorylation. Science 1990; 250: 1253-1256.

38. Mohammadi M, Dionne CA, Li W, et al. Point mutation of FDF receptor eliminates phosphatidylinositol hydrolysis without affecting mitogenesis. Nature 1992; 358: 681-684.

39. Peters KG, Marie J, Wilson E, et al. Point mutation of FGF receptor abolishes phosphatidylinositol turnover and Ca^{2+} flux but not mitogenesis. Nature 1992; 358: 678-681.

40. Carpenter CL, Duckworth BC, Auger KR, Cohen B, Schaffhausen BS, Cantley LC. Purification and characterization of phosphoinositide 3-kinase from rat liver. J Biol Chem 1990; 265: 19704-19711.

41. Shibasaki F, Homma Y, Takenawa T. Two types of phosphatidylinositol 3-kinase from bovine thymus. J Biol Chem 1991; 266: 8108-8114.

42. Cantley LC, Auger KR, Carpenter C, et al. Oncogenes and signal transduction. Cell 1991; 64: 281-302.

43. Coughlin SR, Escobedo JA, Williams LT. Role of phosphatidylinositol kinase in PDGF receptor signal transduction. Science 1989; 243: 1191-1194.

44. Kazlauskas A, Cooper JA. Autophosphorylation of the PDGF receptor in the kinase insert region regulates interactions with cell proteins. Cell 1989; 58: 1121-1133.

45. Auger KR, Serunian LA, Soltoff SP, Libby P, Cantley LC. PDGF-dependent tyrosine phosphorylation stimulates production of novel polyphosphoinositides in intact cells. Cell 1989; 57: 167-175.

46. Hawkins PT, Jackson TR, Stephens LR. Platelet-derived growth factor stimulates synthesis of $PtdIns(3,4,5)P_3$ by activating a $PtdIns(4,5)P_2$-OH kinase. Nature 1992; 358: 157-159.

47. Katzav S, Cleveland JL, Heslop HE, Pulido D. Loss of the amino-terminal helix-loop domain of the *vav* proto-oncogene activates its transforming potential. Mol Cell Biol 1991; 11: 1912-1920.

48. Bustelo XR, Ledbetter JA, Barbacid M. Product of *vav* proto-oncogene defines a new class of tyrosine protein kinase substrates. Nature 1992; 356: 68-71.

49. Margolis B, Hu P, Katzav S, et al. Tyrosine phosphorylation of *vav* proto-oncogene product containing SH2 domain and transcription factor motifs. Nature 1992; 356: 71-74.

50. Berridge MJ. Inositol trisphosphate and diacylglycerol as second messengers. Biochem J 1984; 220: 345-360.

51. Dohlman HG, Caren MG, Lefkowitz RJ. Biochemistry 1987; 26: 2657-2664.

52. Birnbaumer L, Abramowitz J, Brown AM. Biochim Biophys Acta 1990; 1031: 163-224.

53. Nishizuka Y. Studies and perspectives of protein kinase C. Science 1986; 233: 305-12.

54. Nishizuka Y. The molecular heterogeneity of protein kinase C and its implications for cellular regulation. Nature 1988; 334: 661-665.

55. Kariya K, Kawahara Y, Fukuzaki H, et al. Two types of protein kinase C with different functions in cultured rabbit aortic smooth muscle cells. Bichem Biophys Res Comm 1989; 16: 1020-1027.

56. Rosengurt E. Signal transduction pathways in mitogenesis. Br Med Bull 1989; 45: 515-528.

57. Mehmet H, Rosengurt E. Regulation of c-fos expression in Swiss 3T3 cells: An interplay of multiple signal transduction pathways. Brit Med Bull 1991; 47: 76-86.

58. Ohmi K, Yamashita S, Nonomura Y. The effect of K252a, a protein kinase C inhibitor on the proliferation of vascular smooth muscle cells. Biochem Biophys Res Comm 1990; 173: 976-981.

59. Tagaki Y, Hirata Y, Takata S, et al. Effects of protein kinase inhibitors on growth factor-stimulated DNA synthesis in cultured rat vascular smooth muscle cells. Atherosclerosis 1988; 74: 227-230.

60. Davis PD, Hill CH, Keech E, et al. Potent selective inhibitors of protein kinase C. Febs Lett 1989; 259: 61-63.

61. Evans ME, Assender JW, Newby AC. Selective inhibitors of protein kinase C are potent inhibitors of vascular smooth muscle proliferation. Br Heart J 1992; 68: 109.

62. Angel P, Karin M. The role of Jun, Fos and the AP-1 complex in cell proliferation and transformation. Biochim Biophys Acta 1991; 1072: 129-157.

63. Herschman HR. Primary response genes induced by growth factors and tumour promotors. Annu Rev Biochem 1991; 60: 281-319.

64. Southgate KM, Davies M, Booth RFG, Newby AC. Involvement of extracellular matrix degrading metalloproteinases in rabbit aortic smooth muscle cell proliferation. Biochem J 1992; 288: 93-99.

65. Sjölund M. Autocrine stimulation of arterial smooth muscle cells by platelet-derived growth factor . Stockholm: Karolinska Institutet, 1990.

66. Simons M, Edelman ER, De Keyser J-L, Langer R, Rosenberg RD. Antisense c-myb oligonucleotides inhibit intimal arterial smooth muscle accumulation in vivo. Nature 1992; 359: 67-70.

67. Speir E, Epstein E. Inhibition of smooth muscle cell proliferation by an antisense olidodeoxynucleotide targeting the messemger RNA encoding proliferating cell nuclear antigen. Circulation 1992; 86: 538-547.

68. Nabel EG, Plautz G, Nabel GJ. Gene transfer into vascular cells. J Am Coll Cardiol 1991; 17 (SupplB): 189B-194B.

69. Banskota NK, Taub R, Zellner K, Olsen P, King G. Characterization of induction of protooncogene c-myc and cellular growth in human vascular smooth muscle cells by insulin and IGF-1. 1989;

70. Gadeau A-P, Campan M, Desgranges C. Induction of cell cycle-dependent genes during cell cycle progression of arterial smooth muscle cells in culture. J Cell Physiol 1991; 146: 356-361.

71. Campan M, Desgranges C, Gadeau A-P, Millet D, Belloc F. Cell cycle dependent gene expression in quiescent stimulated and asynchronously cycling arterial smooth muscle cells in culture. J Cell Physiol 1992; 150: 493-500.

72. Miano JM, Tota RR, Vlasic N, Danishefsky KJ, Stemerman MB. Early proto-oncogene expression in rat aortic smooth muscle cells following endothelial removal. Am J Pathol 1990; 137: 761-765.

73. Bauters C, DeGroot P, Adamantidis M, et al. Proto-oncogene expression in rabbit aorta after wall injury. First marker of the cellular process leading to restenosis after angioplasty. Eur Heart J 1992; 13: 556-559.

74. Newby AC, Southgate KM, Assender JW. Inhibition of vascular smooth muscle cell proliferation by endothelium-dependent vasodilators. Herz 1992; 17: 291-299.

75. Rink TJ, Sage SO. Calcium signalling in human platelets. Annu Rev Physiol 1990; 52: 431-449.

76. Abe A, Karaki H. Effects of forskolin on cytosolic Ca^{++} level and contraction in vascular smooth muscle. J Pharmacol Exp Ther 1989; 249: 895-900.

77. Assender JWA, Southgate KM, Hallett MB, Newby AC. Inhibition of proliferation but not Ca^{2+} mobilization by cAMP and cGMP in rabbit aortic smooth muscle cells. Biochem J 1992; 288: 527-532.

78. Bennett MR, Evan G, Newby AC. Early down-regulation of c-myc proto-oncogene in inhibition of vascualr smooth muscle proliferation. Eur Heart J 1992; 13(Suppl): 28.

79. Loesberg C, Van Wijk R, Zandbergen J, Van Aken WG, Van Mourik JA, De Groot PHG. Cell cycle-dependent inhibition of human vascular smooth muscle cell proliferation by prostaglandin E_1. Exp Cell Res 1985; 160: 117-125.

80. Fukumoto Y, Kawahara Y, Kariya K, Araki S, Fukuzaki H, Takai Y. Independent inhibition of DNA synthesis by protein kinase C, cyclic AMP and interferon alpha/beta in rabbit aortic smooth muscle cells. Biochem Biophys Res Comm 1988; 157: 337-345.

81. Morisaki N, Kansaki T, Motoyama N, Saito Y, Yoshida S. Cell cycle-dependent inhibition of DNA synthesis by prostaglandin I_2 in cultured rabit aortic smooth muscle cells. 1988; 71: 165-171.

13. Basic FGF's role in smooth muscle cell proliferation: A basis for molecular atherectomy

WARD CASSCELLS, DOUGLAS A. LAPPI and ANDREW BAIRD

Introduction

Migration and proliferation of smooth muscle cells (SMC) in the arterial intima are well recognized features of atherosclerosis [1] and are especially prominent features of transplant atherosclerosis [2], and of restenosis after balloon angioplasty [3,4] or coronary bypass grafting [5]. The proliferation of vascular SMC may also be important in Kaposi's sarcoma [6] and in some types of hypertension [7-10]. In atherosclerosis and in restenosis, factors implicated in the migration and proliferation of SMC include thrombi [11-13], lipoproteins [14-16], stretch [17-21], reduced flow and shear [17-21], and loss of endothelial-derived growth inhibitors [22-26]. In addition, the SMC themselves can express mitogenic vasoconstrictors [27-29], such as angiotensin, and platelet-derived growth factors (PDGFs) [30-35]. Various PDGF dimers are also released by platelets, macrophages and endothelial cells [30-35]. The possibility of a similar role for basic

---

Abbreviations:
aFGF: acidic fibroblast growth factor; bFGF: basic fibroblast growth factor; EGF: epidermal growth factor; PDGF: platelet-derived growth factor; FGF-R1: fibroblast growth factor receptor 1 (also known as flg): IGF1: insulin-like growth factor-1; 3HTdR: tritiated thymidine; SMC: smooth muscle cell(s); TGFß; transforming growth factor beta; TNF alpha: tumor necrosis factor α

fibroblast growth factor (bFGF), a heparin-binding 18 kD peptide best known for its angiogenic, neurotropic, and mesoderm-inducing effects [36-38], has only recently been considered.

Embryonic and cultured vascular smooth muscle cells express and respond to bFGF

In fact, while several reports have described a mitogenic effect of bFGF for vascular SMC in vitro and in vivo [39-43 in other reports neither mitogenicity nor chemotaxis was observed [44,45] We found bFGF to be a potent mitogen for cultured rat aortic SMC in low serum concentrations (submitted for publication). However, in optimal concentration of serum exogenous bFGF exerted almost no additional mitogenic effect, suggesting either that serum mitogens (such as PDGFs, EGF, IGFs, TGF-ßs and vasopressor hormones [46]) are sufficient to maximize proliferation, or that serum stimulates SMC to express sufficient bFGF. Indeed, like others [39-43] we have observed that bFGF is expressed by cultured SMC [47]. However, in freshly isolated adult arterial SMC we found only 14% as much bFGF as in cultured aliquots of the same cells [47], in keeping with the fact that there is very little bFGF mRNA in adult tissues, other than brain [36-38]. We have also recently observed a decline in SMC bFGF immunoreactivity as embryonic arteries mature and proliferation slows [48-49].

Increased bFGF expression after vascular injury

To the extent that injury recapitulates embryogenesis, and to the extent that cells in culture are "wounded", it seemed possible that vascular injury might lead to bFGF expression in proliferating SMC. In experiments recently submitted for publication we found that immunostaining revealed an initial decline in bFGF immunoreactivity between 0 and 12 h after injury, suggesting utilization of the bFGF stored in medial SMC, or proposed by Lindner and Reidy [39-43]. This was followed by an increase in bFGF immunoreactivity from 17 h to at least 10 d. The increase paralleled the increase in SMC thymidine incorporation, which began at 24 hours, and was maximal at 48 to 96 hours, as SMC began to migrate through the internal elastic membrane into the intima. Immunoreactivity for bFGF was most intense in the cells closest to the lumen, which had the highest mitotic index. The increase was also seen by immunoblotting of heparin-Sepharose column fractions. The increase may be post-transcriptional, as no increase in steady state bFGF mRNA levels was seen by RNase protection analysis of vessels injured 24 h or 7 d earlier. As noted in previous studies [52-53], thymidine incorporation by medial SMC began by 24 h and was maximal at 48-96 h. Areas of thrombosis and leukocyte attachment and infiltration were noted from 24-72 h. Subsequently, cells migrated across damaged internal elastic laminae and proliferated in the neo-intima. DNA synthesis declined gradually but had not returned to baseline by 14 days. A neo-intima was noted by 5-7 d and by 14 d was 6-20 cells thick. FGF has a number of non-mitogenic functions and in a few cell types can even inhibit proliferation [36-38]. However, the role of bFGF in SMC of injured vessels is likely to be a mitogenic one, since we also found that intravenous injections of bFGF led to an increase in neo-intimal accumulation, compared to saline or heat-denatured bFGF controls.

Inhibition of smooth muscle cell proliferation by anti-bFGFs and by a bFGF-linked ribosome-inactivating protein

These data raised the possibility of inhibiting SMC pro-liferation with an antibody to bFGF. However, three potential problems were foreseen. First, repeated administrations of antibody often elicit a neutralizing immune response [56,57], which precludes long-term therapy. Second, bFGF may work, in part, by an intracrine mechanism [58-60]. Consistent with this, we have isolated bFGF in the nuclei of proliferating SMC in vitro [47] and nuclear bFGF immunoreactivity is also seen in Figure 2 (see later). If some bFGF goes directly to the nucleus without first leaving the cell, it will not be accessible to antibody therapy. Third, we have evidence that bFGF is not always rate-limiting for SMC growth. In culture, several other mitogens can produce rapid SMC proliferation. In fact, we found that neutralizing anti-bFGF antibodies, which are effective in preventing SMC proliferation in response to added bFGF, have little effect on SMC proliferation in either low or high concentrations of unsupplemented serum (which does not contain detectable bFGF [61,62]) It is quite possible that several growth factor systems are maximally stimulated after injury in vivo, in which case bFGF may be largely redundant.

Because of these concerns, we evaluated an alternative approach: we reasoned that bFGF might serve as a Trojan Horse to carry a toxin into the proliferating SMCs. We developed a cytocidal conjugate of bFGF with saporin, a plant-derived protein that inactivates ribosomes

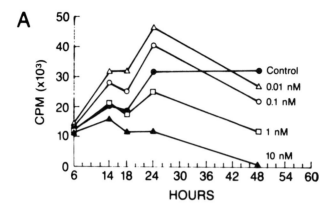

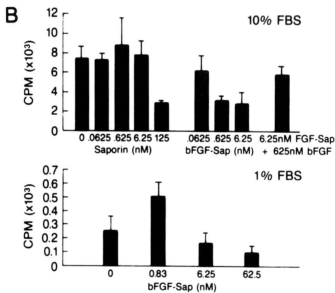

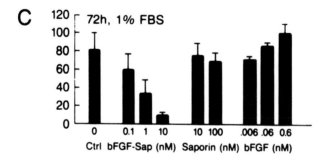

by cleaving adenine from ribose in the 28S RNA of the 60S subunit [61,62]. It seemed likely that bFGF would be good not only at facilitating entry of saporin into cells but also at allowing saporin to have access to ribosomes : bFGF's unusually slow degradation and its transit to the nucleus suggest that much of it does not enter the lysosomes [66,67].

In 10% serum, 10 nM bFGF-saporin inhibited protein synthesis by 14 hours and DNA synthesis by 24 hours (Figure 1). Cell death began by 24 to 48 hours. Cells were killed by as little as one hour exposure to bFGF-saporin. These effects were not seen in the presence of 400-fold excess bFGF, and saporin alone inhibited cell growth only at concentrations 500-fold greater than those required for bFGF-saporin.

By 96 hours after a single exposure to 10 nM bFGF-saporin, only 10% of cells were viable, as indicated by exclusion of trypan blue. The survival of these cells may be due to failure of bFGF-saporin to bind or enter the cells or to resistance to saporin at an intracellular site. Some SMC clones may have few or no FGF receptors, particularly if quiescent. Interestingly, in post-confluent cultures (figure 2) bFGF-saporin had almost no effect, consistent with a low density of

Figure 1. Effects of bFGF-saporin on protein and DNA synthesis and cell number. A. Time course of effect of various concentrations of bFGF-saporin on protein synthesis by smooth muscle cells (SMC). Rat aortic SMC from 8th passage were plated at 30,000 cells/cm^2 in 10% FBS in leucine-free M199. At 20 h cells received .01-10nM bFGF-saporin, conjugated and purified as described [63-65]. At 14, 18 or 24 h cells were pulsed for 2 h and counted by liquid scintillation. For clarity, means are shown without SD, which were $\leq$ 10% of means. Also omitted are the data with 10 and 100 nM saporin, which did not differ from controls. Experiment was repeated twice with similar results, using rabbit aortic SMC. B. Inhibition of DNA synthesis by bFGF-saporin, but not saporin or bFGF-saporin competed by bFGF, in rat aortic smooth muscle cells. Cells were plated in M199/1% FBS at 10,000/cm2 and exposed to additives and 3-HTdR at 24 h, for 24 h more. Bars indicate means + SD of triplicate wells. In 10% FBS (upper panel) no initial enhancement of DNA synthesis was noted even at low doses of bFGF-saporin. However, in 1% FBS (lower panel) there is an initial increase in DNA synthesis with low (but not high) concentrations of bFGF-saporin. DNA synthesis decreases further by 48 and 76 h (not shown). C. Killing of SMC by bFGF-saporin. Cells were plated at 10,000/cm2 in 1% FBS/M199 for 24 h then exposed to the indicated concentrations of bFGF-saporin, saporin or bFGF for 72 h, at which time cells excluding trypan blue were counted in 3 randomly chosen fields of 1.2 mm2 each. Reprinted from Casscells et al., Proc. Natl. Acad. Sci. USA 1992;89:7159-7163, with permission.

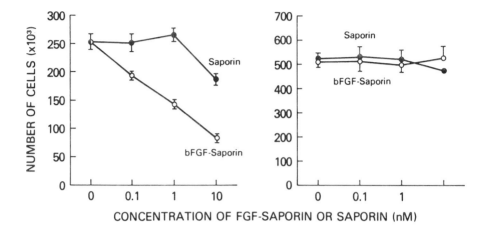

Figure 2. Quiescent smooth muscle cells are not killed by bFGF-saporin. Left panel: Subconfluent ($2 \times 10^4/cm^2$) P_{12} rat aortic SMC in 10% FBS were exposed to indicated concentrations of saporin or bFGF-saporin for 1 h then washed for 10min with 10 μg/ml heparin to remove proteoglycan-bound bFGF-saporin, re-fed 10% FBS/M199 and trypsinized and counted 96 h later. Right panel: Confluent ($2 \times 10^5/cm^2$) cells were made more quiescent by 72 h in serum-free M199, then exposed to bFGF-saporin (open circles) or saporin (closed circles), washed, re-fed, and counted as above. Bars indicate standard deviations of triplicate wells counted by hemacyto-meter. Experiment was repeated once with similar results.

FGF receptors at confluence [68,69]). We also found that the initial response to low (0.1-1 nM) concentrations of bFGF-saporin was an increase in protein and DNA synthesis; with 1 nM doses there was an eventual decline at 48-72 hours. This initial stimulation was best seen under low serum conditions that revealed bFGF's mitogenic capacity. Presumably bFGF exerts its effect sooner and at a lower concentration than saporin. Little initial stimulation was detected in 10% serum with 1 or 10 nM bFGF-saporin. In 0.1 nM bFGF-saporin, incorporation was reduced by 33% with no change in cell number, suggesting that bFGF-saporin can exert a cytostatic effect at sub-cytocidal concentrations.

FGF receptors are expressed by proliferating SMC in injured vessels

These data led us to ask whether quiescent and proliferating SMC differentially express FGF receptors in vivo. If so, and if quiescent cells express fewer receptors, a local application of bFGF-saporin could have therapeutic value. Moreover, we have recently noted that, in vitro, endothelial cells are much more resistant to bFGF-saporin than SMC [70]. In fact, 0.1-1 nM bFGF-saporin stimulated endothelial cells but inhibited SMC. These findings raised the possibility of a selective, self-targeting intravenous therapy to inhibit or ablate SMC, yet enhance endothelial growth.

Recent studies have yielded conflicting data as to the presence of FGF receptors in adult tissues. We found only low affinity binding of radio-labeled FGF in vessels, lungs, liver, heart and kidneys of normal adult rats; high affinity FGF receptors became sparse or undetectable in all but neural tissues after embryogenesis [71-73]. By Northern analysis, mRNA transcripts for *flg* (FGF Receptor 1) [74,75] have been variably reported as detectable in normal adult tissues [76-78], or absent in adult tissues other than brain, but present in embryonic tissues [79-82]. Expression of *bek* (FGF Receptor 2) has been undetectable in cultured rhabdo-myosarcoma and umbilical vein cells [83] but detectable in adult liver, lung, brain and kidney [84]. Recently the distribution of FGF receptors has been further complicated by the discovery of related genes, [85-86] of alternatively spliced *flg* transcripts and of *flg* transcripts which encode truncated secreted receptor sequences [87-88]. Another complicating element is the recent identification of an FGF receptor unrelated to either *flg* or *bek* and of membrane-bound heparan-sulfate proteoglycans that have recently been shown to be required for high affinity bFGF binding [89-95]. Finally, bFGF binding appears to be subject to post-translational regulation [96], and a developmentally regulated discrepancy between *flg* mRNA and bFGF binding, has been described [97]. For these reasons, mRNA analyses at present may not yield physiologically understandable data. Consequently we have focused on bFGF receptor protein and binding assays. In vivo autoradiographic experiments (Figure 3) showed only low affinity, heparin-displaceable binding of ^{125}I-bFGF in normal vessels. We were not able to identify high affinity FGF receptors in normal vessel homogenates by Scatchard analysis, cross-linking or Western blotting (Figure 3).

Moreover, functional evidence of the absence or near-absence of bFGF receptors in normal vessels is that when bFGF was injected in large doses over 1-3 days, no increase in DNA synthesis rates of any cardiovascular tissues was seen with tritiated thymidine autoradiography or by liquid scintillation counting of tissue digests, confirming the recent results of Whalen et al.[98] (see also Lindner et al.[39-43]). In contrast, when we gave repeated subcutaneous injections of bFGF, to injure the tissue and up-regulate FGF receptors, we found increased

234

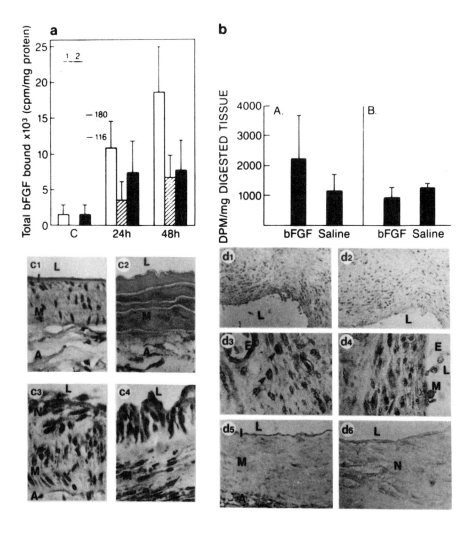

Figure 3. FGF receptors are increased by balloon injury.

a. Detectable binding of bFGF by membranes from balloon-injured adult arteries. Open bars: total cpm bound; hatched: nonspecific cpm; filled: specific cpm. Membranes were prepared as described by Burrus and Olwin [89-95]. Background counts obtained in the absence of membrane protein were $\leq 20\%$ of the total cpm and were subtracted from the samples. Specific counts were determined as above in the presence of a 200-fold molar excess of bFGF. All samples were normalized to ^{125}I-cpm bound per mg membrane protein. The graph and standard deviations represent counts determined twice from the four different protein concentrations with each point assayed in triplicate. Inset: immunoblotting indicates an FGF receptor in injured but not in normal arteries. Normal (lane 1) and 48 h balloon-injured (lane 2) rat carotid arteries were homogenized as described above and supernates boiled in Laemmli buffer with ß-mercaptoethanol prior to SDS-PAGE, transfer to nitrocellulose and blotting. The antiserum was raised against the synthetic peptide, RITGEEVEVRDR, an extracellular domain of the FGF receptor deduced from the chicken and mouse *flg* genes (FGF receptor 1) [87-88].

b. Repeated injections of bFGF increase thymidine incorporation in injured tissue (A) but not in uninjured tissue (B). Rats were injected every 2 h with 2 μg bFGF s.c., or saline, for 10 h then 1 μCi/gm 3HTdR i.p. at 46 h and sacrificed at 48 h. Tissues were subjected to digestion in Protosol (New England Nuclear) according to the manufacturer's instructions, and liquid scintillation counting in Ionic-Fluor (Packard), corrected by quench curves. Despite plasma levels of 0.8 ng/ml 24 h after injection (estimated by mixing 50 ng of ^{125}I-bFGF in 950 ng unlabeled bFGF and gamma counting of trichloroacetic acid-insoluble counts), a level giving nearly maximal mitogenic effect in vitro, only 0.33% of the bFGF tracer bound to the heart and 42% of this was displaceable by heparin. There was no effect on thymidine incorporation in the heart, as shown. Similar results were obtained when heart sections were embedded in paraffin and subjected to autoradiography using NTB-2 emulsion. Labeled capillary nuclei were counted in 2 sections of each of 4 rats treated with bFGF and in 2 rats treated with saline. The average ($\pm$SD) number of labeled nuclei per mm^2 in the bFGF-treated rats was 11.4 ± 5.3, vs. 12.6 ± 4.0 for the saline-treated rats ($p > .1$ by 2-tailed t-test).

In contrast, as shown in A, the tissue injured by repeated injections revealed more local 3HTdR uptake when injected with bFGF than with saline.

c. In vivo autoradiographic evidence that FGF receptors are expressed after vascular injury. Adult rats were subjected to balloon dilation of the carotid artery and injected i.v. 2 d later with 60 ng of either mitogenically active or heat-denatured (90°C,1 h) ^{125}I-bFGF (10^5 cpm/ng iodinated as described[18]) with or without 10 μg unlabeled bFGF, followed 1 h later by i.v. heparin (165 U/kg) then anesthetized by pentobarbital (75 mg/kg) and killed by perfusion with 10% formalin 1 h later. Tissues were dipped in NTB-2 (Kodak), processed for autoradiography and developed 10 d later. Panel C1: Uninjured vessel causes almost no precipitation of silver grains, indicating little or no heparin-resistant (high affinity) binding. Panel C2:

(Figure 3 cont) demonstrates binding of bFGF 48 h after balloon injury. Panel C3: At day 4, bFGF binds preferentially to cells in neointima (N). Panel 4 illustrates competition by excess unlabeled bFGF (no grains over neointima). Magnifications: C1:X280, C2:X464, C3:X464, C4:X464.

<u>d</u>. Immunocytochemical localization of an FGF receptor after vascular injury. d1: Rat aorta, 14 d after de-endothelialization and dilation, stained as in Figure 2 but with a polyclonal antiserum (R129) raised against a synthetic peptide replicate of an intracellular domain deduced from the FGF receptor 2 gene *(flg)* [74-84]. The residues (CSSGEDSVFSHEPLPEEP) were chosen for maximal antigenicity and cross-species homology (100% for chicken, mouse, and human). Many of the proliferating smooth muscle cells exhibit the brown immunoperoxidase reaction product. L = lumen. Methyl green counterstain (X140).

<u>d2</u>. Injured segment of same rat stained with the anti-FGF *(flg)* receptor polyclonal antibody R131 described in Figure 7a. (X140). The similarity of the immunohistological results using antisera directed against different peptides deduced from the same receptor cDNA, as well as the Western analysis

(Fig. 7a), and the lack of stain using peptide-adsorbed (panel d6) or non-immune serum, indicate the specificity of the assay. Same slides at higher power (850X) are shown in d3 and d4. Brown (immunoperoxidase-positive) smooth muscle cells are indicated by arrowheads. Monocyte (M) is immunoreactive but most erythrocytes (E) show only background staining. Normal segment shows little immunoreactivity of the medial layer with R131. The near absence of stain for the *flg* gene product is shown in d5. <u>d6:</u> Normal rabbit serum is unreactive with injured vessels (or normal vessels, not shown); d3-d6:X464. Reprinted from Casscells et al., Proc Natl Acad Sci USA 1992; 89: 7169-7163, with permission.

thymidine incorporation compared to areas repeatedly injected with saline. Similarly, when we gave bFGF intravenously for 3 days to rats subjected 5 days earlier to left carotid balloon injury, neo-intimal growth was accelerated only in the injured left carotid and not in the uninjured right carotid. No stimulation was seen if the animals were injected with heat-denatured bFGF or saline. (Casscells et al., submitted for publication).

These data may reflect: 1) balloon-induced loss of endothelium, permitting direct access of bFGF to medial SMC, 2) down-regulation by injury of some growth inhibitory mechanism(s), and 3) expression of bFGF receptors in response to injury. In fact, upregulation of FGF receptors is supported by several types of data. First, radioligand-binding studies in vessel homogenates revealed that balloon injury stimulated the appearance of high affinity bFGF binding sites. Moreover, autoradiograms of histologic sections revealed high affinity binding of bFGF (i.e., not displaced by heparin) to neo-intimal and medial SMC of injured vessels but not to quiescent smooth muscle of normal vessels (Figure 7c -see below). Similarly, immunoblotting with an antibody raised against a sequence deduced from the mouse *flg* (FGF-R1) gene demonstrated characteristic bands in injured vessels but none in normal vessels. Likewise, using these antibodies in immunohistology, we found few cells in normal vessels to be immunoreactive, but most proliferating mesenchymal cells were immunoreactive for FGF-R1 (and for smooth muscle α actin, not shown). Thus, injuring, like culturing, induces expression of FGF receptors.

We tested bFGF-saporin in several in vivo models of vascular injury. In rats subjected 24 hours earlier to balloon injury of the carotid artery, 1 or 10 μg bFGF-saporin, locally applied, resulted in the death of most medial SMC, and a 75% reduction in neo-intimal cell number 14 days after injury (Figure 4). Rats given 100 μg/kg i.v. at 24, 48, and 72 hours after injury had 83% less neo-intimal accumulation at 7 days than saporin- or saline-treated controls. However, there were some areas of apparent SMC death in the medial layer, implying a risk of aneurysm or rupture. The uninjured right carotids were histologically normal, but an 8% weight loss was noted, suggesting systemic toxicity (the LD50 for saporin in mice is 4-7 mg/kg i.v.[99,100]). Rats given intravenous bFGF-saporin as a single 75 μg/kg dose 24 hours after balloon injury revealed 24% less neo-intimal proliferation at 14 days (Fig. 8e). In this model there was almost no evidence of the necrosis, thrombosis, or inflammation noted in the rats treated by local infusion or with larger amounts of intravenous bFGF-saporin.

We also tested bFGF-saporin in a model of pulmonary vascular smooth muscle proliferation. Endotoxin was used to produce foci of pulmonary vascular injury, thrombosis, inflammation and smooth muscle proliferation [101,102]. Endotoxin is known to cause the death of some endothelial cells [103-105], while others are stimulated to produce leukocyte adhesion molecules [106], pro-coagulant factors [43], and cytokines mitogenic for SMC, such as bFGF [109], interleukin 1 [110], PDGF-B chain [111], TNF α [112], and endothelin [113]. In rats given 40 μg/kg i.v. bFGF-saporin 24 hours after 1 μg i.p. endotoxin, there were fewer foci of smooth muscle proliferation 7 days later, and many vessels in fact appeared thinned. Intravascular thrombi in rats treated with saporin or saline contained SMC, while those in rats treated with bFGF-saporin did not.

Studies are in progress to determine optimum dosing and to exclude the possibility that with milder injury or lower doses the bFGF

238

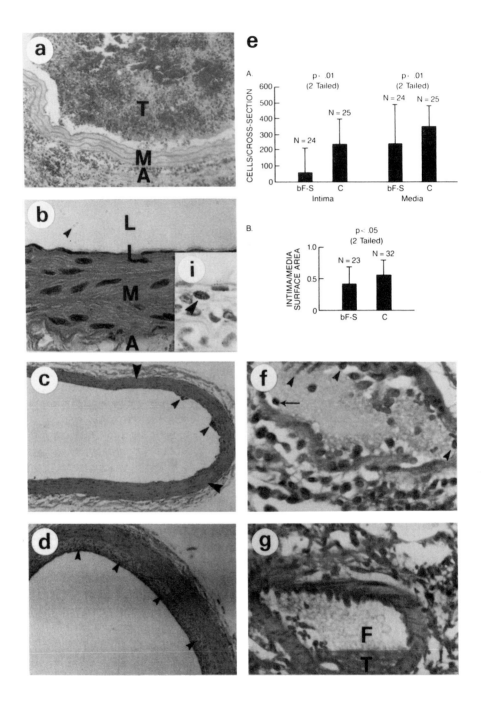

Figure 4. After arterial injury, bFGF-saporin kills proliferating smooth muscle cells (SMC) and inhibits neointimal accumulation. (a) 24 h after balloon injury the carotid artery was occluded by proximal and distal ties and 10 μg of bFGF-saporin in 20 μl saline was instilled for 15min followed by release of the ligatures, and sacrifice 11 d later. In panel (a) the medial (M) smooth muscle cells are lysed, and the layers of elastica are collapsed. The lumen is largely occluded by organizing thrombus (T). Some hemorrhage and inflammatory cells are noted in the adventitia (A) (H and E, X200). Saporin alone was non-toxic (not shown) and bFGF-saporin was not toxic to the uninjured right carotid of a rat subjected to left carotid balloon injury and bFGF-saporin 75 μg/kg i.v. (panel b). The intimal endothelium (I) and medial SMC (M) appear normal and no cells are synthesizing DNA, as illustrated by the absence of silver grains (small arrowhead) over the cell nuclei. The inset (i) illustrates an S-phase SMC from a ballooned artery treated with saline (H and E, X800). Panel (c) illustrates the dramatic inhibition by bFGF-saporin (75 μg/kg i.v. at 24, 48, 72 h after balloon injury) of neointimal SMC accumulation (small arrowheads): 83% less than in animals injected with 40 μg/kg (equimolar) saporin (panel d) or saline, as determined by Zeiss Videoplan 2 planimetry of neointimal areas normalized to medial areas. All samples were coded for "blinded" morphometry. By 2-tailed unpaired t-test, p = 0.004. However, toxicity was indicated by an 8% weight loss and by a few areas of medial SMC lysis (large arrowheads in panel c). For this reason, lower doses were tested and gave the results graphed in panel e: Effects of lower doses of bFGF-saporin on injured arteries. Upper panel A: The numbers of intimal and medial cells from the central (non-endothelialized) segments of carotid artery from μats treated 24 h after balloon injury with a 15min local application of 1 μg bFGF-saporin (bF-S) or saline (C), followed by sacrifice 10 d later. The samples were coded for "blind" counting by 2 observers with intra- and inter-rater reproducibilities of 92%. Lower panel B: Rats were given a single dose of 75 μg/kg bFGF-saporin or 40 μg/kg i.v. saporin (an equimolar dose) 24 h after carotid balloon injury and sacrificed 12 d later. Data are given as ratio of neointimal to medial surface areas. The t-test for unpaired samples was used. Panels f,g: Photomicrographs of rat lung vessels injured by 1 μg lipopolysaccharide i.p. (2X10^4 endotoxin units/μg, Ribi Immunochem, Hamilton, MT), followed at 24 h by 10 μg saporin or bFGF-saporin, i.v., and sacrifice on d 7. (f): pulmonary artery of control rat treated with saporin is filled with thrombus caused by endotoxin. In addition to trapped erythrocytes and a polymorphonuclear neutrophil (arrow) apparent smooth muscle cells (arrowheads) have migrated into the clot. In contrast, the vessel of a rat treated with bFGF-saporin (g) contains no smooth muscle cells either in the loose fibrin (F) or organized thrombus (T); magnifications: a(X464), b(X224), c(X140), d(X140), f(X464), g(X224).

moiety could exert a greater effect than the saporin moiety, and thereby enhance SMC proliferation. It will also be important to determine if cytocidal therapy merely delays the proliferative response, or permanently ablates the subpopulation that responds to the balloon stimulus. We are also investigating the cause of the weight loss. Conceivably, with optimal dosing, there may be no toxicity. Moreover, toxicity may be minimized by bFGF-saporin mutants, by using a heparin chase, or using glutathione or N-acetyl cysteine to reduce the disulfide linkage.

Clinical potential

Attempts to prevent or reverse atherosclerosis, and the rapid smooth muscle proliferation which contributes importantly to pulmonary hypertension [7-10], transplant rejection [2] and restenosis after angioplasty [3,4] or bypass grafting [5], include the use of adrenergic antagonists and other antihypertensives [7-10], cholesterol-lowering agents [114,115], fish oils [116,117], corticosteroids [118,119] cyclosporin A [120], heparin and non-anticoagulant heparin fragments [22-26], inhibitors of angiotensin-converting enzyme [121,122], calcium antagonists [123,124], aspirin, prostacyclin and other modulators of platelet and smooth muscle eicosanoid metabolism [129-131], colchicine [132], terbinafine [133], triazolopyrimidine [134], analogs of somatostatin [135], and seeding with endothelial cells [136,137]. Also being tested are intravascular stents, to maintain patency and flow (which is anti-thrombotic and growth-inhibiting), and laser angioplasty and atherectomy, which might, once optimized, produce less vascular trauma than balloon angioplasty [138-142]. Preliminary results in experimental animals and in humans show promise for some of these therapies. The attractiveness of the bFGF-saporin conjugate is that it would in theory require only a few treatments and could be self-targeting. However, it would be contraindicated in pregnancy, or in patients with recent cerebral vascular injury, as defects in the blood-brain barrier could result in death of those neurons expressing receptors for bFGF. Wound healing might be delayed by bFGF-saporin if fibroblasts or activated leukocytes express bFGF receptors. Thus, while local delivery of bFGF can be contemplated, intravenous therapy may not be feasible, at least with this first generation conjugate. Conceivably, the targeting of saporin could be made even more selective using a monoclonal antibody specific for some internalized antigen on the surface of activated smooth muscle cells. An alternative possibility is suggested by the unprecedented

	C–C	C–C	C–C					
R1(*flg*) vs. R2 (*bek*)	38%	81%	79%	66%	88%	50%	92%	60%
R1 vs. R3	21%	66%	82%	41%	83%	43%	91%	44%
R1 vs. R4	2½%	63%	74%	32%	75%	14%	86%	38%
R2 vs. R3	27%	72%	81%	45%	87%	50%	92%	56%
R2 vs. R4	21%	70%	72%	31%	78%	29%	84%	48%
R3 vs. R4	26%	78%	74%	34%	78%	36%	80%	46%

Figure 5 . Schematic diagram of the reported FGF receptor families (R1, R2, R3, R4). The disulfide-bonded Ig-like loops represent the extracellular domains, which diverge substantially in the most N-terminal loop, as indicated by the % of identical amino acid residues. The rectangles represent the split tyrosine kinases, which exhibit considerable sequence similarity. The insert region, the transmembrane domain and the C- and N- termini diverge substantially.

diversity of the FGF receptor family: at least 4 distinct genes, each of which give rise to dozens of alternatively spliced isoforms (Fig. 5). Evidence from several labs, including our own, indicates varying degrees of ligand-specificity and cell-specificity. Thus it is quite possible that activated vascular smooth muscle cells express a unique isoform that could be targeted using a monoclonal antibody. An additional inference from these studies is that [99]technetium-labeled bFGF (or labeled antibodies against activated smooth muscle cells or against a putative SMC-specific FGF receptor isoform) could be used as an imaging agent to predict the development of restenosis--currently a difficult problem--and to detect areas of bFGF receptor activity that would contra-indicate use of bFGF-saporin.

Abstract

Multiple therapies have largely failed to inhibit restenosis. Thus there is increasing interest in the roles of vascular growth factors. In this report we describe recent, as well as new data suggesting that injury of rat

242

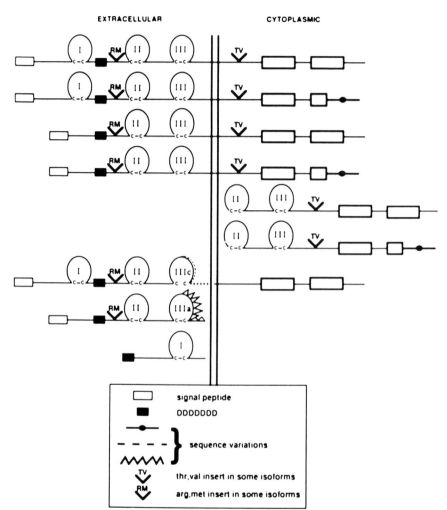

Figure 6. Predicted structures of FGF-R1 isoforms deduced from reported cDNAs. The alternatively spliced variants in loop III confer a degree of ligand specificity such that some forms bind aFGF but bFGF, for example, while other forms bind multiple members of the FGF family. Note also the putative secreted forms, which may serve to export FGFs from the cell or to bind up extracellular FGFs. Putative cytosolic forms are also shown.

arteries leads to an increase in bFGF, and FGF receptors. Administration of bFGF enhanced SMC proliferation. A conjugate of bFGF with saporin (a ribosome- inactivating protein) proved superior to anti-bFGF antibodies in inhibiting SMC DNA synthesis. The conjugate killed proliferating, but not quiescent SMC in vitro. In vivo, one to three doses inhibited neointimal proliferation. The activation of the FGF system in vascular injury suggests new diagnostic and therapeutic possibilities.

References

1. Ross R, Masuda J, Raines E. Ann NY Acad Sci 1990; 598: 103.
2. Billingham ME. Transplant Proc 1989; 21: 3665.
3. McBride W, Lange RA, Hillis LD. N Engl J Med 1988; 318: 1734 (1988).
4. Waller BF et al, Am J Card 1984; 53 (Suppl C): 42C.
5. Bulkley BH, Hutchins GM, Circulation 1977; 50: 163.
6. Weich HA, Salahuddin S-Z, Gill P, Nakamura S, Gallo RC, Folkman J. Am J Path 1991; 139; 1251.
7. Jones RC, Reid LM, Current Pulmonol 1987; 8, 175.
8. VanKleef EM et al. Circ. Res 1992; 70: 1122.
9. Owens GK, Circ Res 1985; 56; 525.
10. Willerson JT et al. Proc Nat AcadSci USA 1991; 88: 10624.
11. Gajdusek C, Carbon S, Ross R, Nawroth P, Stern D, J Cell Biol 1986; 103: 419.
12. Chesebro JH et al. N Engl J Med 1982; 307: 73.
13 Schwartz CJ, Valente AJ, Kelly JL, Sprague EA, Edwards EH. Sem Thromb Hemost 1988; 14: 189.
14. Steinberg D. Ann NY Acad Sci 1990 598: 125.
15 Libby P, Miao P, Ordovas JM, Schaefer EJ, J Cell Physiol 1985; 124: 1.

16. Brown MS, Goldstein JL, Nature 1987; 330: 113.
17. Ku DN, Giddens DP, Zarins CK, Glagov S. Arteriosclerosis 1985; 5: 292.
18. Davies PF Jr., Kemuzzi A, Gordon EJ, Dewey CF Jr, Gimbrone MA Jr. Proc Natl Acad Sci USA 1986; 83: 2114.
19. Langille BL, Bendeck MP, Kelley FW, Amer J Physiol 1989; 256: H931.
20. Ingber DE, Folkman J. J Cell Biol 1989; 109: 317.
21. Sachs F. Fed Proc 1987; 46: 12.
22. Clowes AW, Clowes MM. Transplant Proc 1989; 21: 3700.
23. Clowes AW, Reidy MA, Clowes MM. Lab Invest 1983; 49. 327.
24. Herman IM, Castellot JJ Jr. Arteriosclerosis 1987; 78: 463.
25. Edelman, ER Adams DH, Karnovsky MJ. Proc Natl Acad Sci USA 1990; 82: 3773.
26. Fritze LMS, Reilly CF, Rosenberg RD. J Cell Biol 1985; 100: 1041.
27. Bell L, Madri JA. Circ Res 1989; 65: 1057.
28. Daemen MJAP, Lombardi DM, Bosman FT, Schwartz SM. Circ Res 1991; 68: 450.
29. Owens GK. Amer J Physiol 1989; 252: H1755.
30. Barrett TB, Benditt EP. Proc Natl Acad Sci USA 1987; 84: 1099.
31. Walker LN, Bowen-Pope DF, Ross R, Reidy M. Proc Natl Acad Sci USA 1986; 83: 7311.
32. Terracio L et al. J Cell Biol 1988; 107: 1947.
33. Rubin K et al. Lancet 1988; 2: 1353.
34. Libby P, Warner SJC, Solomon RN, Birinyi LK. N Engl J Med 1988; 318: 1493.
35. Wilcox JN, Smith KM, Williams LT, Schwartz SM, Gordon D. J Clin Invest 1988; 82: 1134.
36. Gospodarowicz D. Crit Rev Oncogen 1989; 1: 1.
37. Baird A, Bohlen P. In: Sporn MB, Roberts AB, editors. Handbook of Experimental Pharmacology. Peptide Growth Factors and Their Receptors. Springer, Berlin, 1990; 369-418.
38. Rifkin DB, Moscatelli D. Cell 1989; 109 1.
39. Gospodarowicz D, Hirabayashi K, Giguere L, Tauber, JP J. Cell Biol. 1981; 89: 568.
40. Chen J-K, Hoshi, McKeehan HWL. In Vitro 1988; 24: 199.
41. Weich HA, Iberg N, Klagsbrun M, Folkman J. Growth Factors 1990; 2: 313.

42. Klagsbrun M, Edelman ER. Arteriosclerosis 1989; 9: 269.
43. Lindner V, Lappi DA, Baird A, Majack RA; Reidy MA. Circ Res 1991; 68: 106.
44. Risau W. Proc Natl Acac Sci USA 1986; 83: 3855.
45. Grotendorst GR, Chang T, Seppa HEJ, Kleinman HK, Martin GR. J Cell Physiol 1982; 113: 261.
46. Thyberg J, Hedin U, Sjolund M, Palmberg L, Bottger BA. Arteriosclerosis 1991; 10: 966.
47. Speir EH, Sasse J, Shrivastav S, Casscells W. J Cell Physiol 1991; 147: 362.
48. Spirito P, Fu Y-M, Yu Z-X, Epstein SE, Casscells W. Circulation 1991; 84: 322.
49. Casscells W et al. J Clin Invest 1990; 85: 433.
50. Fu Y-M et al. J Cell Biol (in press).
51. Casscells W. Prog Growth Factor Res 1991; 3: 177.
52. Clowes AW, Schwartz SM. Circ Res 1985; 56: 139.
53. Steele PM et al. Circ Res 1985; 57: 105.
54. Manderson JA, Mosse PRL, Safstrom JA, Young SB, Campbell GR: Arteriosclerosis 1989; 9, 289.
55. Ferns GAA, Ready MA, Ross R. Am J Path 1991; 138: 1045.
56. Fitzgerald D, Pastan I. J Natl Cancer Inst 1989; 81: 145.
57. Vitetta E, Thorpe PE. In: DeVita V, Hellman S, Rosenberg S editors. Biologic Therapy of Cancer: Principles and Practice, Lippincott, Philadelphia, 1991 (in press).
58. Renko M, Quarto N, Morimoto T, Rifkin DB. J Cell Physiol 1990; 144: 108.
59. Baldin V, Roman A-M, Bosc-Bierne I, Amalric F, Bouche G. EMBO J 1990; 9: 1511.
60. Dell'Era P, Presta, M Ragnotti G. Exptl Cell Res 1991; 192: 505.
61. Zimering MB et al. J Clin Endocrinol Metab 1990; 70: 149.
62. Casscells W et al. J Clin Invest 1990; 85: 433.
63. Lappi DA, Martineau D, Baird A. Biochem Biophys Res Commun 1989; 160: 917.
64. Stirpe F, Bailey S, Miller SP, Bodley JW. Nucl Acids Res 1990; 16: 1349.
65. Lappi DA et al. J Cell Physiol 1991; 147: 17.
66. Moscatelli D. J Cell Biol 1988; 107: 753.
67. Bikfalvi A et al. Exp Cell Res 1989; 181: 75.
68. Neufeld G, Gospodarowicz D. J Biol Chem 1985; 260: 13860.

69. Veomett G, Kuszynski C, Kazakoff P, Rizzino A. Biochem Biophys Res Commun 1989; 159: 694.
70. Biro S, Casscells W, manuscript in preparation.
71. Rosengart TK et al. J Vasc Surg 1988; 7: 311.
72. Olwin BB, Hauschka SD. J Cell Biol 1990; 110: 503.
73. Ledoux D, Mereau A, Dauchel MC, Courty J. Biochem Biophys Res Commun 1989; 159: 290.
74. Ruta M et al. Proc Natl Acad Sci USA 1989; 86: 5722.
75. Lee PL, Johnson DE, Cousens LS, Fried VA, Williams LT. Science 1989; 245: 57.
76. Mansukhani A, Moscatelli D, Talarico D, Levytska V, Basilico C. Proc Natl Acad Sci USA 1990; 87: 4378.
77. Safran A et al. Oncogene 1990; 5: 635.
78. Friesel R, Dawid I. Mol Cell Biol 1991; 11: 2481.
79. Pasqauale EB, Singer SJ. Proc Natl Acad Sci USA 1989; 86: 5449.
80. Reid HH, Wilks AF, Bernard O. Proc Natl Acad Sci USA 1990; 87: 1596.
81. Imamura T, Tokita Y, Mitsui Y. Biochem.Biophys Res Commun 1988; 155: 583.
82. Mereau A, Pieri I, Gamby C, Courty J, Barritault D. Biochimie 1989; 71: 865.
83. Dionne CA et al. EMBO J 1990; 9: 2685.
84. Kornbluth S, Paulson KE, Hanafusa H. Mol Cell Biol 1988; 8: 5541.
85. Houssaint E et al. Proc Natl Acad Sci USA 1990; 87: 8180.
86. Alitalo R et al. J Cell Biochem 1991; 15 F: 88.
87. Johnson DE, Lee PL, Lu J, Williams LT. Mol Cell Biol.1990; 10: 4728.
88. Hou J et al. Science 1991; 251: 665.
89. Burrus LW, Olwin BB. J Biol Chem 1989; 264: 18647.
90. Saunders S, Jalkaren M, O'Farrell S, Bernfield M. J Cell Biol 1989; 108: 1547.
91. Kiefer MC, Stephans JC, Crawford K, Okino K, Barr PJ. Proc Natl Acad Sci USA 1990; 87: 6985.
92. Sakaguchi K, Yanagishita M, Takeuchi Y, Aurbach GD. J Biol Chem 1991; 266: 7270.
93. Yayon A, Klagsbrun M, Esko JD, Leder P, Ornitz DM. Cell 1991; 64:841.
94. Rapraeger AC, Krufka A, Olwin BB. Science 1991; 252: 1705.

95. Klagsbrun M, Baird A. Cell 1991; 67: 299.
96. Savona C, Feige J-J. Ann NY Acad Sci 1991; in press.
97. Musci TJ E, Amaya, Kirschner MW. Proc Natl Acad Sci USA 1990; 87: 8365.
98. Whalen GF, Shing Y, Folkman J. Growth Factors 1989; 1: 157.
99. Tazzari PL et al. Cancer Immunol Immunother 1988; 26: 231.
100. Blakey DC et al. Cancer Res 1988; 48: 7072.
101. Kirton OC, Jones R. Lab Invest 1987; 56: 198.
102. Prescott MF, McBride CK, Court M. Am J Path 1989; 135: 835.
103. Sage H, Tupper J, Bramson R. J Cell Physiol 1986; 127: 373.
104. Smedly LA et al. J Clin Invest 1986; 77: 1233.
105. Reidy M, Schwartz SM. Exp Mol Pathol 1984; 41: 419.
106. Bevilacgua MP, Pober JS, Mendrick DL Cotran RS, Gimbrone MA Jr. Proc Natl Acad Sci USA 1987; 84: 9238.
107. Scheef RR, Loskutoff DJ. Haemostasis 1988; 18: 328.
108. Crutchley DJ, Conanan LB, Ryan US. Biochem Biophys Res Commun 1987; 148: 1346.
109. Gajdusek CM, Carbon S. J Cell Physiol 1989; 139: 570.
110. Libby P, Warner SJC, Friedman GB. J Clin Invest 1988; 81: 487.
111. Albelda SM, Elias JA, Levine EM, Kern JA. Am J.Physiol 1989; 257: L65 .
112. Han J, Brown T, Beutler B. J Exp Med 1990; 171: 465 .
113. Sugiura M, Inagami T, Kon V. Biochem Biophys Res Commun 1989; 161: 1220.
114. Blankenhorn D et al. JAMA 1987; 257: 3233.
115. Backman JJ, Badimon L, Fuster V. J Clin Invest 1990; 85: 1234.
116. Reis GJ et al. Lancet 1989; 2: 177.
117. Dehmer GJ et al., N Engl J Med 1988; 319: 733.
118. Pepine CJ et al. Circulation 1990; 81: 1753.
119. Munro JM, Cotran RS. Lab Invest 1988; 58: 249.
120. Wengrovitz M, Selassie LG, Gifford RRM, Thiele BL, J Vasc Surg 1990; 12: 1.
121. Powell JS et al. Science 1989; 245: 186.
122. Multicenter European Research Trial with Cilazapril After Angioplasty to Prevent Transluminal Coronary Obstruction and Restenosis, Circulation 1992; 86: 100.
123. Henry PD, Bentley KI, J Clin Invest 1981; 68: 1366.
124. Watanabe N et al. Artery 1987; 14: 283.

125. Block LH, et al. Proc Natl Acad Sci USA 1989; 86: 2388.
126. Tilton GD et al. J Amer Coll Cardiol 1985; 16: 141.
127. Blumlein SL, Sievers R, Kida P, Parmley WW. Amer J Cardiol 1984; 54: 88.
128. Lichtlen PR et al. Lancet 335, 1109.
129. Chesebro JH et al., N Engl J Med 1984; 310: 209.
130. Schwartz L, Bourassa MA, Lesperance J, Aldridge HE, Kazim F, N Engl J Med 1988; 318: 1714.
131. Pomerantz KB, Hajjar DP. Arteriosclerosis 1989; 9: 413.
132. Thyberg J, Blomgren K. Virchow's Arch Cell Pathol 1990; 59: 1.
133. Nemecek GM et al. J Pharmacol Exp Ther 1989; 248: 1167.
134. Tiell ML, Sussman II, Gordon PB, Saunders RN. Artery 1983; 12: 33.
135. Lundergan C et al. Atherosclerosis 1989; 80: 49.
136. Dichek DA et al. Circulation 1989; 80: 1347.
137. Nabel EG, Plautz G, Nabel GJ. Science 1990; 249: 1285.
138. Ip JH et al. J Amer Coll Cardiol 1990; 15: 1667.
139. Liu MW, Roubin GS, King SB III. Circulation 1989; 79: 1374.
140. Serruys P et al. N Engl J Med 1991; 324: 13.
141. Block PC. N Engl J Med 1991; 324: 52.
142. Leon MBet al. Circulation 1990; 81: 143.

14. Role of transforming growth factor ß in cardioprotection of the ischemic-reperfused myocardium

ALLAN M. LEFER

TGFß is produced in significant amounts by virtually every cell type within the circulatory system including cardiac myocytes, arterial and venous vascular smooth muscle cells, fibroblasts, endothelial cells, leukocytes and platelets [1]. This broad distribution of TGFß within the circulation clearly is consistent with the variety of effects of this homodimeric peptide on the development and maturation of many systems including the circulatory system. Thus, TGFß binds to specify membrane receptors on over 150 cells types generally at concentrations of this regulatory peptide in the picomolar to nanomolar range [2].

Recently, TGFß has been categorized as a biological switch [3] which has the potential to modify an interaction, between a cell and its environment or with another cell, in either a positive (i.e., a potentiating) or a negative (i.e., an inhibitory) manner. Thus, TGFß can act as either an accelerator or a brake on a wide variety of molecular processes. In this framework, TGFß exerts very interesting cardiovascular effects, despite its short half-life in the circulatory system. The circulating half-life of TGFß may not yield the complete picture of its pharmacokinetics since this half-life can be greatly extended when TFGß complexes with its latency associated peptide (LAP) [4]. Moreover, TGFß may bind to surface proteins or receptors (e.g., on the endothelium) so that it is protected from degradation and clearance from circulation.

A few years ago, TGFß was shown to be present in normal

cardiac myocytes and endothelial cells [5], but disappears from the myocardium after acute myocardial infarction except at the border zone of injured myocardial tissue, where increased amounts of TFGß were present [6]. This intriguing finding led to the speculation that TGFß may exert some ameliorating effect on injured cardiac myocytes. An extension of this hypothesis is that exogenously administered TGFß can exert cardioprotective effects in myocardial ischemia-reperfusion. This supposition was clearly shown to be the case by Lefer et al [7] in rats both in vitro and in vivo, and is the primary subject of this review. TGFß given administered 1 to 24 hours prior to ischemia-reperfusion exerted a significant cardioprotective effect in a perfused rat heart model of ischemia-reperfusion as evidenced by preservation of EDRF release from the coronary vascular endothelium [7]. This endothelial preservation effect in ischemic reperfused rat hearts occurred at dose of TFGß ranging from 100 ng to 10 mg per rat. This calculates to be effective TGFß plasma concentration of about 1 to 100 nM. When applied to the intact rat, 10 mg of TGFß either injected intravenously 24 hours prior to ischemia or 10 min post-ischemia (i.e., just a reperfusion), exerted a significant cardioprotective effect. Myocardial injury was assessed by loss of creatine kinase activity from the ischemic reperfused myocardium. TFGß attenunated CK loss from the injured myocardium by 50 to 55%, 24 hours after reperfusion (p<0.02). This significant cardioprotective effect was associated with reduced circulating concentrations of the cytokine, TNF α [7]. This was not totally surprising since TGFß is known to oppose the cytotoxic actions of cytokines including TNF α [8]. The protective effect of TGFß in rats during myocardial ischemia was the first demonstration of a cardioprotective effect of TGFß in vivo, and has stimulated further studies on this subject.

Reperfusion of a previously ischemic vascular bed results in significant enhancement of tissue injury, the so called "reperfusion injury" effect. In addition to the effects of TGFß in myocardial ischemia-reperfusion in the rat, TGFß has been studied in several ischemic-reperfusion stated including myocardial ischemia-reperfusion in the cat [9], splanchnic ischemia-reperfusion in the cat [10], and cerebral ischemia-reperfusion in the pig [11]. In each case, TGFß$_1$ was the isoform of TGFß studied. The common finding in all these studies is that TGFß$_1$ exerts significant cytoprotective effects resulting in reduced tissue injury upon reperfusion of an ischemic vascular bed. Moreover, in all these cases, TGFß$_1$ preserved endothelial cell integrity. Endothelial cell cytoprotection thus becomes an important mechanism for the protection against reperfusion injury by TGFß$_1$.

One important question that remained to be answered was: Does TGFß actually retard ischemic injury when indexed to the area-at-risk (i.e., that region of the tissue actually under jeopardy)? Since collateral blood flow can alter the apparent mass of jeopardized tissue, the actual area-at-risk helps define the "jeopardized region". In the previous study employing TGFß during ischemia-reperfusion in the rat, it was assumed that the entire organ or region was "at-risk". In the cat study, the exact area of myocardium at-risk was measured and the degree of necrosis was indexed to this reference point. Thus, by expressing myocardial damage as % necrosis/area-at-risk, $TGFß_1$ reduced myocardial necrosis by 60% expressed as % necrosis indexed to area-at-risk [8]. This represents a highly significant cardioprotective effect, and was similar to the 50% reduction in ischemic injury observed in the rat study.

In addition to endothelial dysfunction as a prominent feature of reperfusion injury [12], polymorphonuclear neutrophil (PMN) adherence to the endothelium and subsequent activation of these PMNs plays an important role in the ultimate pathogenesis of reperfusion injury. Thus, an important feature of the cat study was to ascertain the effect of $TGFß_1$ on PMN adherence to the coronary vascular endothelium in ischemic-reperfusion, and to determine if $TGFß_1$ exerts any anti-adherence action. $TGFß_1$ did exhibit a marked anti-adherence effect. Adherence of autologous PMNs were measured on the coronary endothelium of the ischemic-reperfused left anterior descending coronary artery. LAD coronary arteries from the occluded-reperfused vessel, exhibited markedly enhanced PMN adherence compared to the non-ischemic circumflex coronary artery. However, injection of $TGFß_1$ to the cat 10 min prior to reperfusion markedly inhibited this increased PMN adherence to its endothelial lining

$TGFß_1$ failed to exert any significant systemic hemodynamic effect on either mean arterial blood pressure (MABP), heart rate (HR) or on its product, the pressure-rate index (PRI) at a dose of 20mg kg given intravenously to cats 10 min prior to reperfusion. Therefore, the cardioprotective effect of $TGFß_1$ observed in cats was not due to an effect on myocardial oxygen demand. Previous studies on isolated cat coronary arteries have ruled out any direct coronary vasodilator effect [13], and studies on isolated cat cardiac muscle have ruled any direct inotropic effects [13]. Thus, it is unlikely that $TGFß_1$ protects the ischemic reperfused myocardium via a hemodynamic effect. Figure 1 illustrates the lack of an effect of $TGFß_1$ on coronary vasoactivity at concentrations of 10, 100 and 1000 nM in isolated cat coronary artery rings either in presence or absence of humorally induced vascular tone.

Cat Coronary Artery Rings

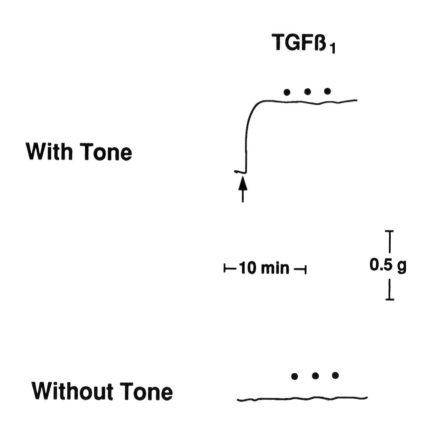

Figure 1. Representative recordings of isolated cat coronary artery rings to TGFß, at 10,100 and 1000 ng/ml at the dots, in the presence of tone induced by 9, 11-methanoepoxy-PGH$_2$ at (10 nM) (arrow) or in the absence of tone. No vasoactive effect of TGFß$_1$ was observed.

Clearly, TGFß does not have a significant coronary vasodilator effect.

A major effect of TGFß$_1$ in feline myocardial ischemia-reperfusion is its endothelial preservation effect. TGFß markedly preserved the ability of the ischemic-reperfused coronary vascular endothelium to release endothelium-derived relaxing factor (EDRF) now identified as nitric oxide [14]. This is consistent with the earlier reports that TGFß$_1$ preserves nitric oxide release in the rat coronary vascular endothelium [7] as well as the cat splanchnic vascular endothelium following ischemia-reperfusion [9]. Moreover, it helps to explain the anti-TNFα and anti-superoxide radical effects of TGFß since both TNF α and superoxide radicals acutely oppose the actions of endothelium-derived nitric oxide [15]. Figure 2 illustrates the inhibitory effects of TNF α on the ability of the coronary endothelium to release EDRF in response to acetylcholine (ACh). This anti-EDRF effect was prevented by addition of 10 nM TGFß$_1$. The significance of preserving nitric oxide extends far beyond maintaining the ability of the vasculature to dilate, since endothelium-derived nitric oxide also exerts anti-aggregatory actions in platelets [16], anti-adherent effects in neutrophils [17], and quenches superoxide radicals [18]. Thus maintaining nitric oxide at control levels, on or near the endothelial surface, promotes a variety of anti-thrombotic and anti-inflammatory effects which could be of significant value in attenuating reperfusion injury. Moreover, since nitric oxide synergizes with prostacyclin [19], and since prostacyclin also inhibits platelet aggregation, reduces neutrophil adherence and retards endothelial leakiness, endothelial protection is an important action of TGFß. It appears that TGFß$_1$ exhibits preservation of reperfused myocardial tissue as a result of endothelial protection.

In the cat myocardial ischemia reperfusion study, data were obtained on the role of neutrophils in myocardial reperfusion injury since PMNs have been shown to contribute to the post-reperfusion endothelial dysfunction [20,21]. In this connection, cardiac myeloperoxidase activity was measured as an index of PMN infiltration into the post-reperfused myocardium [22]. Ischemic non-necrotic myocardial tissue (i.e., the area-at-risk) as well as necrotic myocardial tissue exhibited a significant increase in cardiac MPO activity in cats subjected to ischemia and reperfusion. However, TGFß$_1$ treated ischemic-reperfused cats showed significantly lower MPO activity in both cardiac regions, indicating an anti-neutrophil effect of TGFß$_1$.

Not only does TGFß$_1$ inhibit adherence of PMNs to endothelial cells, but TGFß$_1$ also inhibits adherence of PMNs to isolated cardiac

Cat Coronary Artery Rings

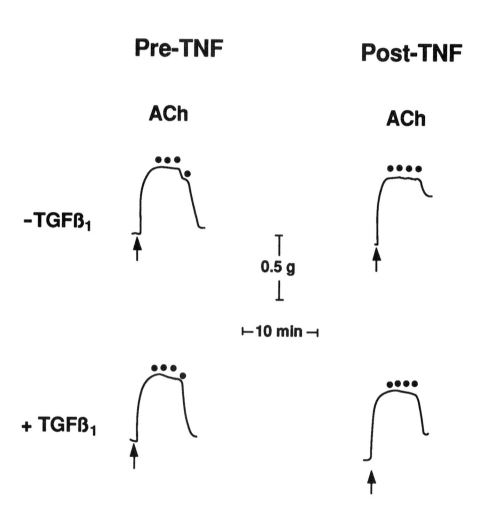

Figure 2. Representative recordings of isolated cat coronary artery rings to acetylcholine (ACh) given at concentrations of 0.1, 1, 10 and 100 nM (dots) to 9, 11-methanoepoxy-PGH$_2$ (10 nM) contracted rings. TNFα was added at 2 mg/ml two hours prior to addition of TGFβ_1 or its vehicle (Na acetate buffer). Note the preservation of the ACh induced vasorelaxation by TGFβ_1.

myocytes. This may be important in blocking the effects of activated neutrophils after they undergo transendothelial migration and adhere to cardiac myocytes [23] where they release their cytotoxic mediators (i.e. oxygen derived free radicals, cytokines, proteases, lipid mediators) in very close proximity to the myocyte. Figure 3 illustrates the inhibitory action of TGFß$_1$ at 100 ng/ml on the adherence of rat PMNs to isolated rat myocytes. In contrast to TGFß$_1$, TGFß$_2$ did not exert this anti-adherence effect on cardiac myocytes.

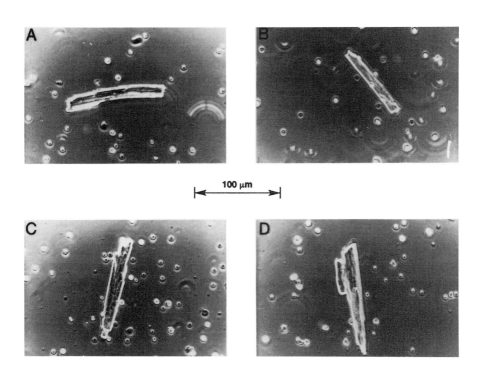

Figure 3. Photomicrograph under phase contract microscopy of isolated adult rat myocytes in the present of PMNs. The myocytes were stimulated by 100 U/ml IL-Iß and the PMNs by 100 nM leukotriene B$_4$ (LTB$_4$). (A) Control myocytes and control PMNs (no stimulation), (B) stimulated myocytes and PMNs, (C) Stimulated myocytes and PMNs in the presence of 100 ng/ml TGFß$_2$, (D) Stimulated myocyts and PMNs in the presence of 100 ng/ml of TGFß$_1$.

Figure 4 illustrates the action of TGFß[1] on the adherence of rat PMNs to rat endothelial cells (EC) in the left panel and to adult rat cardiac myocytes (MC) in the right panel. In the former case, only the EC were stimulated by IL-1ß, whereas in the latter situation, the myocytes were stimulated by IL-1ß and the PMNs by LTB[4] to induce a significant increase in adherence. In both cases, 100 ng/ml of TGFß[1] attenuated adherence of PMNs almost completely. This anti-adherence effect of TGFß[1] may be an important feature of its cardioprotective effect. Moreover, it is an endothelial effect of TGFß[1] rather than a direct effect on neutrophils. If TGFß[1] is incubated only with PMNs, and the TGFß is washed out, there is no inhibtion of adherence of these PMNs to endothelial cells [9].

In summary, TGFß[1] exerts marked cardioprotective effects in murine and feline myocardial ischemia-reperfusion injury. TGFß[1] exerts these cardioprotective effects in the absence of a significant effect on cardiac afterload or on cardiac inotropic state (i.e. without reducing myocardial oxygen demand). Moreover, TGFß protects the heart in the absence of an effect on coronary blood flow (i.e., without increasing myocardial oxygen supply). Thus, TGFß does not operate via an overt systemic hemodynamic effect.

There are however, several potentially important cellular effects of TGFß[1] that may help explain its cardioprotective actions. These are (a) anti-cytokine effects of TGFß [7, 8] in which TGFß inhibits the formation or opposes the deleterious actions of cytokines like TNF α and 1L-1ß, including their anti-EDRF effect, [24] (b) anti-free radical effect of TGFß[1] particularly with regard to inhibiting the formation of superoxide radicals [7] rather than by scavenging uperoxide radicals, (c) protection of the endothelium, partcularly including preservation of EDRF [7, 9, 10, 11] and prostacyclin [11, 25] release from the endothelium, (d) anti-adherence effects of neutrophils including inhibition of adherence of PMNs to the endothelium [9, 26, 27, 28] and to cardiac myocytes [29]. Moreoever, TGFß[1] appears to be more active in its endothelial regulatory role than TGFß[2] [30)]and was found to be more effective in inhibiting adherence of PMNs to endothelial or

Figure 4. Inhibition of adherence of rat PMNs to rat endothelial cells (EC) and rat cardiac myocytes (MC). All values are means SEM; numbers at bottom of the bars indicate numbers of experiments studied. Concentrations of agents are the same as in Figure 3. LTB[4] is not required for PMN adherence to EC.

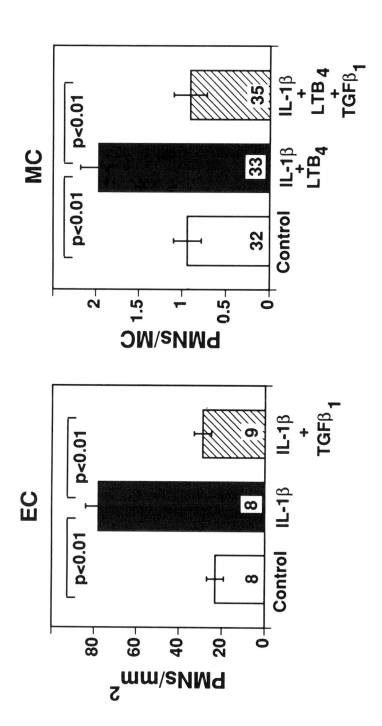

myocardila cells than TGFß$_2$. In addition to its endothelial preserving and cardioprotective effects followng acute myocardial ischemia and reperfusion, TGFß has been shown to preserve endothelial function and protect against tissue injury following splanchnic [10] and cerebral [11] ischemia-reperfusion. Thus, common protective mechanisms of TGFß appear to exist in a variety of forms of reperfusion injury. Future work will be needed to clarify and integrate these findings so as to obtain a comprehensive and accurate mechanism of the cytoprotective effect of TGFß.

Acknowledgements

Supported in part by Research Grant No. GM-45434 from the National Institute of General Medical Sciences of the NIH

References

1. Sporn MB, Roberts AB. The transforming growth factor-ßs. In: Sporn MB, Roberts AB. Peptide Growth Factors and Their Receptors I. Springer, New York.1990; 419-472.
2. Massague J, Like B. Cellular receptors for type ß transforming growth factor. Ligand binding and affiity labeling in human and rodent cell lines. J Biol Chem 1985; 260: 2636-2645.
3. Sporn MB, Roberts AB. TGF-ß: problems and prospects. Cell Regulation 1990; 1: 875-882.
4. Wakefield LM, Winokur TS, Hollands RS, Christopherson K, Levinson AD, Sporn MB. Recombinant latent transforming growth factor ß$_1$ has a longer plasma half-life in rats than active transforming growth factor ß$_1$, and a different tissue distribution. J Clin Invest 1990; 86:1976-1984.
5. Eghbali M. Cellular origin and distribution of transforming growth factor-ß$_1$ in the normal rat myocardium. Cell Tissue Res 1989; 256:553-558.
6. Thompson NL. Bazoberry F, Speir EH, Casscells W, Ferrans VJ, Flanders KC. Kondaiah P, Geiser AG, Sporn MB. Transforming growth factor beta-1 in acute myocardial infarction in rats. Growth Factors 1988; 1: 91-99.
7. Lefer AM, Tsao P, Aoki N, Palladino MA Jr. Mediation of cardioprotection by transforming growth factor-ß. Science 1990; 249: 61-64.

8. Espevik T, Figari I, Ranges GE, Palladino MA Jr. Transforming growth factor-ß1 (TGF-ß$_1$) and recombinant human tumor necrosis factor-alpha reciprocally regulate the generation of lymphokine-activated killer cell activity. Comparison between natural porcine platelet-derived TGF-ß$_1$ and TGF-ß$_1$ and recombinant human TGF-ß$_1$. J Immunol 1988; 140: 2312-2316.

9. Lefer AM, Ma X-I, Weyrich AS, Scalia R. Mechanisms of the cardioprotective effect of transforming growth factor-ß$_1$ in feline myocardial ischemia and reperfusion. 1992; Submitted.

10. Karasawa A, Guo J-p, Ma X-I, Lefer AM. Beneficial effects of transforming growth factor-ß and tissue plasminogen activator in splanchnic artery occlusion and reperfusion in cats. J Cardiovasc Pharmacol 1991; 18: 95-105.

11. Armstead WM, Mirro R, Suckerman S, Shibata M, Leffler, CW. Transforming growth factor ß attenuates ischemia-induced alterations in cerebrovascular responses. Circulation 1991; 84: 11-77.

12. Lefer AM, Tsao PS, Lefer DJ, Ma X-I. Role of endothelial dysfunction in the pathogenesis of reperfusion injury after myocardial ischemia. FASEB J 1991; 5: 2029-2034.

13. Lefer AM. Mechanisms of the protective effects of transforming growth factor-ß in reperfusion injury. Biochem Pharmacol 1991; 42: 1323-1327.

14. Palmer RMJ, Ferridge AG, Moncada S. Nitric oxide release accounts for the biological activity of endothelium-derived relaxing factor. Nature 1987; 327:524-526.

15. Stewart DJ, Pohl U, Bassenge E. Free radicals inhibit endothelium-dependent dilation in the coronary resistance bed. Am J Physiol 1988; 255: H765-769.

16. Radomski MW, Palmer RMJ, Moncada S. Comparative pharmacoloy of endothelium-derived relaxing factor, nitric oxide and prostacyclin in platelets. Br J Pharmacol 1987; 92: 181-187.

17. McCall T, Whittle BJR, Boughton-Smith NK, Moncada S, Inhibition of FMLP-induced aggregation of rabbit neutrophils by nitric oxide. Br J Pharmacol 1988; 95: 517P.

18. Rubanyi GM, Vanhoutte PM. Superoxide anions and hyperoxia in inactive endothelium-derived relaxing factor. Am J Physiol 1986; 250: H822-H827.

19. Moncada S, Palmer RMJ, Higgs EA. Nitric oxide: physiology, pathophysiology and pharmacology. Pharmacol Rev 1991; 43: 109-142.

20. Weissman G. The role of neutrophils in vascular injury: a summary of signal transduction mechanisms in cell/cell interactions. Springer Semin Immunopath 1989; 11: 235-258.

21. Ma X-I, Tsao PS, Viehman GE, Lefer AM. Neutrophil-mediated vasoconstriction and endothelial dysfunction in low-flow perfusion-reperfused cat coronary artery. Circ Res 1991; 69: 95-106.

22. Mullane KM, Kraemer, Smith B. Myeloperoxidase activity as an assessment of neutrophil infiltration into the ischemic myocardium. J Pharmacol Meth 1985; 14: 157-167.

23. Entman ML, Youker K, Shappell SB, Siegel C, Rothlein R, Dreyer WJ, Schmalstieg FC, Smith CW. Neutrophil adherence to isolated adult canine myocytes. Evidence for a CD 18-dependent mechanism. J Clin Invest 1990; 85: 1497-1506.

24. Aoki N, Siegfried M, Lefer AM. Anti-EDRF effect of tumor necrosis factor in isolated, perfused cat carotid arteries. Am J Physiol 1989; 256: H1509-H1512.

25. Ristimaki A, Ylikorkala O, Viinikka L. Effect of growth factors on human vascular endothelial cell prostacyclin production. Arteriosclerosis 1990; 10: 653-657.

26. Gamble JR, Vadas MA. Endothelial adhesiveness for blood neutrophils is inhibited by transforming growth factor ß. Science 1988; 242: 97-99.

27. Gamble JR, Vadas MA. Endothelial cell adhesiveness for human T lymphocytes is inhibited by transforming growth factor-ß. J Immunol 1991; 146: 1149-1154.

28. Cai J-p, Falanga V, Chin Y-h. Transforming growth factor-ß regulates the adhesive interactions between mononucleur cell and microvascular endothelium. J Invest Dermatol 1991; 97: 169-174.

29. Weyrich AS, Lefer AM. Transforming growth factor-ß$_1$ attenuates neutrophil adherence to ischemic-reperfused cardiac myocytes. Circulation 1992; abstract submitted.

30. Chaudhury RA, D'Amore PA. Endothelial cell regulation by transforming growth factor-beta. J Cell Biochem 1991; 47: 224-229.

15. Platelet-derived growth factor release after angioplasty

P. MACKE CONSIGNY

Introduction

The purpose of this chapter is to examine the role of platelet-derived growth factor (PDGF) in the vascular smooth muscle (VSMC) hyperplastic response that occurs in the intima of arteries after balloon angioplasty. This proliferative response results in the reappearance of stenoses in approximately 40% of the patients undergoing coronary balloon angioplasty. To place into perspective the role of PDGF in restenosis, the evidence implicating VSMC proliferation as the cause of restenosis and the approaches that have been used but have failed to resolve the problem are presented. Thereafter, recent cell and molecular biology studies which provide a foundation for the understanding of sources and possible roles of PDGF in restenosis are presented. Finally, PDGF release after angioplasty is described.

Balloon angioplasty

The concept of angioplasty was first introduced by Dotter and Judkins [1] who demonstrated that the lumen of an artery could be enlarged by introducing into the lumen successively larger coaxial catheters. However, angioplasty did not become popular until after the introduction of the balloon angioplasty technique by Gruentzig in 1978 [2]. In balloon angioplasty, a balloon-tipped catheter is positioned in an artery at the site of a hemodynamically significant stenosis. The artery is then irreversibly stretched and the lumen enlarged by inflating the balloon.

Restenosis

After several years of experience with angioplasty, it became apparent that one of the most severe long-term side effects of angioplasty was the reappearance of the stenosis several months after the dilatation, a phenomenon referred to as restenosis [3]. Restenosis occurs often and quickly. For example, in a recent study, Nobuyoshi et al [4] performed repeated coronary angiography on 229 patients that had undergone coronary angioplasty. They found that 1, 3, 6, and 12 months after angioplasty the restenosis rates were 13%, 43%, 49%, and 53%, respectively.

Histologic studies of necropsy specimens [5] and specimens of restenotic lesions obtained by atherectomy [6] have both implicated intimal VSMC hyperplasia and extracellular matrix deposition as primary causes of restenosis in man. VSMC hyperplasia after angioplasty has also be observed in other species including rabbits [7] and pigs [8]. However, restenosis need not always be the result of VSMC hyperplasia. Waller et al [9], in their study of restenotic human coronary arteries obtained 1 -24 months after successful dilatation, found that 40% of the arteries had no evidence of a previous angioplasty and inferred that restenosis, in these cases, was the result of arterial elastic recoil.

Prevention of restenosis

Pharmacologic interventions

Once the pathologic changes produced by angioplasty were understood and restenosis had been identified as a clinical problem, PDGF was presumed to be involved. Facts implicating PDGF included the finding of platelets adherent to the luminal surfaces of balloon-dilated arteries shortly after angioplasty [8,10] and prior knowledge that PDGF is one of the factors released from alpha-granules upon platelet adhesion, that PDGF is a potent chemoattractant and mitogen for VSMCs, and that PDGF had been implicated as a factor involved in the genesis of atherosclerosis (the response-to-injury hypothesis) [11]. Based upon the presumption that platelet deposition and PDGF release were intimately involved in restenosis, several clinical studies were performed using drugs with antiplatelet properties. Unfortunately, no studies to date have demonstrated any inhibition of restenosis by antiplatelet agents. [3,12] However, Chesebro et al [13] did report that aspirin and dipyridamole reduced acute complications after angioplasty from 20% to

11% even through there was no effect on the rate of restenosis.

Alternative interventional devices

As angioplasty gained in popularity, its weaknesses (inability to dilate totally occluded vessels, the development of acute thromboses or occlusions after dilatation, arterial recoil after dilatation, and long term restenosis) became more apparent. In an attempt to alleviate these problems and also to extended angioplasty to vessels that could not otherwise be treated, alternative techniques were developed. These techniques and their purported advantages included laser angioplasty developed to recanalize totally occluded arteries and debulk arteries of plaque, atherectomy developed to debulk arteries of plaque without overdilating the artery, and arterial stenting developed to prevent elastic recoil. Unfortunately, as with balloon angioplasty, restenosis was a problem for all of these interventions [14-17].

Application of cell and molecular biology to the problem of restenosis

When it became apparent that neither anti-platelet therapies nor other interventional methods would solve the problem of restenosis, investigators began to look for other explanations. It was at this time that several facts brought the role of the platelets as the sole source of PDGF into question. These facts included: (1) the observation that platelet adhesion occurred within the first 24 hours after balloon angioplasty and yet VSMC proliferation did not begin until 2-4 days after angioplasty [10,18]; (2) VSMC proliferation was observed 14 to 28 days after angioplasty, a period when platelet adhesion to the arterial wall was not apparent [18], (3) indium-111 platelet deposition at balloon angioplasty sites did not correlate with the occurrence of restenosis [19], and (4) cells other than platelets, including endothelial cells [20-23], VSMCs [24-28] and macrophages [29-31] had the capacity to release PDGF. The fact that cells other than platelets could release PDGF renewed interest in PDGF but broadened the search for its sources and how its release was controlled.

PDGF: Our current understanding is that PDGF is secreted as a dimer of two chains linked by disulfide bonds. The two chains that make up PDGF can be either of two forms, the A chain or the B chain. As a result, there are three possible PDGF dimers, PDGF-AA, PDGF-AB, and PDGF-BB. The synthesis of the A and B chains are controlled by separate genes so it is possible for different cell types to release different forms of PDGF and for the same cell type to release different forms and amounts of PDGF under different conditions [32].

Some of the conditions known to alter PDGF gene expression and release include changes in phenotype associated with tissue culture [27] and stimulation by growth factors such as PDGF and TGF-ß [27,33], cytokines such as IL-1 [34], and hormones such as norepinephrine and angiotensin [35,36].

PDGF Receptors: For PDGF to elicit an effect, the PDGF must bind to a PDGF receptor on the cell's surface. It is currently thought that each PDGF receptor consists of two subunits which dimerize upon receptor occupation. There are two subunits that can make up a PDGF receptor, an α subunit and a ß subunit. As a result, there are three possible receptor types - the aa receptor, the α-ß receptor, and the ßß receptor. The α and ß receptor subunits have different affinities for the A and B chains of PDGF; the α subunit will bind either the A or the B chains of PDGF whereas the b subunit will only bind the B chain. The different PDGF isoforms and their different binding affinities to the different PDGF receptors are summarized in Table 1. From this table it is apparent that cells expressing only the α subunit will respond to all three forms of PDGF, whereas cells expressing only the b subunit will respond only to PDGF-BB. [37,38]

Table 1. Interactions between different forms of PDGF and different PDGF receptors.

		PDGF RECEPTOR		
		α-α	α-ß	ßß
	AA	+	-	-
PDGF LIGAND	AB	+	+	-
	BB	+	+	+

The PDGF ligand-receptor interactions summarized in Table 1 are important because they demonstrate that the response of a cell to PDGF is dependent upon (1) the forms and concentration of PDGF presented to the cell and (2) the type and number of PDGF receptors present on the cell membrane. For example, human dermal fibroblasts, which express α and ß PDGF receptor subunits at a 20:1 ratio, respond readily to PDGF-BB but respond poorly to PDGF-AA. In contrast, NIH 3T3 cells, which express α and β subunits at a 1:1 ratio, respond equally to PDGF-AA and PDGF-BB [38].

Like PDGF A and B-chain gene expression, the expression of the genes for the α and ß subunits of the PDGF receptor are under individual control. Factors known to alter the expression of these genes include tissue culture [39], inflammation [40], exposure to the growth factor TGF-ß1 [41] and the hormones angiotensin II and norepinephrine [42].

PDGF release after angioplasty

The PDGF that can promote intimal VSMC hyperplasia and thereby promote restenosis most likely originates from two sources, the platelets and the cells within the dilated artery.

Platelet release of PDGF

Upon platelet adhesion, platelets release their α granules. One of the constituents of these granules is PDGF. Because platelet adhesion occurs primarily within the first 24 hours after angioplasty, it seems likely that platelets are the source of PDGF for early cell proliferation. It is impossible to know the amount of active PDGF that enters the arterial wall and stimulates the cells therein. However, the total mount of PDGF activity released by platelets and the isoforms released have been determined by Bowen-Pope et al [43] and are summarized in Table 2. PDGF in species other than man is primarily the B-B homodimer form. In contrast, in man the A-B heterodimer predominates [44].

Table 2. Platelet PDGF: Type and Amount Released

SPECIES	PDGF-BB ACTIVITY (%)	TOTAL PDGF ACTIVITY (ng/ml)
human	15	13.
baboon	54	2.6
monkey	63	4.5
dog	76	.3
rat	100	1.4
pig	100	0.6

Plaque release of PDGF

A second source of PDGF after angioplasty is that PDGF produced by cells within the dilated arterial wall, particularly the endothelium that lines the lumen, the VSMCs and macrophages that make up the plaque, and the VSMCs within the media. Barrett and Benditt [44,45] examined carotid endarterectomy specimens for the expression of PDGF A and B chains using Northern hybridization. They found PDGF B-chain gene transcripts were 5 times higher in human carotid plaques than in normal arteries and that these transcripts correlated with the presence of *f*ms oncogene transcripts, a marker of macrophages. PDGF A-chain transcripts were also found in plaque and normal artery and their presence correlated with smooth muscle α-actin transcripts.

Wilcox et al [46] examined human carotid endarterectomy specimens using in situ hybridization. They found that PDGF A-chain mRNA was expressed primarily in mesenchymal-appearing intimal cells whereas B-chain mRNA was expressed in endothelial cells lining the arterial lumen and capillaries within the plaque. B-chain mRNA was not localized in macrophages to any great extent as suggested by Barrett and Benditt [45].

Libby et al [47] demonstrated that PDGF gene expression results in the release of PDGF mitogenic activity. They found that cultured VSMCs from human carotid plaque expressed PDGF A-chain but not PDGF B-chain mRNA. Furthermore, they found that culture media conditioned by these cells was able to stimulate bovine aortic VSMC replication. This replication was due, in part, to the presence of PDGF in the media as determined by anti-PDGF antibody neutralization. The rate of PDGF production, determined by radioreceptor competition assay, averaged 355 pg/ml/48 hrs.

Angioplasty-induced release of PDGF

Perhaps our best understanding of the PDGF release after angioplasty comes from experiments by Majesky et al [48] who used Northern and in situ hybridization to characterize PDGF A and B-chain, and α and ß-receptor subunit expression in balloon denuded rat carotid arteries. Although the injury elicited by balloon denudation is not exactly the same as the injury produced by angioplasty balloon inflation, the model is similar enough to provide important insights. They found PDGF A-chain transcripts present at low levels in the carotid artery prior to angioplasty. However, balloon denudation increased A-chain transcription 3-fold, 10 to 12-fold and 4-fold at 4 hours, 6 hours and 24 hours after injury, respectively. At 1 week A-chain transcription was only slightly elevated and by 2 weeks only neointimal cells adjacent to the lumen stained positive for A-chain mRNA by situ hybridization.

Transcripts for the B-chain of PDGF were present in normal and balloon denuded rat carotid arteries. However, the levels were low and did not change over the 2 week post-injury period, suggesting that B-chain PDGF of arterial origin may not play a role in post-injury VSMC proliferation.

α-receptor transcripts were present in the uninjured rat carotid artery and remained constant over the first week after injury. However, by two weeks after denudation, α-receptor expression was 2 to 3-fold greater in the media than in the intima. The presence of α-receptor transcripts suggests that the VSMCs in the media and neointima have the α-receptors needed to respond to the PDGF A-chain produced by cells within the arterial wall (Table 1). Furthermore, since these α-receptors can also bind B-chain PDGF, the VSMC can respond to rat platelet PDGF, which is a B-chain homodimer (Table 2).

ß-receptor transcripts were also present in the uninjured rat carotid artery. However, unlike the α-receptor transcripts, the ß-receptor transcripts were reduced 2 hours and 4 hours after balloon denudation by 50% and by 80%, respectively. One week after balloon denudation, ß-receptor transcripts were 2-fold greater than normal. Similar changes were observed by Fingerle et al [49] after gentle denudation of the rat carotid artery. Since the PDGF that is released by platelets can bind to ß-receptors and since ß-receptor transcripts were low at a time when platelet adhesion to the arterial wall was high, the results of these two studies suggest that the early decreases in β-receptor transcripts were the result of platelet PDGF-induced ß-receptor down regulation.

Consigny and Bilder [50] have studied the expression and release of PDGF mitogens by arteries that have undergone conventional balloon angioplasty. In their studies, balloon angioplasty was performed on one iliac artery in normal rabbits; the contralateral iliac artery served as an undilated control. Four days after angioplasty, the dilated and control arteries were removed and placed in co-culture with quiescent rabbit aortic VSMC in order to bioassay for the presence of VSMC mitogens.

After four days in co-culture, VSMC number increased only 1% in the presence of control arteries but increased an average of 93% in the presence of dilated arteries. In parallel experiments, PDGF A and B-chain gene expression were measured by Northern hybridization. Compared to control arteries denuded of endothelium, the mRNA concentrations for the A and B chains were unchanged in dilated arteries removed 4 hours after angioplasty but were increased 8.7 fold and 1.7 fold, respectively, in dilated arteries removed 4 days after angioplasty. These experiments demonstrated that arteries removed 4 days after angioplasty release VSMC mitogen(s) and suggest that the mitogen(s) may be A and B-chain PDGF.

Additional experiments were performed to further characterize the mitogens released by the dilated arteries [51] In these experiments, normal and dilated arteries were removed 4 days after angioplasty and placed in tissue culture. After 4 days in culture, the media "conditioned" by the arteries was collected and tested for its ability to stimulate rabbit aortic VSMC proliferation. Media conditioned by the dilated arteries (DCM) stimulated VSMC proliferation, whereas the media conditioned by the normal arteries (NCM) did not. (Change in cell number: NCM: $-9.5\% \pm 6.2$; DCM: 26.4 ± 6.9, $p < 0.05$, n=10) Two additional experiments were performed to identify the mitogens present in the media. In the first series of experiments, DCM was heated to $90^{o}C$ for 10 minutes, since this treatment does not denature PDGF but does denature bFGF, another potential mitogen [52]. The mitogenicity of the DCM was not destroyed by heating (Change in cell number: unheated DCM: $42.6 + 10.7$; heated DCM: $55.2 + 13.7$, $p < 0.05$, n=5) suggesting that the mitogen may be PDGF. In the second series of experiments, DCM was again heated and its mitogenicity measured in the presence and absence of an anti-PDGF antibody. In 4 of 6 experiments, 10 ug of goat anti-human PDGF completely blocked the mitogencity of the heated DCM. However in the other two experiments, the mitogenicity was not affected. The results of these two series of experiments indicate that heat-insensitive mitogen(s) are released from dilated arteries and that one of the mitogens is PDGF-like.

One particularly interesting finding in the above experiments was that heat treatment increased the mitogenicity of DCM. This findings suggests that a heat-sensitive inhibitor was released by the dilated arteries while in culture. Recently, Raines et al [53] reported that the glycoprotein SPARC (secreted protein, acidic and rich in cysteine), also called osteonectin, is present in both normal and atherosclerotic arteries. This protein has the ability to bind the AB and BB isoforms of PDGF but not the AA isoform. This binding prevents PDGF from binding to PDGF receptors on fibroblasts. Since the binding of PDGF to SPARC is reversed by denaturation, it is possible that the heat-sensitive inhibitory activity observed in conditioned media was SPARC.

Summary

Restenosis after angioplasty is a complicated problem involving a number of factors, as summarized in numerous review articles [54-57]. PDGF is one of these factors. Obviously, platelets are an important source of PDGF and it is this PDGF that most likely contributes to VSMC proliferation in the early stages of restenosis. However, the studies of Majesky, Linder, and Consigny [48-51] suggest that angioplasty can induce the release of PDGF from cells within the arterial wall and it is presumably this PDGF which stimulates VSMC proliferation is the later stages of restenosis. It is important to note that mitogens other than PDGF are also likely to be involved in this proliferation, particularly bFGF [58,59] and IGF-1[60].

REFERENCES

1. Dotter CT, Judkins MP. Transluminal treatment of arteriosclerotic obstruction. Description of a technique and preliminary report of its application. Circulation 1964; 30: 654-670.
2. Gruentzig AR. Transluminal dilatation of coronary artery stenosis. Lancet 1978; 1: 263-266.
3. Holmes DR, Vlietstra RE, Smith HC, Vetrovec GW, Kent KM, Cowley MJ, Faxon DP, Gruentzig AR, Kelsey SF, Detre KM. Restenosis after percutaneous transluminal coronary angioplasty (PTCA): a report from the PTCA registry of the National Heart, Lung and Blood Institute. Am J Cardiol 1984; 53: 77C-81C.
4. Nobuyoshi M, Kimura T, Nosaka H, Mioka S, Ueno K, Yokoi H. Hamasaki N, Horiuchi H, Ohishi H. Restenosis after successful coronary angioplasty: serial angiographic follow-up of 229 patients. J Am Coll Cardiol 1988; 12: 616-623.
5. Austin GE, Ratliff NB, Hollman J, Tabei S, Phillips DF. Intimal proliferation of smooth muscle cells as an explanation for recurrent coronary artery stenosis after percutaneous transluminal coronary angioplasty. J Am Coll Cardiol 1985; 6: 369-375.

6. Johnson DE, Hinohara T, Selmon MR, Braden LJ, Simpson JB. Primary peripheral arterial stenoses and restenoses excised by transluminal atherectomy: a histopathologic study. J Am Coll Cardiol 1990; 15: 419-425.

7. Faxon DP, Sanborn TA, Weber VJ, Haudenschild C, Gottsman SB, McGovern WA, Ryan TJ. Restenosis following transluminal angioplasty in experimental atherosclerosis. Arteriosclerosis 1984; 4: 189-195.

8. Steele PM, Chesebro JH, Stanson AW, Holmes DR Jr, Dewanjee MK, Badimon L, Fuster V. Balloon angioplasty. Natural history of the pathophysiological response to injury in a pig model. Circ Res 1985; 57: 105-112.

9. Waller BF, Pinkerton CA, Orr CM, Slack JD, VanTassel JW, Peters T. Restenosis 1 to 24 months after clinically successful coronary balloon angioplasty: A necropsy study of 20 patients. J Am Coll Cardiol 1991; 17: 58B-70B.

10. Wilentz IR, Sanborn TA, Haudenschild CC, Valeri CR, Ryan TJ, Faxon DP. Platelet accumulation in experimental angioplasty: time course and relation to vascular injury. Circulation 1987; 75: 636-642.

11. Ross R. The pathogenesis of atherosclerosis - an update. N Engl J Med 1986; 314: 488-500.

12. Ip JH, Fuster V, Israel D, Badimon L, Badmon J, Chesebro JH. The role of platelets, thrombin and hyperplasia in restenosis after coronary angioplasty. J Am Coll Cardiol 1991; 17: 77B-88B.

13. Chesebro JH, Webster MWI, Reeder GS, Mock MB, Grill DE, Bailey KR, Steichen S, Fuster V. Coronary angioplasty: Antiplatelet therapy reduces acute complications but not restenosis. 1989; Circ 80: II-64.

14. Perler BA, Osterman FA, White RI Jr., Williams GM. Percutaneous laser probe femoropopliteal angioplasty: a preliminary experience. J Vasc Surg 1989; 10: 351-357.

15. Buchwald AB, Werner GS, Unterberg C, Voth E, Kreuzer H, Wiegand V. Restenosis after excimer laser angioplasty of coronary stenoses and chronic total occlusions. Am Heart J 1992; 123: 878-885.

16. Schatz RA, Goldberg S, Leon M, Baim D, Hirshfeld J, Cleman M, Ellis S, Topol E. Clinical experience with the Palmaz-Schatz coronary stent. J Am Coll Cardiol 1991; 17: 155B-159B.

17. Umans VA, Beatt KJ, Rensing BJ, Hermans WR, deFeyter PJ, Serruys PW. Comparative quantitative angiographic analysis of directional coronary atherectomy and balloon coronary angioplasty. Am J Cardiol 1991; 68: 1556-1563.

18. Hanke H, Strohschneider T, Oberhoff, Betz E, Karsch KR. Time course of smooth muscle cell proliferation in the intima and media of arteries following experimental angioplasty. Circ Res 1990; 67: 651-659.

19. Minar E, Ehringer H, Ahmadi H. Platelet deposition at angioplasty sites and its relation to restenosis in human iliac and femoropopliteal arteries. Radiology 1989; 170: 767-772.

20. Barrett TB, Gajdusek CM, Schwartz SM, McDougall JK, Benditt EP. Expression of the sis gene by endothelial cells in culture and in vivo. Proc. Natl. Acad Sci. USA 1984; 81: 6772-6774.

21. Collins T, Pober JS, Gimbrone MA Jr, Hammacher A, Betsholtz C, Westermark B, Heldin CH. Cultured human endothelial cells express platelet-derived growth factor A chain. Am J Pathol 1987; 126: 7-12.

22. Sitaras NM, Sariban E, Pantazis P, Zetter B, Antoniades HN. Human iliac artery endothelial cells express both genes encoding the chains of platelet-derived growth factor (PDGF) and synthesize PDGF-like mitogen. J Cell Physiol 1987; 132: 376-380.

23. Limanni A, Fleming T, Molina R, Hufnagel H, Cunningham RE, Cruess DF, Sharefkin JB. Expression of genes for platelet-derived growth factor in adult human venous endothelium. A possible non-platelet-dependent cause of intimal hyperplasia in vein grafts and perianastomotic areas of vascular prostheses. J Vasc Surg 1988; 7: 10-20.

24. Nilsson J, Sjolund M, Palmberg L, Thyberg J, Heldin CH. Arterial smooth muscle cells in primary culture produce a platelet-derived growth factor-like protein. Proc Natl Acad Sci USA 1985; 82: 4418-4422.

25. Sejersen T, Betsholtz C, Sjolund M, Heldin C-H, Westermark B, Thyberg J. Rat skeletal myoblasts and arterial smooth muscle cells express the gene for the A-chain but not the gene for the B-chain (c-sis) of platelet derived growth factor (PDGF) and produce a PDGF-like protein. Proc Natl Acad Sci USA 1986; 83: 6844-6848.

26. Walker LN, Bowen-Pope DF, Ross R, Reidy MA. Production of platelet-derived growth factor-like molecules by cultured arterial smooth-muscle cells accompanies proliferation after arterial injury. Proc Natl Acad Sci USA 1986; 83: 7311-7315.

27. Sjolund M, Helin U, Sejerson T, Heldin C-H, Thyberg J. Arterial smooth muscle cells express platelet-derived growth factor (PDGF) A chain mRNA, secrete a PDGF-like mitogen, and bind exogenous PDGF in a phenotype- and growth state-dependent manner. J Cell Biol 1988; 106: 403-413.

28. Valente AJ, Delgado R, Metter JD, Cho C, Sprague EA, Schwartz CJ, Graves DT. Cultured primate aortic smooth muscle cells express both PDGF-A and PDGF-B gene but do not secrete mitogenic activity or dimeric platelet-derived growth factor protein. J Cell Physiol 1988; 136: 479-485.

29. Shimokado K, Raines EW, Madtes DK, Barrett TB, Benditt EP, Ross R. A significant part of macrophage-derived growth factor consists of at least two forms of PDGF. Cell 1985; 43: 277-286.

30. Martinet Y, Bitterman PB, Mornex JF, Grotendorst GR, Martin GR, Crystal RG. Activated human monocytes express the c-sis proto-oncogene and release a mediator showing PDGF-like activity. Nature 1986; 319: 158-160.

31. Ross R, Masuda J, Raines EW, Gown AM, Katsuda S, Sasahara M, Malden LT, Masuko H, Sato H. Localization of PDGF-B protein in macrophages in all phases of atherogenesis. Science 1990; 248: 1009-1012.

32. Ross R, Raines EW, Bowen-Pope DF. The biology of platelet-derived growth factor. Cell 1986; 46: 155-169.

33. Majack RA, Majesky MW, Goodman LV. Role of PDGF-A expression in the control of vascular smooth muscle cell growth by transforming growth factor-ß. J Cell Biol 1990; 111: 239-247.

34. Raines EW, Dower SK, Ross R. Interleukin-1 mitogenic activity for fibroblasts and smooth muscle cells is due to PDGF-AA. Science 1989; 243:393-396.

35. Naftilan AJ, Pratt RE, Dzau VJ. Induction of platelet-derived growth factor A-chain and c-myc gene expressions by angiotensin II in cultured rat vascular smooth muscle cells. J. Clin Invest 1989; 83: 1419-1424.

36. Majesky MW, Daemen MJAP, Schwartz SM. α1-adrenergic stimulation of platelet-derived growth factor A-chain gene expression in rat aorta. J Biol Chem 1990; 265: 1082-1088.

37. Hart CE, Bowen-Pope DF. Platelet-derived growth factor receptor: current views of the two-subunit model. J Invest Dermatol 1990; 94: 53S-57S.

38. Ross R, Bowen-Pope DF, Raines EW. Platelet-derived growth factor and its role in health and disease. Phil Trans R Soc Lond 1990; 327: 155-169.

39. Terracio L, Ronnstrand L, Tingstrom A, Rubin K, Claesson-Welsh L, Funa K, Heldin C-H. Induction of platelet-derived growth factor receptor expression in smooth muscle cells and fibroblasts upon tissue culturing. J Cell Biol 1988; 107: 1947-1957.

40. Rubin K, Hansson GK, Ronnstrand L, Claesson-Welch L, Fellstrom B, Tingstrum A, Larsson E, Klareskog L, Heldin C-H, Terracio L. Induction of B-type receptors for platelet-derived growth factor in vascular inflammation: possible implications for development of vascular proliferative lesions. Lancet (June 18) 1988; i: 1353-1356.

41. Janat MF, Liau G. Transforming growth factor $\beta 1$ is a powerful modulator of platelet-derived growth factor action in vascular smooth muscle cells. J Cell Physiol 1992; 150: 232-242.

42. Bobik A, Grinpukel S, Little PJ, Grooms A, Jackman G. Angiotensin II and noradrenalin increase PDGF-BB receptors and potentiate PDGF-BB stimulated DNA sysnthesis in vascular smooth muscle. Biochem Biophys Res Comm 1990; 166: 580-588.

43. Bowen-Pope DF, Hart CE, Weifert RA. Sera and conditioned media contain different isoforms of platelet-derived growth factor (PDGF) which bind to different classes of PDGF receptor. J Biol Chem 1989; 264: 2502-2508.

44. Barrett TB, Benditt EP. sis (platelet-derived growth factor B chain) gene transcript levels are elevated in human atherosclerotic lesions compared to normal artery. Proc Natl Acad Sci USA 1987; 84: 1099-1103.

45. Barrett TB, Benditt EP. Platelet-derived growth factor gene expression in human atherosclerotic plaques and normal arterial wall. Proc Natl Acad Sci USA 1988; 85: 2810-2814.

46. Wilcox JN, Smith KM, Williams LT, Schwartz SM, Gordon D. Platelet-derived growth factor mRNA detection in human atherosclerotic plaques by in situ hybridization. J Clin Invest 1988; 82: 1134-1143.

47. Libby P, Warner SJC, Salomon RN, Birinyi LK. Production of platelet-derived growth factor-like mitogen by smooth-muscle cells from human atheroma. N Eng J Med 1988; 318: 1493-1498.

48. Majesky MW, Reidy MA, Bowen-Pope DF, Hart CE, Wilcox JN, Schwartz SM. PDGF ligand and receptor gene expression during repair of arterial injury. J Cell Biol 1990; 111: 2149-2158.

49. Fingerle J, Au YPT, Clowes AW, Reidy MA. Intimal lesion formation in rat carotid arteries after endothelial denudation in absence of medial injury. Arteriosclerosis 1990; 10: 1082-1087.

50. Consigny PM, Bilder GE. Expression and release of smooth muscle cell mitogens in the arterial wall after balloon angioplasty. J Vasc Med Biol 1992; In press.

51. Consigny PM, O'Reilly TM, Fernandez AM. Bioassay for smooth muscle cell mitogens released from arteries after angioplasty. Arteriosclerosis and Thrombosis 1991; 1444a.

52. Vlodavsky I, Fridman R, Sullivan R, Sasse J, Klagsbrun M. Aortic endothelial cells synthesize basic fibroblast growth factor which remains cell associated and platelet-derived growth factor which is secreted. J Cell Physiol 1987; 131: 402-408.

53. Raines EW, Lane TF, Iruela-Arispe ML, Ross R, Sage EH. The extracellular glycoprotein SPARC interacts with platelet-derived growth factor (PDGF)-AB and -BB and inhibits the binding of PDGF to its receptors. Proc Natl Acad Sci USA 1992; 89: 1281-1285.

54. Liu MW, Roubin GS, King SB III. Restenosis after coronary angioplasty. Potential biologic determinants and role of intimal hyperplasia. Circ 1989; 79: 1374-1387.

55. Habenicht AJR, Salbach P, Janssen-Timmen U, Blattner C, Schettler G. Platelet-derived growth factor - a growth factor with an expanding role in health and disease. Klin Wochenschr 1990; 68: 53-59.

56. Forrester JS, Fishbein M, Helfant R, Fagin J. A paradigm for restenosis based on cell biology: Clues for the development of new preventative therapies. J Am Coll Cardiol 1991; 17: 758-769.

57. Cercek B, Sharifi B, Barath P, Bailey L, Forrester JS. Growth factors in pathogenesis of coronary arterial restenosis. Am J Cardiol 1991; 68: 24C-33C.

58. Lindner V, Reidy MA: Proliferation of smooth muscle cells after vascular injury is inhibited by an antibody against basic fibroblast growth factor. Proc Natl Acad Sci USA 1991; 88: 3739-3743.

59. Lindner V, Majack RA, Reidy MA: Basic fibroblast growth factor stimulates endothelial regrowth and proliferation in denuded arteries. J Clin Invest 1990; 85: 2004-2008.

60. Cercek B, Fishbein MC, Forrester JS, Helfant RH, Fagin JA. Induction of insulin-like growth factor-1 mRNA in rat aorta after balloon denudation. Circ Res 1990; 66: 1755-1769.

16. Platelet-derived growth factor (PDGF) receptor induced by vascular injury

GLENDA E. BILDER

Introduction

The platelet-derived growth factor receptor (PDGFr) belongs to the protein tyrosine kinase family of membrane receptors. Central to cellular signal transduction by the PDGF ligand is activation of the tyrosine kinase activity intrinsic to the PDGFr. In the cardiovascular system it is hypothesized that inappropriate PDGFr activity may result in undesirable vascular changes leading to development of the atherosclerotic plaque and restenosis following the clinical procedure of angioplasty. The importance of PDGFr protein tyrosine kinase in cell signaling and the influence of vascular injury on this receptor activity is discussed.

The PDGF receptor: member of the protein tyrosine kinase family of receptors

Within the past several years, the PDGFr has been extensively characterized [see reviews 1,2,3,4]. Major advances in understanding the PDGFr followed from results of receptor ligand binding studies, cloning and sequencing of receptors and receptor deletion mutation experiments [5,6,7,8,9,10]. The existence of two polypeptide PDGF receptors termed α and β subunits, each a product of a separate, independently regulated gene, is now established. Both exhibit an external ligand binding domain of five immunoglobulin-like structures, a single short transmembrane region, and a cytoplasmic catalytic domain containing the tyrosine kinase. Unique to the PDGF receptor subunits, and related proteins, i.e. colony stimulating factor-1 receptor and the c-Kit gene product, is the kinase insert (KI), a 104 amino acid sequence splitting the cytoplasmic kinase catalytic domain. Whereas sequence homology between the α and ß-subunits with respect to the kinase domain is 70-80%, sequence homology in the KI, a region implicated in receptor-protein recruitment of signal transmission, is 35% [10]. Thus signaling through the two subunits need not be identical.

PDGF-receptor tyrosine kinase: role in signal transduction

Signal transduction through the PDGFr is incompletely understood. The dimeric PDGF ligand exists in three isoforms comprised of two similar but nonidentical chains, termed A and B [see reviews 3,11]. High affinity α and ß PDGF receptor subunits bind PDGF ligands in an isoform-specific manner (β subunit combines with B-chain; α subunit combines with both A- and B-chain) [7,8]. Mismatch of ligand isoform (AA,BB,AB) and appropriate receptor subunits would negate a potential PDGF-dependent effect. Ligand binding results in dimerization of subunits, induction of conformational change and activation of the intrinsic protein tyrosine kinase activity of the receptor subunits [3,4,9]. Activation of the PDGF receptor protein tyrosine kinase (PDGFr-PTK) activity is key to signal transduction as it leads to tyrosine phosphorylation of the receptor (autophosphorylation), subsequent recruitment and tyrosine phosphorylation of cytoplasmic proteins and postulated receptor substrates, e.g. phosphatidyl-inositol(PI)-3'Kinase(PI3K), phospholipase Cγ, GTPase activating protein and P74c-raf protein (see review 12) and a cascade of events directed to nuclear signaling and PDGF-dependent effects [13].

Results of studies which utilized mutated PDGFr have emphasized the importance of autophosphorylation at specific receptor sites. It is established that in the absence of a functional PDGFr kinase, the PDGFr can not transmit a cellular signal when stimulated by ligand [14,15,16]. PDGF receptors with partial, full or point deletions of the KI region fail to associate with various cytoplasmic enzymes [14,15,16,17,18]. Specifically modification of the kinase insert region in which the tyrosine phosphorylation site 751 (of human ß subunit) is omitted, inhibited, or substituted to phenylalanine, prevented association of the PDGFr with the P85 regulatory protein of PI3K, an enzyme which catalyzes the phosphorylation of the 3D-inositol position of PI to generate novel phospholipids. Significantly modification of the PDGFr as above prevented PDGF-induced DNA synthesis [19]. Other PDGF-associated cellular activities such as an increase in calcium uptake, cytoplasmic alkalization, PDGFr downregulation and PI turnover were unaffected [19]. Results of experiments with mutated receptors are supported by those which use a chimeric receptor. Addition of the PDGF kinase insert to the FGF receptor, a tyrosine kinase receptor of another subclass, conferred on the chimeric receptor the ability to associate with PI3K and enhanced ligand-induced mitogenic activity [20]. Of importance to the cardiovascular system, novel lipids phosphorylated at the 3D position of inositol, products of PI3K activity, have been isolated from PDGF-stimulated human vascular smooth muscle cells; furthermore the time course of appearance of these phosphorylated lipids is consistent with their possible role as second messengers [21].

Expression of the PDGF receptor in atherosclerosis and restenosis.

PDGF receptors are expressed on a variety of cells, mostly of mesenchymal origin eg smooth muscle cell, fibroblast, glial. PDGFr activation culminates in a variety of actions relevant to the cardiovascular system such as vasoconstriction, chemotaxis, mitogenesis and extracellular matrix formation [see reviews 11,22]. If inappropriately initiated, such effects may contribute to abnormal cardiovascular activity of vasospasm, restenosis following angioplasty and atherosclerotic plaque formation [22,23]. The latter phenomena are forms of vascular remodeling in which migration and proliferation of smooth muscle cells within the subendothelial space result in compromised arterial function [22,23].

It is postulated that vascular injury in the adult reactivates an arrested but previously developmentally-active PDGF ligand/receptor growth regulatory network [24,25]. Proof that a PDGF autocrine/paracrine mode of injury-dependent growth is the exclusive mediator of smooth muscle cell migration and proliferation promoting intimal hyperplasia, is lacking. Available evidence, however, points to a major role, but perhaps not exclusive role, for the PDGF ligand/receptor system in intimal hyperplasia of restenosis and atherosclerosis. Clearly both receptors and ligands are important in vascular injury. Whereas our focus is on the PDGFr, it is noted that PDGF ligand has been convincingly implicated in affecting injury-induced migration of medial smooth muscle cells. Intimal hyperplasia induced by balloon catheter denudation was inhibited by administration of antiplatelet antiserum to rabbits [26] and rats [27]and by antiPDGF antiserum to nude rats [28]. In these experiments [27,28], medial DNA synthesis remained elevated suggesting that the predominant effect of platelet PDGF was on smooth muscle migration. Since the PDGF ß-subunit tyrosine kinase tranduces a chemotactic signal [29], a crucial role of tyrosine kinase of the PDGF ß-subunit in smooth muscle cell migration is indicated. It is important to note that while smooth muscle cell migration is essential for development of intimal hyperplasia in the rat and rabbit, the presence of intimal smooth muscle cell masses in normal human arteries suggest that phenomena of smooth muscle cell migration may not be as important in man as in animal models.

In normal arteries low levels of functional PDGF receptors exist as demonstrated by the ability of isolated rat aortic rings to vasocontract in response to exogenous PDGF [31] and presence of low levels of PDGFr transcripts and protein [33,34]. In contrast, results of in situ immunocyto-chemisty and hybridization of human carotid endarterectomy sections show enhanced expression of the PDGF ß-receptor protein [32] and mRNA [33] respectively. The latter was localized to "modified" smooth muscle cells of the intima [33]. In a well-characterized experimental model of intimal hyperplasia induced by balloon catheter denudation of the rat carotid artery, the ß-subunit mRNA transiently decreased (within 2 hours of injury) but increased by two fold within one week in the injured artery compared to the contralateral control [33]. There were no dramatic or consistent changes in the α-subunit mRNA levels, although gene expression in the media exceeded that in the intima [34]. In a model of intimal hyperplasia induced by chronic electrode cuff stimulation, ß-subunit mRNA in rat carotid arteries increased rapidly within 1-2 days of daily electrical stimulation [36] and remained above contralateral control levels for an additional two weeks (Bilder et al., submitted). Unlike balloon catheter denudation, electrical stimulation produces subtle alterations in endothelial permeability but the endothelium as a layer remains intact [35].

The mechanism(s) responsible for increased expression of the PDGFr induced by vascular injury is unknown. Results of extensive cell culture experiments suggest that expression of α and ß-subunits depends on the phenotype and growth state of the vascular smooth muscle cell [24,25]. Specifically, as rat aortic smooth muscle cells changed from contractile to synthetic phenotype by cell culture manipulation, a situation analogous to vascular injury [37], gene expression of the ß-subunit increased and the transcripts for the α-subunit appeared for the first time. With addition of ligand, further modulation of the PDGFr occurred, production of the PDGF A-chain increased and an autocrine-dependent DNA synthesis was established [25]. A comprehensive approach at the organ or in vivo level analogous to cell culture studies [25] is now needed to complement and confirm these ideas.

Receptor tyrosine kinase in cuff injury and balloon denudation

Because of the central role of PDGFr tyrosine kinase in signal transduction, an assay was developed to measure PDGFr autophosphorylation in injured arteries. It was reasoned that since PDGFr mRNA increased rapidly with electrode cuff injury [35] and at a slower pace with balloon catheter denudation injury [34] and since PDGFr expression could be modulated by cell culture manipulations which influenced smooth muscle cell phenotype and growth state [24,25] then PDGFr level should be sufficiently elevated to detect PDGFr-PTK activity if indeed arterial PDGF receptors were functionally active. Injury was induced either perivascularly and chronically by placement of a flexible tygon cuff around the left carotid artery of the rat or luminally and acutely by balloon catheter denudation of the rat aorta. The procedure for perivascular injury followed that previously reported for the rabbit in which intimal hyperplasia was induced by a hypoxia-dependent mechanism generated by compression of the vasa vasorum [38,39]. PDGFr-PTK activity was measured by incubating the exised, manually denuded cuffed, contralateral and normal, nonmanipulated arteries with exogenous PDGF in a tissue bath environment. This was followed by rapid homogenization in Laemmli buffer containing protease and phosphatase inhibitors and western blotting with antiphosphotyrosine/antiPDGFr antibody. Characteristics of PDGFr PTK activity in injury arteries are summarized in Table 1. In control arteries, PDGFr-PTK activity (determined from the density of scanned autoradiographs normalized to standard amount of phosphorylated receptor) was minimally stimulated by PDGF-BB isoform and unaffected by PDGF-AA isoform; constitutive PDGFr-PTK activity (without exogenous PDGF) was barely detectable. In contrast, constitutive PDGFr-PTK activity of the cuffed artery was increased 2 fold compared to controls, and elevated 7 and 3 fold in the presence of homodimers, PDGF-BB and PDGF-AA respectively.

Table 1. PDGF-Receptor Tyrosine Kinase Activity in Injured Arteries

Artery	Constitutive	Response to PDGF-BB	Response to PDGF-AA	Maximal Expression	Response to other mitogens
Normal Carotid	+/-	2 fold (120 ng/ml)	-		
Cuffed Carotid	+	7 fold (90-360 ng/ml)	3 fold (180 ng/ml)	4 days	EGF - FCS - FGF -
Normal Aorta	-	-	ND		
Balloon Catheter Denuded Aorta	++	3 fold (180 ng/ml)	ND	18-30 hrs	ND

PDGF-receptor tyrosine kinase activity was measured in arteries removed at various times from rats (a) implanted with a flexible tygon cuff (cuffed left carotid) or (b) subjected to balloon catheter denudation(aorta, 2F Fogerty catheter, 0.3 cc air, three times).
(+) signifies a low but measurable level of activity
(-) signifies activity below detection
(ND) indicates not done but experiment planned.
Epidermal growth factor (EGF), fibroblast growth factor (FGF), fetal calf serum (FCS)

These effects were maximal at 4-5 days after cuff placement. Interestingly, perivascular injury also induced similar changes in the contralateral artery suggesting a secondary injury propagated by hemodynamic changes, circulating factors or by cell communication as suggested by others [40]. AntiPDGFr immunoblots showed that the tyrosine phosphorylated protein detected in antiphosphotyrosine immunoblots was the PDGFr. Whether injury increased receptor number or accessibility to ligand cannot be determined with the present methods. Western blots revealed the presence of cytoplasmic proteins (kDa: 80-90 and 112-119) which were dose-relatedly tyrosine phosphorylated in cuffed arteries in response to exogenous PDGF. The identity of these proteins is unknown. Neither EGF, FGF nor fetal calf serum produced consistent and dose-related tyrosine phosphorylation patterns in cuffed arteries related to known receptors, suggesting that perivascular injury was specific to PDGF.

In rats subjected to aortic balloon catheter denudation by procedures which produce intimal hyperplasia [41], constitutive PDGFr PTK activity, measured as above, was elevated above control levels at 18 hours post denudation and declined thereafter (30 hours). High concentrations of PDGF-BB were ineffective in stimulating PDGFr-PTK at 18 hours but produced a 3 fold increase (180 ng/ml) at 30 hours at a time when constitutive PDGFr-PTK activity was low. The early elevation of constitutive PDGFr-PTK activity may be a consequence of endogenous stimulation from platelet PDGF as this model unlike perivascular injury is more dependent on platelet PDGF [27,28]. In both perivascular injury and balloon catheter denudation, elevated PDGFr-PTK activity preceded the maximal increase in thymidine incorporation (5-8 days in perivascular injury and 48 hours in balloon catheter denudation).

Although our data show that PDGFr-PTK activity is elevated with vascular injury, our findings do not prove that PDGFr-PTK activity is the necessary event for smooth muscle cell migration and proliferation. It seemed possible that the synthetic low molecular weight tyrphostins [42] could be useful tools to probe this issue. Several tyrphostins have recently been shown to inhibit PDGFr-PTK activity in situ in vascular smooth muscle cells and at similar concentrations to inhibit PDGF-dependent proliferation and growth in cultured vascular smooth muscle cells [43]. One available tyrphostin, RG 50864, was administered to cuffed rats (slow 24 hour infusion, total dose 42 mg/kg). PDGFr-PTK activity of the cuffed artery stimulated with PDGF was inhibited 50%. It is, therefore, possible to inhibit in vivo injury-induced PDGFr-PTK activity.

Conclusions and future research

The PDGFr-PTK activity is a major determinant of the PDGF-signal transduction pathway. Depending on the vascular injury, mRNA and protein for at least one receptor subunit has been found to increase above normal. Functional capacity of the PDGFr as measured by receptor autophosphorylation is increased with both perivascular and luminal type injury. Additionally with perivascular injury, PDGFr-PTK activity can be significantly reduced with in vivo administration of a tyrosine kinase inhibitor.

Many unanswered questions remain. It seems worthwhile to ask the nature of the elevated constitutive PDGFr-PTK in injury, and the contribution of the α and b-subunits to injury. Does the α subunit appear with perivascular injury as antiphosphotyrosine immunoblots suggest and as reported in cell culture experiments? Is there an increase in PDGFr number per cell with injury or is the increase in PDGFr-PTK activity dependent on other receptor changes? Finally, will specific blockade of vascular PDGFr-PTK activity result in inhibition of injury-related events of smooth muscle cell migration and proliferation, which determine the extent of vascular remodeling in restenosis and atherosclerosis.

Acknowledgement

The author is grateful to Dr. Mark Perrone for his critical review of this chapter and to Ms. Rosalie Ratkiewicz for her expert secretarial skills.

References

1. Deuel T. Polypeptide growth factors: roles in normal and abnormal cell growth. Annu Rev Cell Biol 1987; 3: 433-492.
2. Yarden Y, Ullrich A. Growth factor receptor tyrosine kinases. Annu. Rev. Biochem 1988; 57: 443-478.
3. Heldin C-H, Westermark B. Platelet-derived growth factor: Three isoforms and two receptor types. Trends in Genetics 1989; 5: 108-11.
4. Ullrich A, Schlessinger J. Signal transduction by receptors with tyrosine kinase activity. Cell 19900; 61: 203-212.
5. Yarden Y, Escobedo JA, Kuang W-J, Yang-Feng TL, Daniel TO, Tremble PM, Chen EY, Ando ME, Harkings RN, Francke U, Freid VA, Ullrich A, Williams LT. Structure of the receptor for platelet-derived growth factor helps define a family of closely related growth factor receptors. Nature 1986; 323: 226-232.

6. Matsui T, Heidaran M, Miki T, Popescu N, LaRochelle W, Kraus M, Pierce J, Aaronson S. Isolation of a novel receptor cDNA establishes the existance of two PDGF receptor genes. Science 1989; 243:800-804.

7. Hart CE, Forstrom JW, Kelly JD, Seifert RA, Smith RA, Ross R, Murray MJ, Bowen-Pope DF. Two classes of PDGF receptor recognize different isoforms of PDGF. Science.Wash. DC 1988; 240: 1529-1531.

8. Seifert RA, Hart CE, Phillips PE, Forstrom JW, Ross R,Murray MJ, Bowen-Pope DF. Two different subunits associate to create isoform-specific platelet-derived growth factor receptors. J Biol Chem 1989; 264: 8771-8778.

9. Williams TL. Signal transduction by platelet-derived growth factor receptor. Science Wash, DC 1989; 243: 1564-1570.

10. Claesson-Welsh L, Eriksson A, Westermark B, Heldin C-H. cDNA cloning and expression of the human A-type platelet-derived growth factor (PDGF) receptor establishes structural similarity to the B-type PDGF receptor. Proc Natl Acad Sci USA 1989; 86: 4917-4921.

11. Hannink M, Donoghue DJ. Structure and function of platelet-derived growth factor (PDGF) and related proteins. Biochim Biophys Acta 1989; 989: 1-10.

12. Cantley LC, Auger KR, Carpenter C, Duckworth B, Graziani A, Sapeller R, Soltoff S. Oncogenes and signal transduction. Cell 1991; 64: 281-302.

13. Rozengurt E. Early signals in mitogenesis. Science 1986; 234: 161-166.

14. Severinsson L, Ek B, Mellstrom K, Cleasson-Welsh L, Heldin C.-H. Deletion of the kinase insert sequences of the platelet-derived growth factor B-receptor affects kinase activity and signal transduction. Mol. Cell. Biol 1990; 10: 801-809.

15. Escobedo JA, Williams LT. A PDGF receptor domain essential formitogenesis but not for many other responses to PDGF. Nature 1988; 335: 85-87.

16. Escobedo JA, Barr PJ, Williams LT. Role of tyrosine kinase and membrane-spanning domains in signal transduction by the platelet-derived growth factor receptor. Mol Cell Biol 1988; 8: 5126-5131.

17. Kazlauskas A, Cooper JA. Autophosphorylation of the PDGF receptor in the kinase insert region regulates interactions with cell proteins. Cell 1989; 58: 1121-1122.

18. Escobedo JA, Kaplan DR, Kavanaugh W M, Turck CW, Williams, LT. A phosphatidylinositol-3 kinase binds to platelet-derived growth factor receptors through a specific receptor sequence containing phosphotyrosine. Mol Cell Biol 1991; 11: 1125-1132.

19. Coughlin SR, Escobedo JA, Williams LT. Role of phosphatidyl-inositol kinase in PDGF receptor signal transduction. Science Wash DC 1989; 243: 1191-1193.

20. Wennstrom S, Lendgren E, Blume-Jensen P, Claesson-Welsh L. The platelet-derived growth factor ß-receptor kinase insert confers specific signaling properties to a chimeric fibroblast growth factor receptor. J Biol Chem 1992; 267: 13749-13756.

21. Auger, KR, Serunian LA, Soltoff SP, Libby P, Cantley LC. PDGF-dependent tyrosine phosphorylation stimulates production of novel polyphosphoinositides in intact cells. Cell 1989;57: 167-175.

22. Ross R, Raines EW, Bowen-Pope DF. The biology of platelet-derived growth factor. Cell 1986; 46: 155-169.

23. Munroe JM, Cotran RS. The pathogenesis of atherosclerosis: atherogenesis and inflammation. Lab Invest 1988; 58: 249-261.

24. Sjolund M, Hedin U, Sejersen T. Heldin C-H, Thyberg J.Arterial smooth muscle cells express platelet-derived growth factor (PDGF) A chain mRNA, secrete a PDGF-like mitogen and bind exogenous PDGF in a phenotype-and growth state-dependent manner. J Cell Biol 1988; 106: 403-413.

25. Sjolund M, Rahm M, Claesson-Welsh L, Sejersen T, Heldin C.-H, Thyberg J. Expression of PDGF a and b-receptors in rat arterial smooth muscle cells is phenotype and growth state dependent. Growth Factors 1990; 3: 191-203.

26. Friedman RJ, Stemerman MB, Weng B, Moore S, Gauldie J, Gent M, Tiell ML, Spaet TH. The effect of thrombocytopenia on experimental arteriosclerotic lesion formation in rabbits. J Clin Invest 1977; 60: 1191-1201.

27. Fingerle J, Johnson R, Clowes AW, Majesky MW, Reidy MA. Role of platelets in smooth muscle cell proliferation and migration after vascular injury in rat carotid artery. Proc Natl Acad Sci USA 1989; 86: 8412-8416.

28. Gordon A, Ferns A, Raines EW, Sprugel KH, Motani AS, Reidy MA, Ross R. Inhibition of neointimal smooth muscle accumulation after angioplasty by an antibody to PDGF. Science 1991; 253: 1129-1132, 1991.

29. Westermark B, Siegbahn A, Heldin C-H, Claesson-Welsh L. B-type receptor for platelet-derived growth factor mediates a chemotactic response by means of ligand-induced activation of the receptor protein-tyrosine kinase. Proc. Natl. Acad. Sci., USA 1990; 87: 128-132.

30. Velican C, Velican D. Intimal thickening in developing coronary arteries and its relevance to atherosclerotic involvement. Atheroscl 1976; 23: 345-355.

31. Berk BC, Alexander RW, Brock JA, Gimbroni MA, Webb RC. Vasoactive effects of growth factors. Biochem Pharmacol 1989; 38: 219-225.

32. Rubin K, Hansson GK, Ronnstrand L, Claesson-Welsh L, Fellstrom B, Tingstrom A, Larsson E, Klareskog L, Heldin C-H, Terracio L. Induction of B-type receptors for platelet-derived growth factor in vascular inflammations: possible implications for development of vascular proliferative lesions. Lancet 1988; 1: 1353-1356.

33. Wilcox JN, Smith KM, Williams LT, Schwartz SM, Gordon D. Platelet-derived growth factor mRNA detection in human atherosclerotic plaques by in situ hybridization. J Clin Invest 1988; 82: 1134-1143.

34. Majesky MW, Reidy MA, Bowen-Pope DF, Hart CE, Wilcox JN, Schwartz SM. PDGF ligand and receptor gene expression during repair of arterial injury. J Cell Biol 1990; 111: 2149-2158.

35. Betz E, Schlote W. Responses of vessel walls to chronically applied electrical stimuli. Basic Res Cardiol 1979; 74: 10-20.

36. Bilder GE, Kasiewski CJ, Hodge TG, Perrone MH. Electrically-induced fibroma is sensitive to Diltiazem and exhibits early expression of PDGF-beta chain mRNA. Circ 80: Suppl. II-331.

37. Campbell JH, Manderson JA, Harrigan S, Rennick RE. Arterial smooth muscle. A multifunctional mesenchymal cell. Arch Pathol Lab Med 1988; 112: 979-986.

38. Booth RFG, Martin JF, Honey AC, Hassel DG, Bessley JE,Moncada S. Rapid development of atherosclerotic lesions in the rabbit carotid artery induced by perivascular manipulation. Atherosclerosis 1989; 76: 257-268.

39. Martin JF, Booth RFG, Moncada S. Arterial wall hypoxia following thrombosis of the vasa vasorum is an initial lesion in atherosclerosis. Eur J Clin Invest 1991; 21: 355-359.

40. Reidy MA. Proliferation of smooth muscle cell at sites of distant vascular injury. Arterioscl Thromb 1990; 10: 298-305.

41. Bettmann DS, Stemerman MB, Ransil BJ. The effect ofhypophysectomy on experimental endothelial cell regrowth and intimal thickening in the rat. Circ Res 1981; 48: 907-912.

42. Levitzki A. Tyrphostins-potential antiproliferative agents and novel molecular tools. Biochem Pharm 1990; 40: 913-918.

43. Bilder GE, Krawiec JA, McVety K, Gazit A, Gilon C, Lyall R,Zilberstein A, Levitzki A, Perrone MH, Schreiber AB. Tyrphostins inhibit PDGF-induced DNA synthesis and associated early events in smooth muscle cells. Amer J Physiol 1991; 260: C721-C730.

17. Growth factors and hypertension: Implications for a role in vascular remodelling

ABDEL-ILAH K. EL AMRANI, FRANCINE EL AMRANI and
PETER CUMMINS

Introduction

It is now well established that whatever the mechanisms that initiate elevation of blood pressure, a significant increase in arterial wall thickness is always observed in hypertension. This structural change in the arterial wall is considered to be an adaptive response to the elevated arterial blood pressure that plays a major role in the increase in vascular resistance responsible for chronic hypertension [1]. The structural remodelling of blood vessels in hypertension may involve important changes in the arterial intima, extracellular matrix and arterial media. Alterations in the shape of endothelial cells and an increase in their number may be observed, for example in the deoxycorticosterone acetate-salt (DOCA-salt) hypertension model, probably in response to the increase in arterial diameter [2]. The extracellular matrix expansion is mainly due to increases in arterial collagen, elastin and proteoglycans presumably as a result of stimulation of their production by smooth muscle cells. In the medial layer which normally constitutes most of the arterial wall thickness, the number of lamellar units (which are usually composed of smooth muscle cells surrounded by a dense network of connective tissue), remains relatively constant in large vessels. However, the increased wall thickness in hypertension is mainly due to the alteration in cellular mass that is accompanied by significant changes in connective tissue content including collagen, elastin proteoglycans and fibronectin. Therefore, hypertension could be considered as a disease of abnormal growth of the arterial media. The increase in cellular mass in the arterial wall during hypertension is still a matter of debate, in particular whether there is a true cell proliferation or only cellular hypertrophy. This controversy is due in part to differences in the animal species, model of hypertension, arterial vessel (i.e. small or large arteries) and the technical difficulties in investigating these processes, since an increase in DNA synthesis, which could be considered as cell proliferation, might simply be a smooth muscle cell polyploidy. Similar controversy also exists for cardiac tissue since myocyte mitotic division has been described in long-term cardiac hypertrophy and in ageing rats [3,4]. However, many studies have demonstrated that in several slowly-developing chronic models of hypertension, such as the renovascular model (i.e. two kidney, one clip) or in spontaneously hypertensive rats, the major increase in cellular mass in the large arteries is due to smooth muscle cell hypertrophy rather than hyperplasia, and can be associated with nuclear hyperploidy [5,6]. In contrast, a real process of aortic smooth muscle cell proliferation (i.e. hyperplasia) without hypertrophy or polyploidy has been clearly demonstrated in aortic stenosis-induced hypertension in a variety of animal species [7]. Owens and Reidy [7] demonstrated that DNA replication in smooth muscle cells was 25-fold increased in the thoracic aorta after coarctation in the rat (i.e. partial ligation of the abdominal aorta between the renal arteries) compared to sham-operated animals, while no differences were observed in cells in the abdominal segment 1cm. distal to the ligature. These results clearly demonstrate that the growth response of smooth muscle cells within a given blood vessel can be different depending on the model of hypertension.

Moreover, Mulvany et al.[8] have shown an increase in medial smooth muscle cell number in small arteries and in resistance vessels. Indeed sound evidence in favour of an increase in the number of smooth muscle cells in mesenteric resistance vessels of spontaneously hypertensive rats was demonstrated [8,9]. This may be of considerable importance since small blood vessels play a major role in the regulation of arterial blood flow. Therefore, whether there is hyperplasia and / or hypertrophy would not necessarily in our opinion be the vital question for at least two reasons; 1. Both hyperplasia or hypertrophy lead to an increase in wall thickness and vascular resistance and 2. Despite the considerable controversy regarding the relative role of smooth muscle cell hypertrophy vs. hyperplasia in the increase in cellular mass, at present there is no clear evidence in the literature that these processes are initiated by distinct intrinsic factors. Peptide growth factors acting through autocrine or paracrine mechanisms may be important in growth responses of the vessel wall which could include the stimulation of cell divison or hypertrophy.

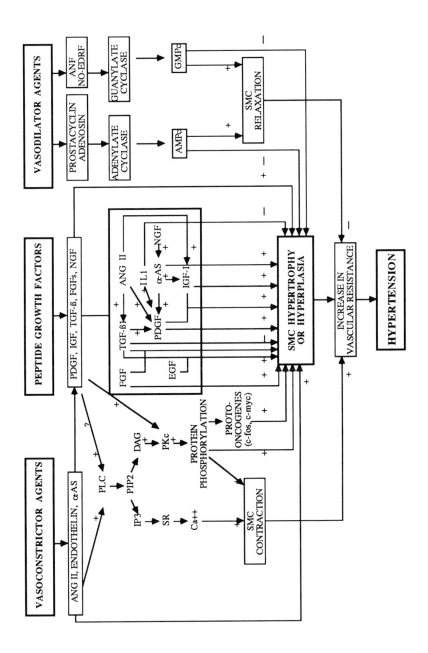

Figure 1. A proposed scheme for peptide growth factors and vasoactive agents in the increase in arterial wall growth during hypertension.

ANGII: angiotensin II, α-AS: α-adrenergic stimulation, IGF-1: insulin-like growth factor 1, NGF: nerve growth factor, PDGF: platelet-derived growth factor, FGFs: fibroblast growth factors, TGFß: transforming growth factor ß, EGF: epidermal growth factor, IL-1: interleukin-1, SMC: vascular smooth muscle cells, PLC: phospholipase C, SR: sarcoplasmic reticulum, PKc: protein kinase C, PIP2: phosphoinositide lipids, DAG: diacyl glycerol, IP3: inositol 1,4,5-triphosphate, +: stimulation, -: inhibition.

In hypertension, the increase in vascular resistance may be due to an increase in smooth muscle cell contraction or growth promotion (Figure 1) (for review see [10]). While the role of some of the peptide growth factors in increasing cell numbers is less well established, their direct effect in enhancing cell contraction is now clear. Moreover, some agents, such as angiotensin II, endothelin and catecholamines may have dual effects on smooth muscle cells, i.e. contraction and growth promotion. This review will be primarily focused on the growth mechanisms of the arterial wall in hypertension.

Vasoactive agents as growth promoters

Growth promoters, such as angiotensin II, endothelin and α-adrenergic agents, are not yet classified as growth factors. These promoters have several biological and physiological effects in common: 1) they possess powerful vasoconstrictor properties; 2) they induce an increase in myocardial contractility (positive inotropic effect) [11,12,13]; 3) at high concentrations they improve myocardial relaxation in vitro (positive lusitropic effect) [11,14]; 4) they possess a chronotropic effect; 5) they act through the hydrolysis of polyphosphoinositide lipids that liberate two second messengers namely inositol-1,4,5-triphosphate (IP3) and 1,2-diacylglycerol (DAG) [15]; 6) and importantly they stimulate the processes of growth or proliferation [16,17,18]. The common breakdown of inositol lipid has been suggested as the precursor of cell growth or proliferation [19]. In addition, some evidence in favour of a close relationship between phosphoinositide lipids and certain proto-oncogenes has been described in the literature [20]. For example, angiotensin-II may induce vascular hypertrophy (or hyperplasia) by hydrolysis of inositol lipids and stimulation of nuclear proto-oncogene expression [21]. Naftilan et al, [22] have shown that this hypertrophic response is associated with an increase in mRNA levels of proto-oncogenes, c-fos, c-jun and c-myc and the autocrine growth factors, platelet-derived growth factor A (PDGF A) chain and TGF-ß1. In addition, a further direct effect of angiotensin-II has been suggested in which it induces the gene expression of other growth factors such as PDGF that possess potent vasoconstrictor and mitogenic properties. In fact, antisense oligonucleotides to PDGF mRNA have been shown to reduce vascular hypertrophy induced by angiotensin-II [23]. Endothelin has also been reported as a regulator of gene expression. In fact, Komuro et al., [18] have shown that endothelin stimulates c-fos and c-myc expression and proliferation of smooth muscle cells.

It is suggested that these vasoactive agents and growth factors could act through the same signal transduction pathways. Both classes of agents can activate phospholipase C resulting in the production of IP3 and DAG (see Figure 1), an increase in intracellular calcium and cellular alkalinization (for review see [24]). Other vasoconstrictor agents such as vasopressin, serotonin, leukotrienes and thromboxane have also been described as promoters of vascular smooth muscle cell growth and could act through the same intracellular mechanisms. Interestingly, some endogenous vasodilators which act either via adenylate cyclase stimulation (prostacyclin and adenosine) or by guanylate cyclase activation (atrial natriuretic peptide and nitric oxide-endothelium-derived relaxing factor [NO-EDRF]) inhibit vascular smooth muscle cell growth [25,26] (Figure 1).

The endothelium plays an important role in the process of vascular remodeling, since biological mediators are synthesized at this level and may directly or indirectly participate in the abnormality of the endothelium itself during hypertension [27,28,29,30]. In fact, some of the agents described previously are produced by the endothelium, although other factors, considered as growth factors are also produced here at this level.

Peptide growth factors

Growth factors such as fibroblast growth factor (FGF), insulin-like growth factor (IGF), transforming growth factor ß (TGFß) and platelet-derived growth factor (PDGF) are extensively described in the literature as major modulators of smooth muscle cell proliferation. The expression of these growth factors in the rat aorta has been demonstrated [31]. Others such as nerve growth factor (NGF) may also be implicated, especially in genetic hypertension. In addition, the possibility that other growth factors, both known and unknown may play a direct or indirect role in the process of proliferation cannot be excluded. Also, some vasoactive agents may act on cell growth via specific growth factors. One example of this is the association of the increased expression of PDGF and of the proto-oncogene c-myc in the hypertrophic effect of angiotensin-II on cultured smooth muscle cells [22]. It is for reasons of clarity only that these factors will be dealt with separately in the following sections. The involvement of more than one growth factor in the same biological effect cannot be excluded. We describe here some of the more important results during the last five years which either directly or indirectly implicate a role for peptide growth factors in increasing vascular resistance and developing chronic hypertension.

Transforming growth factor-β (TGF-β)

TGF-ß is one of the most widespread growth factors and is characterized by paradoxical effects on a variety of cells. TGF-ß stimulates in vitro production of fibronectin [32,33], proteoglycan [34], thrombospondin [35], collagen [32,33], and elastin [36]. Increased TGF-ß has been observed in models of vascular remodeling including development of pulmonary hypertension after air embolism [37], repair of arterial injury after carotid endarterectomy [38] and development of systemic hypertension after salt and mineralocorticoid administration [31]. At least five differents isoforms of TGF-ß (TGFß1-5) have been described.

TGF-ß1 has been shown to be capable of either stimulating or inhibiting the growth of cultured smooth muscle cells depending on culture conditions [39,40]. TGF-ß1 also stimulates the expression and synthesis of several extracellular matrix proteins. It acts as a modulator of vascular smooth muscle cells [32,35], inhibits serum-or PDGF-mediated proliferation at low cell density and potentiates proliferation at high cell density [39,41]. TGF-ß1 has a bifunctional effect on vascular smooth muscle cell growth. It inhibits vascular smooth muscle cell proliferation and stimulates extracellular matrix production but stimulates the proliferation of these cells when mediated by the autocrine production of PDGF AA (Figure 1) [42]. Sarzani et al [31] have demonstrated a significant increase in TGF-ß1 mRNA in aorta of DOCA hypertensive rats. These findings suggest a link between synthesis and release of growth factors from vascular smooth muscle cells and their autocrine / paracrine role in vivo. Hamet et al. [43]

demonstrated an increased accumulation of c-fos mRNA in calf serum-stimulated spontaneously hypertensive rat (SHR) vascular smooth muscle cells but only at a high cell density. The expression of TGF-ß1 mRNA was enhanced in growing SHR cells at every density studied, with stimulation as early as 24 hours after inoculation with calf serum,with a further increase at later times. At low cell density TGF-ß1 had no effect on DNA synthesis (evaluated by 3H thymidine incorporation) in either Wistar-Kyoto (WKY) or SHR vascular smooth muscle cells, but at a high cell density, there was a significant increase in DNA synthesis in response to TGF-ß1 in SHR cells without any effect in WKY cells. These findings demonstrate an abnormal expression and response to TGF-ß1 and suggest that the autoinduction of TGF-ß1 is particularly enhanced in growing vascular smooth muscle cells from SHR. Such a defect in feed-back regulation of an endogenous growth factor may be involved in the expression of abnormal growth phenotypes in SHR animals resulting in greater vascular smooth muscle cell proliferation and increased peripheral vascular resistance.

TGF-ß1 also induces an increase in the levels of both PDGF A and B chain mRNA in microvascular endothelium, probably through a transcriptional mechanism, which is also inhibited by stimulators of adenylate cyclase [44,45]. TGF-ß1 has been shown to induce the expression of PDGF-A mRNA in vascular smooth muscle cells (Figure 1) and increase the secretion of PDGF-like protein [46]. Further studies are required to determine whether TGF-ß1 exerts its growth stimulatory effect directly or indirectly via PDGF-like molecules.

Botney et al. [47] have investigated pulmonary hypertension in hypoxic new-born calves which is also associated with a profound remodeling of the pulmonary arterial wall [48] and increased extracellular matrix synthesis and deposition in the medial layer of large vessels [49]. They demonstrated a progressive age-dependent increase in normotensive pulmonary artery TGF-ß1 mRNA after birth, whereas TGF-ß1 mRNA remained at low, basal levels in hypertensive remodelled pulmonary arteries. Therefore, the local expression of TGF-ß1 is not associated with increased extracellular matrix protein synthesis in this model. However, these results differ from in vivo experiments that have shown a positive correlation between TGF-ß1 levels and extracellular matrix production [50,51]. Furthermore, an age-related progressive increase in steady state mRNA for TGF-ß1 in aorta has been described in normotensive rats which is further increased in SHR animals [52].

TGF-ß1 which is secreted by both endothelial and smooth muscle cells can act in a paracrine or autocrine fashion [53] resulting in cell hypertrophy and polyploidy [42]. Furthermore, using vascular smooth muscle cells from 10 to 12 week-old SHR, Saltis et al. [54] have shown that TGF-ß1 acts synergistically with epidermal growth factor to stimulate vascular smooth muscle cell proliferation. This would suggest that even in the absence of major changes in the level of growth factor, TGF-ß1 may stimulate the proliferation of smooth muscle cells resulting in vascular hypertrophy [54].

Platelet-derived growth factor (PDGF)

Studies based on cultured cells have shown that platelet-derived growth factor (PDGF) is the major mitogen for smooth muscle cells. Biologically active PDGF consists of two subunits: A and B. The PDGF AA and BB dimers are synthesised by macrophages, endothelial cells and vascular smooth muscle cells [55,56]. Two receptors have been described for PDGF dimers: α-receptor that binds both PDGF A and B chains and ß-receptor that binds the B chain only with high affinity [57,58]. The α and ß receptors are activated when dimerized in the $\alpha\alpha$, ßß or αß form [57,58]. Variations in the absolute or relative proportion of α- and ß-receptor could explain some of the differences in the effects of PDGF AA and BB dimers [58].

While the PDGF α-receptor has not been found to be influenced by age or by the level of blood pressure, an age-related progressive increase in steady state mRNA for PDGF ß-receptor in aorta has been described in normotensive rats although this is greatest in spontaneously hypertensive rats [59]. In the heart however a decrease in both receptor mRNA's has been observed. Increased aortic PDGF ß-receptor expression has also been shown in DOCA-salt hypertensive rats [59]. Interestingly, a partial reversion of the increased PDGF ß-receptor expression was observed after the normalization of blood pressure in DOCA-salt hypertension [59]. The increased PDGF ß-receptor expression in hypertension could in part explain the fact that cultured aortic smooth muscle cells from SHR [59] and DOCA-salt hypertensive animals [60] have a greater proliferation rate in comparison with WKY and normotensive controls respectively. However, Sarzani et al. [31] have shown that PDGF A and B mRNA expression in aorta is not changed in DOCA-salt hypertensive rats.

In cultured smooth muscle cells, it has been clearly shown that cell hypertrophy (with or without polyploidy) can be initiated by cathecholamines [61], angiotensin [62] and arginine vasopressin [63].

It has been suggested that one of the mediators of the expression of these biological vasoactive agents is PDGF (Figure 1). In fact in smooth muscle cells, both angiotensin II and α-adrenergic stimulation induce an increase in the expression of PDGF A-chain mRNA [22,64]. In addition, both angiotensin II and α-adrenergic stimulation induced a significant increase in binding sites for PDGF BB-chain dimers in cultured smooth muscle cells [65]. Therefore, PDGF dimers which can be produced by the endothelium [56] induce smooth muscle cell proliferation [55].

PDGF secretion by endothelial cells may also be promoted by interleukin-1 (IL-1), which is also an endothelium-derived growth factor [66] (Figure 1). IL-1 induces a decrease in cell proliferation that can be reversed by antisense oligonucleotides against IL-1 [67]. However, the specific role of IL-1 in vascular remodelling is still poorly understood.

Insulin-like growth factor-I (IGF-I)

Insulin-like growth factor-I (IGF-I) is a 70 residue peptide which shares 48% amino acid sequence homology with human pro-insulin [68]. IGF-I has been found to be synthesized in the liver under growth hormone regulation [69]. However recent studies have shown that IGF-I may be also synthesized in the heart and in skeletal muscle [70] with a paracrine / autocrine mechanism. Engelman et al. [71] have demonstrated the presence of IGF-I mRNA in neonatal ventricles of normotensive rats with a relatively high abundance in hypertensive rats. Moreover, IGF-I mRNA expression determined by in-situ hybridization was localized in myocytes and occasionally in endothelial cells.

An important question has been posed as to whether there is vascular cell synthesis or internalization of IGF-I [72]. Using ribonuclease protection assays, northern hybridization and protein-binding techniques, Delafontaine et al. [72] have found strong evidence that both endothelial and rat aortic vascular smooth muscle cells secrete IGF-I.

In vitro, IGF-I and PDGF are potent co-mitogens acting in synergy to promote vascular smooth muscle cell growth [73]. Similar synergism implicating both PDGF and IGF-I has been shown to result in a high connective tissue division within the wound and re-epithelialization after injury [74]. IGF-I stimulates vascular smooth muscle cell hypertrophy and matrix production [75].

Delafontaine et al. [76] have demonstrated the presence of IGF-I mRNA transcript in cultured rat aortic smooth muscle and in bovine aortic endothelial cells. They have also shown that cultured rat aortic smooth muscle deprived of serum for 48 hours demonstrates a marked reduction in IGF-I mRNA and that the exposure of quiescent cultured rat aortic smooth muscle to PDGF AB or BB induces a rapid and sustained increase in IGF-I mRNA. This is accompanied by an increase in IGF-I release into cultured rat aortic smooth muscle conditioned medium. This suggests that IGF-I mRNA levels in vascular smooth muscle cells are regulated by serum and by PDGF.

Certain forms of hypertension such as that induced by abdominal coarctation in the rat are thought to represent a form of acute vessel wall injury and are accompanied by endothelial cell and vascular smooth muscle cell hyperplasia [7]. Fath et al. [77] have demonstrated a marked increase in IGF-I gene expression in aortic endothelial and vascular smooth muscle cells in their model. These results are consistent and imply a role for IGF-I in the hypertensive remodelling of the vessel wall. Other data from Cercek et al. [78] have shown an increase in IGF-I mRNA levels in rat aorta after balloon injury. Since the response to vessel wall de-endothelialization includes platelet aggregation, one could speculate on the importance of PDGF release from activated platelets and subsequent induction of IGF-I gene expression [79].

Enhancement of IGF-I mRNA levels and IGF-I protein has also been detected in the left ventricle in two-kidney, one-clip Goldblatt hypertension [80]. The main localisation of IGF-I has been found in the subendocardial layers. The increased wall stress in this model has been suggested as the primary stimulus for the increase of IGF-I [80]. However, enhancement of IGF-I expression in vascular tissue has not been reported in this investigation, a finding supported by Sarzani et al., [31] have shown that IGF-I and IGF-II mRNA expression in aorta is not significantly changed in DOCA-salt hypertensive rats.

It has been suggested that IGF-I is a final common pathway for pressure and hormonal signals and that increased pressure and growth factors act directly on vessels to produce hypertrophy. A related possibility is that they act indirectly via IGF-I [81] (Figure 1).

Fibroblast growth factors (FGFs)

The FGFs are a widely distributed family of growth factors that affect the growth and function of a remarkable number of cell types including vascular and capillary endothelial cells, smooth muscle cells, fibroblasts and chondrocytes. Acidic (aFGF) and basic (bFGF) fibroblast growth factors induce important stimuli for cell components of the vascular wall [82]. They are chemotactic and mitogenic for endothelial cells. bFGF is also a mitogen for vascular smooth muscle cells and may play a very important role in pathologies as different as atherosclerosis and hypertension (see Section Four). bFGF might also have important therapeutic clinical applications where an enhancement of vascularisation is beneficial. bFGF is considered as a potent mitogen for smooth muscle cells and a potent autocrine growth factor for endothelial cells [83,84]. It plays an important role in cell migration, endothelial cell proliferation and matrix production [84,85]. Although its role in angiogenesis during myocardial infarction is clearly established [84,86] (see Section Three), its specific role in vascular remodelling and the regulation of its function during hypertension are still poorly understood.

It has been demonstrated that both aFGF and bFGF are expressed in rat aorta, but no difference has been found between normotensive and DOCA-salt hypertensive rats [31]. In cell culture, aFGF has been found in smooth muscle cells, but not in endothelial cells [87]. Others authors, however, have found that both vascular cell types can produce bFGF in culture [88].

Lindner et al. [89] have shown that systemic administration of bFGF can significantly restimulate quiescent endothelial cells in an incomplete endothelial monolayer in a denuded artery. Moreover, contineous administration of bFGF leads to a significant increase in the area of re-endothelization and complete regrowth can be achieved. These results showed that; 1.bFGF is a potent mitogen for large vessel endothelium (carotid artery) in vivo and 2. that quiescent endothelial cells can be restimulated by bFGF to grow into denuded areas where re-endothelization would not normally occur. One possible implication is that complete re-endothelization of synthetic vascular grafts might be achieved after bFGF treatment.

Medial smooth muscle cell proliferation, migration to the intima and subsequent intimal proliferation are characteristic responses to balloon catheter injury of the rat carotid artery. Recents studies have suggested that bFGF may play an important role in the proliferation of the smooth muscle cell in the injured artery. It has been shown that not only is bFGF synthesized by arterial smooth muscle cells in vivo but also that exogenous bFGF is a potent mitogen for smooth muscle cells in the de-endothelialized rat carotid artery [90]. McNeil et al.,[91] and Gajdusek and Carbon [92] have suggested that bFGF is released after cellular injury. Lindner and Reidy [93] have shown that the administration of an antibody to bFGF inhibits the smooth muscle cell proliferation which occurs 48 hours after injury and also after baloon catheter injury. However the role of bFGF in the intima in the chronic proliferation of smooth muscle cells is not yet clear.

Olson et al. [94] have shown by immunocytochemical staining, the presence of bFGF in the injured arterial wall which was decreased after balloon injury. Similar results were observed in bFGF protein and mRNA. The administration of antibody to bFGF 4-5 days after injury had no effect on intimal smooth muscle cell proliferation. These authors concluded that an increase in bFGF is not necessary for chronic smooth muscle cell proliferation. One interpretation is that after injury, bFGF could be released from storage sites and interacts with its receptors to stimulate smooth muscle cell proliferation. After injury bFGF would be released by the action of proteases such as plasmin [85]. This could explain the decrease in the amount of bFGF protein and mRNA.

In immunoblotting with bFGF antibodies a new band of 18 Kd appears after injury in addition to one of 23 Kd but the significance of this is still unknown [94]. The failure of antibody to bFGF to inhibit intimal smooth cell proliferation demonstrates that bFGF is not the most important factor controlling smooth muscle cell proliferation. Olson's results [94] suggest that even if bFGF is an important mitogen for medial smooth muscle cells immediately after injury, the fact that its synthesis subsequently decreases coupled to the inability of bFGF antibody to stop intimal smooth muscle cell proliferation suggests that it does not play a key role in smooth muscle cell proliferation several days after injury.

Nerve growth factor (NGF)

Nerve growth factor (NGF) which acts as a neurotrophic factor for peripheral sympathetic neurons [95,96], may play an important role in the development and maintainance of genetic hypertension. In fact strong positive correlation between tissue NGF protein or mRNA and norepinephrine content has been demonstrated [97,98]. An increase in norepinephrine content has been demonstrated in arteries of both young and adult spontaneously hypertensive rats (SHR) [99,102]. NGF content in vascular tissue has also been found to be increased in young SHR [103,104]. However in adult rats, no difference has been shown between SHR and WKY [104]. This would suggest that NGF may play an important role in initiating the increase in arterial blood pressure during genetic hypertension. The role of NGF in other models of hypertension is still poorly understood. However, one of the most important examples of evidence for the role of NGF (see Figure 1) in enhancing sympathetic nervous innervation and contributing to the pathogenesis of hypertension, was provided by Lee et al., [105] who showed that neonatal sympathectomy of SHR rats treated with guanethidine and antiserum against NGF prevented the development of hypertension.

Clinical implications

Growth factors may play an important role not only in hypertension but also in a large number of clinical diseases in which growth mechanisms are involved, including cancer and acquired immunodeficiency syndrome (AIDS) [106]. In a very recent investigation, the proteoglycan decorin, which is a natural inhibitor of TGF-ß, has been proposed as a clinical treatment in lung, liver and especially kidney disease [107].

The role of peptide growth factors in the increase in vascular smooth muscle cell mass is an important factor in understanding pathogenic processes such as hypertension, atherosclerosis, ageing, or restenosis after coronary angioplasty. Hypertension is well recognized as a major risk factor for the development of atherosclerosis. Both hypertension and atherosclerosis are characterized by trophic changes in the vascular wall. In hypertension, an increase in smooth muscle cell mass leads to an increase in vascular resistance. In atherosclerosis, intimal hyperplasia may lead to reduced blood flow and clinical symptoms due to ischemia.

Hypertension is associated with a decrease in compliance of the arterial system [108]. Levy et al. [108] have clearly demonstrated that treatment with converting enzyme inhibitor completely reversed the rigidity of large arteries and aortic media thickness in two-kidney, one-clip Goldblat hypertensive rats. This effect was not associated with regression of the increased absolute collagen content [108]. However, antihypertensives drugs appear to be unable to correct the structure of small arteries despite a normalization of blood pressure [for review 109].

The specific factors that initiate and probably maintain the processes of cellular hyperplasia or hypertrophy are not clearly understood. Knowedge of such factors could provide the opportunity to reverse the processes of vascular remodelling simultaneously with the normalization of arterial blood pressure. This is because as mentioned above, while antihypertensive treatment is an incomplete answer to "hypertensive disease" per se, correction of the arterial wall thickness in parallel with anti-hypertensive treatment could be an adequate solution. Moreover, there is as yet no firm evidence that the reversal of cardiac hypertrophy following treatment with some anti-hypertensive drugs such as the angiotensin-I converting enzyme inhibitors [110,111] increases survival even with the normalization of blood pressure [112]. In addition, with some of these anti-hypertensive drugs, such as the arterial vasodilatators, there is no reversal effect on cardiac hypertrophy [113,114].

It is essential to understand the role of peptide growth factors, vasodilatator agents, such as nitric oxide (NO) and atrial natriuretic factor (ANF), and vasoconstrictor agents such as endothelin, α-adrenergic stimulation and angiotensin II [115] in stimulating cell hypertrophy and / or cell proliferation leading to increasing arterial wall thickness (Figure 1). This is important not only at the arterial level but also at that of the myocardium itself [116,117,118] since an increase in arterial blood pressure also leads to cardiac hypertrophy. Interestingly, a true process of cell proliferation has been clearly demonstrated in ageing mammalian heart [4] and in long-term cardiac hypertrophy [3]. Also, during ageing the remodelling of blood vessels is similar to that observed in hypertension including intimal and medial thickening, intimal accumulation of smooth muscle cells and macrophages and increase in arterial connective tissue content [119-122]. In addition, the number of polyploid smooth muscle cells increases relatively with age in both rat [123] and human arteries [124]. The concept that hypertension accelerates the arterial changes associated with ageing has found further support in the finding of Sarzani et al. [52] described previously. Therefore, one could suggest an attractive hypothesis whereby the increase in vessel wall thickness and cardiac hypertrophy are initiated by the same intrinsic factors. However, this is not the case for the genes for PDGF chains and receptors and for TGF-ß1 which undergo differential regulation in aorta and heart [52]. However, the same growth factor could have different biological effects on different tissues, for example TGF-ß1 could increase or decrease cell proliferation [39]. In addition, cardiac NGF content has been shown to be slightly lower in young SHR, but higher in adult SHR than in age-matched WKY rats. This would also suggest that genes encoding for NGF undergo differential regulation in vascular tissue and myocardium. Furthermore, a dissociation between high arterial blood pressure and cardiac hypertrophy has recently been reported. In a new model of hypertension induced by chronic inhibition of nitric oxide (NO) synthase, Arnal et al. [125] have demonstrated an intruiging absence of cardiac hypertrophy after four weeks of treatment. Therefore a real dissociation between cardiac hypertrophy and increased arterial wall thickness could be observed in this experimental model of hypertension. One may speculate that chronic inhibition of NO synthase could prevent the expression of specific growth factors that are implicated in cardiac hypertrophy during hypertension, independently of their effect on vascular remodelling.

Conclusion

The variability of the findings presented in this review is mainly due to animal species, different models of hypertension, size of arterial vessels and specific effects of growth factors per se. These parameters have to be taking into consideration in interpretating much of the published data. Further investigations are needed to clarify the specific role of peptide growth factors in human hypertension. The absence of reversion of vascular remodeling might explain, at least in part, the limited effectiveness of conventional antihypertensive therapy in preventing cardiovascular morbidity and mortality. Therefore we speculate that agents that could reduce vascular tone as well as correcting vascular remodeling would be more efficient in the future treatment of hypertension. This could lead to a new generation of drugs, which may or may not be associated with the anti-hypertensive compounds currently used in therapy, for reducing the risk factors for most patients.

Acknowledgements

The authors' work is supported by Grants from the British Heart Foundation.

References

1. Folkow B. "Structural factor" in primary and secondary hypertension. Hypertension 1990; 16: 89-101.
2. Chobanian AV. Adaptative and maladive rsponses of the arterial wall to hypertension. Hypertension 1990; 15: 666-674.
3. Olivetti G, Ricci R, Anversa P. Hyperplasia of myocyte nuclei in long-term cardiac hypertrophy in rats. J Clin Inv 1987; 1818-1821.
4. Anversa P, Fitzpatrick D, Argani S, Capasso JM. Myocyte mitotic division in the aging mammalian rat heart. Circ Res 1991; 69:1159-1164.

5. Owens GK, Schwartz SM. Alterations in vascular smooth muscle mass in the spontaneous hypertensive rat. Role in cellular hypertrophy, hyperploidy and hyperplasia. Circ Res 1982; 51: 280-289.

6. Leitschuh Mand Chobanian AV. Inhibition of nuclear polyploid by propranolol in aortic smooth muscle cells of hypertensive rats. Hypertension 1987; 9 (supll III): III-106-III-109.

7. Owens GK, Reidy MA. Hyperplastic growth response of vascular smooth muscle cells following induction of acute hypertension in rats by aortic coarctation. Circ Res 1985; 57: 695-705.

8. Mulvany MJ, Baandrup U, Gundersen HJG. Evidence for hyperplasia in mesenteric resistance vessels of spontaneously hypertensive rats using a three-dimensional disector. Circ Res 1985; 57: 794-800.

9. Mulvany MJ, Hansen PK, Aalkjaer C. Direct evidence that the greater contractility of resistance vessels in spontaneously hypertensive rats is associated with a narrowed lumen, a thickened media, and an increased number of smooth muscle cell layers. Circ Res 1978; 43: 854-864.

10. Bohr DF, Dominiczak AF, Webb RC. Pathophysiology of the vasculature in hypertension. Hypertension 1991; 18 (suppl III): III-69-III-75.

11. El Amrani A-I.K, Lecarpentier Y, Riou B, Pourny JC. Lusitropic effect and modifications of contraction-relaxation coupling induced by alpha-adrenergic stimulation in rat left ventricular papillary muscle. J Mol Cell Cardiol 1989; 21: 669-680.

12. El Amrani A-I.K. Dual effect of angiotensinn II and load on intrinsic myocardial contractility. Heart failure 7 1991; 3: 97-103.

13. Moravec S-C, Reynolds EE, Stewart RW, Bond M. Endothelin is a positive inotropic agent in human and rat heart in vivo. Biochem Biophys Res Commun 1989; 159:14-18.

14. El Amrani A-I.K, El Amrani F, Michel JB, Lecarpentier Y. Effets de l'angiotensine II sur la contractilite intrinseque du myocarde de cobaye. Arch Mal Coeur 1992; 85: 1587-1592.

15. Vigne P, Ladzunski M, Frelin C. The inotropic effect of endothelin-1 on rat atria involves hydrolysis of phosphatidyl-inositol. FEBS Lett 1989; 249: 143-146.

16. Campbell-Boswell M, Robertson LA Jr. Effects of angiotensin II and vasopressin on human smooth muscle cells in vitro. Exp Mol Pathol 1981; 35: 265-276.

17. Simpson P. Norepinephrine-stimulated hypertrophy of cultured rat myocardial cells is an alpha1-adrenergic response. J Clin Invest 1983; 72: 732-738.

18. Komuro Y Kurihara H, Sugiyama T, Takaku F, Yazaki Y: Endothelin stimulates c-fos and c-myc expression and proliferation of vascular smooth muscle cells. FEBS Lett 1988; 238: 249-252.

19. Berridge MJ. Inositol lipids and cell proliferation. Biochim Biophys Acta 1987; 907: 33-45.

20. Mulvagh SL, Roberts R, Schneider MD. Cellular oncogenes in cardiovascular disease. J Mol Cell Cardiol 1988; 20: 657-662.

21. Moalic JM, Bauters C, Himbert D, Swynghedauw B. Phenylephrine, vasopressine, and angiotensin II as determinants of protooncogenes and heat shock proteine genes expression in adult rat heart and aorta. J Hypertens 1989; 7: 195-201.

22. Naftilan AJ, Pratt RE, Dzau VJ. Induction od platelet-derived growth factor A-chain and c-myc gene expressions by angiotensin II in cultured rat vascular smooth muscle cells. J Clin Invest 1989; 83: 1419-1424.

23. Itoh H, Pratt RE, Dzau VJ. Antisense oligonucleotides complementary to PDGF mRNA attenuate angiotensin II-induced vascular hypertrophy (Abstract). Hypertension 1990: 16: 325.

24. Dzau VJ, Gibbons GH. Endothelium and growth factors in vascular remodelling of hypertension. Hypertension 1991, 18 (suppl III): III-115-III-121.

25. Jonzon B, Nilsson J, Fredholm BB. Adenosine receptor-mediated changes in cyclic AMP production and DNA synthesis in cultured arterial smooth muscle cells. J Cell Physiol 1985; 124: 451-456.

26. Garg UC, Hassid A. Nitric oxide-generating vasodilators and 8-bromo-cyclic guanosine monophosphate inhibit mitogenesis and proliferation of cultured rat vascular smooth muscle cells. J Clin Invest 1989; 83: 1774-1777.

27. Lüscher TF, Vanhoutte PM, Raij L. Antihypertensive treatment normalizes decreased endothelium dependent relaxation in rats with salt-induced hypertension. Hypertension 1987; 9 (suppl III): III-193-III-197.

28. Vanhoutte PM. Endothelium and control of vascular function. Hypertension 1989; 13: 658-667.

29. Panza JA, Quyyumi AA, Brush JE, Epstein SE. Abnormal endothelium-dependent vascular relaxation in patients with essential hypertension. N Engl J Med 1990; 323 22-27.

30. Clozel M, Kuhn H, Helft F. Effects of angiotensin converting enzyme inhibitors and of hydralazine on endothelial function in hypertensive rats. Hypertension 1990; 16: 532-540.

31. Sarzani R, Brecher P, Chobanian AV. Growth factor expression in aorta of normotensive and hypertensive rats. J Clin Inv 1989; 83: 1404-1408.

32. Ignotz RA, Massague J. Transforming growth factor-ß stimulates the expression of fibronectin and collagen and their incorporation into the extracellular matrix. J Biol Chem 1986; 261: 4337-4345.

33. Ignotz RA, Endo T, Massague. Regulation of fibronectin and type I collagen mRNA levels by transforming growth factor. J Biol Chem 1987; 262: 6443-6446.

34. Chen JK, Hoshi H, McKeehan WL. Transforming growth factor type ß specifically stimulates synthesis of proteoglycan in human adult arterial smooth muscle cells. Proc Natl Acad Sci USA 1987; 84:5287-5291.

35. Penttinen RP, Kobayashi S, Bornstein P. Transforming growth factor ß increases mRNA for matrix proteins both in the presence and in the absence of changes in mRNA stability. Proc Natl Acad Sci USA 1988; 85:1105-1108.

36. Liu JM, Davidson JM. The elastogenic effect of recombinant transforming growth factor-beta on porcine aortic smooth muscle cells Biochem Biop-hys Res Commun 1988; 154: 895-901.

37. Perkett EA, Lyons RM, Moses HL, Brigham KL, Meyrick B. Transforming growth factor-ß activity in sheep lung lymph during the development of pulmonary hypertension. J Clin Invest 1990; 86: 1459-1464.

38. Majesky MW, Lindner V, Twardzik DR, Schwartz SM, Reidy MA. Production of transforming growth factor ß1 during repair of arterial injury. J Clin Invest 1991; 88: 904-910.

39. Majack RA. Beta-type transforming growth factor specifies organizational behavior in vascular smooth muscle cell cultures. J Cell Biol 1987 105: 465-471.

40. Moses HL. The biological actions of transforming growth factor ß. Growth factors: From genes to clinical applications, edited by Vicki R, Sara et al, Raven Press, New York, 1990.

41. Goodman LV, Majack RA. Vascular smooth muscle cells express distinct transforming growth factor-ß receptor phenotypes as a funcion of cell density in culture. J Biol Chem 1989; 264: 5241-5244.

42. Owens GK, Geistetrfer AT, Yang YW, Komoriya A. Transforming growth factor-ß-induced growth inhibition and cellular hypertrophy in cultured vascular smooth muscle cells. J Cell Biol 1988; 107: 771-780.

43. Hamet P, Hadrava V, Kruppa U, Tremblay J. Transforming growth factor ß1 expression and effect in aortic smooth muscle cells from spontaneously hypertensive rats. Hypertension 1991; 17: 896-901.

44. Starksen NF, Harsh GR, Gibbs VC, Williams LT. Regulated expression of the platelet-derived growth factor A chain gene in microvascular endothelial cells. J Biol Chem 1987; 262: 14381-14384.

45. Daniel TO, Gibbs VC, Milfay DF, Williams CT. Agents that increase cAMP accumulation block endothelial C-SIS induction by thrombin and transforming growth factor-ß. J Biol Chem 1987; 262: 11893-11896.

46. Majack RA, Majesky MW, Goodman LV. Role of PDGF-A expression in the control of vascular smooth muscle cell growth by transforming growth factor-ß. J Cell Biol 1990; 111:239-247.

47. Botney MD, Parks WC, Crouch EC, Stenmark K, Mecham RP. Transforming growth factor-ß1 is decreased in remodeling hypertensive bovine pulmonary arteries. J Clin Inv 1992; 89: 1629-1635.

48. Wagenvoort CA, Wagenvoort N. Pathology of pulmonary hypertension. John Wiley & Sons, Inc., New York 1977.

49. Poiani GJ, Tozzi CA, Yohn SE, Pierce RA, Belsky SA, Berg RA, Yu SY, Deak SB, Riley DJ. Collagen and elastin metabolism in hypetensive pulmonary arteries of rats. Circ Res 1990; 66: 968-978.

50. Roberts AB, Sporn MB, Assoian RK, Smith JM, Roche NS, Wakefield LM, Heine UI, Liotta LA, Falanga V, Kerhl JH, Fauci AS. Transforming growth factor type b: rapid induction of fibrosis and angiogenesis in vivo and stimulation of collagen formation in vitro. Proc Natl Acad Sci USA 1986; 83: 4167-4171.

51. Khalil N, Bereznay O, Sporn M, Greenberg AH. Macrophage production of transforming growth factor ß and fibroblast collagen synthesis in chronic pulmonary inflammation. J Exp Med 1989; 170: 727-735.

52. Sarzani R, Arnaldi G, Takasaki I, Brecher P, Chobanian AV. Effects of hypertension and aging on platelet-derived growth factor and platelet-derived growth factor receptor expression in rat aorta and heart. Hypertension 1991; 18 (suppl III): III-93-III-99.

53. Antonelli-Orlidge A, Saunders KB, Smith SR, D'Amore PA. An activated form of transforming growth factor ß is produced by cocultures of endothelial cells and pericytes. Proc Natl Acad Sci USA 1989; 86: 4544-4548.

54. Saltis J, Agrotis A, Bobik A. Transforming growth factor-beta$_1$ enhances the proliferative effects of epidermal growth factor on vascular smooth muscle from the spontaneously hypertensive rat. J Hypertens 1991, 9 (suppl 6): S184-S185.

55. Ross R, Raines EW, Bowen-Pope DF. The biology of platelet-derived growth factor. Cell 1986; 46: 155-169.

56. Sitaras NM, Sariban E, Pantazis P, Zetter B, Antoniades HN. Human iliac artery endothelial cells express both genes encoding the chains of platelet-derived growth factor (PDGF) and synthetize PDGF-like mitogen. J Cell Physiol 1987; 132: 376-380.

57. Hammacher A, Mellstrom K, Heldin C-H, Westermark B. Isoform-specific induction of actin reorganization by platelet-derived growth factor suggests that the functionally active receptor is a dimer. EMBO J 1989; 8: 2489-2495.

306

58. Seifert RA, Hart CE, Phillips PE, Forstrom JW, Ross R, Murray MJ, Bowen-Pope DF. Two different subunits associate to create isoform-specific platelet-derived growth factor receptors. J Biol Chem 1989; 264: 8771-8778.

59. Sarzani R, Arnaldi G, Chobanian AV. Hypertension-induced changes of platelet-derived growth factor receptor expression in rat aorta and heart. Hypertension 1991; 17: 888-895.

60. Haudenschild CC, Grunwald J, Chobanian AV. Effects of hypertension on migration and proliferation of smooth muscle in culture. Hypertension 1985; 7 (suppl I): I-101-I-104.

61. Printseva OY,Tjurmin AV, Rudchenko SA, Repin VS. Noradrenaline induces the polyploidization of smooth muscle cells: the synergism of second messengers. Exp Cell Res 1989; 184: 342-350.

62. Geisterfer AAT, Peach MJ, Owens GK. Angiotensin II induces hypertrophy, not hyperplasia, of cultured rat aortic smooth muscle cells. Circ Res 1988; 62: 749-756.

63. Geisterfer AAT, Owens GK. Arginine vasopressin-induced hypertrophy of cultured rat aortic smooth muscle cells. Hyprtension 1989; 14: 413-420.

64. Majesky MW, Daemen MJAP, Schwartz SM. a1-adrenergic stimulation of platelet-derived growth factor A-chain gene expression in rat aorta. J Biol Chem 1990; 265: 1082-1088.

65. Bobik A, Grinpukel S, Little PJ, Grooms A, Jackman G. Angiotensin II and noradrenaline increase PDGF BB receptors and potentiate PDGF BB stimulated DNA synthesis in vascular smooth muscle. Biochem Biophys Res Commun 1990; 166: 580-588.

66. Hajjar KA, Hajjar DP, Silverstein RL, Nachman RL. Tumor necrosis factor-mediated release of platelet-derived growth factor from cultured endothelial cells. J Exp Med 1987; 166: 235-245.

67. Maier JAM, Voulalas P, Roeder D, Maliag T. Extension of the lifespan of human endothelial cells by an interleukin-1 alpha antisense oligomer. Science 1990; 249: 1570-1574.

68. Rinderknecht E, Humbel RE.The amino acid sequence of human insulin-like growth factor I and its structural homology with proinsulin. J Biol Chem 1978; 253: 2769-2776.

69. Salmon WD Jr, Daughaday WH. A hormonally controlled serum factor which stimulates sulfate incorporation by cartilage in vitro. J Lab Clin Med 1957; 49: 825-836.

70. D'Ercole AJ, Stiles AD, Underwood LE. Tissue concentrations of somatomedin-C: further evidence for multiple sites of synthesis and paracrine or autocrine mechanisms of action. Proc Natl Acad Sci USA 1984; 81: 935-939.

71. Englemann GL, Boehm KD, Haskell JF, Khairallah PA, Ilan J. Insulin-like growth factors and neonatal cardiomyocyte development: ventricular gene expression and membrane receptor variations in normotensive and hypertensive rats. Mol Cell Endocrinol 1989; 63: 1-14.

72. Delafontaine P, Bernstein KE, Alexander RW. Insulin-like growth factor I gene expression in vascular cells. Hypertension 1991; 17: 693-699.

73. Clemmons DR. Exposure to platelet-derived growth factor modulates the porcine aortic smooth muscle cell response to somatomedin-C. Endocrinology 1985; 117: 77-83.

74. Calvin RB, Antoniades HN. Role of platelet-derived growth factor in wound healing: synergistic effects with other growth factors. Proc Natl Acad Sci USA 1987; 84: 7696-7700.

75. Badesch DB, Lee PDK, Parks WC, Stenmark KR. Insulin-like growth factor I stimulated elastin synthesis by bovine pulmonary arterial smooth muscle cells. Biochem Biophys Res Commun 1989; 160: 382-387.

76. Delafontaine P, Lou H, Alexander RW. Regulation of insulin-like growth factor I messager RNA levels in vascular smooth muscle cells. Hypertension 1991; 18: 742-747.

77. Fath KA, Hanson MC, Delafontaine P, Alexander RW. Hypertension induces insulin-like growth factor I gene expression in rat aorta (abstract). Circulation 1990; 82 (suplIIII): III-761.

78. Cercek B, Fishbein MC, Forrester JS, Helfant RH, Fagin JA. Induction of insulin-like growth factor-I mRNA in rat aorta after balloon denudation. Circ Res 1990; 66: 1755-1760.

79. Bondjers G, Glukhova M, Hansson GK, Postnov YV, Reidy MA, Scharwtz SM. Hypertension and atherosclerosis. Cause and effect, or two effects with one unknown cause? Circulation 1991; 84 (supll VI); VI-2-VI-16.

80. Wahlander H, Isgaard J, Jennische E, Friberg P. Left ventricular insulin-like growth factor I increases in early renal hypertension. Hypertension 1992; 19: 25-32.

81. Lever AF. Slow pressor mechanisms in hypertension: a role for hypertrophy of resistance vessels? J Hypertension 1986; 4: 515-524.

82. Esch F, Baird A, Ling N at al.. Primary structure of bovine pituitary basic fibroblast growth factor (FGF) and comparaison with tha amino-terminal sequence of bovine brain acidic FGF. Proc Natl Acad Sci USA 1985; 82: 6507-6511.

83. Burgess WH, Maciag T. The heparin-binding (fibroblast) growth factor family of proteins. Annu Rev Biochem 1989; 58: 575-606.

84. Mignatti P, Tsuboi R, Robbins E, Rifkin DB. In vitro angiogenesis on human amniotic membrane: Requirement for basic fibroblast growth factor-induced proteinases. J Cell Biol 1989; 108: 671-682.

85. Saksela O, Rifkin DB. Release of basic fibroblast growth factor-heparan sulfate complexes from endothelial cells by plasminogen activator-mediated proteolytic activity. J Cell Biol 1990; 110: 767-775.

86. Yanagisawa-Miwa A, Uchida Y, Nakamura F, Tomaru T, Kido H, Kamijo T, Sugimoto T, Kaji K, Utsuyama M, Kurashima C, Ito H. Salvage of infarcted myocardium by angiogenic action of basic fibroblast growth factor. Science 1992; 257: 1401-1403.

87. Winkles JA, Friesel R, Burgess WH, Howk R, Mehlman T, Weinstein R, Maciag T. Human vascular smooth muscle cells both express and respond to heparin-binding growth factor I (endothelial cell growth factor). Proc Natl Acad Sci USA 1987; 84: 7124-7128.

88. Gospodarowicz D, Ferrara N, Haaparanta T, Neufeld G. Basic fibroblast growth factor: expression in cultured bovine vascular smooth muscle cells. Eur J Cell Biol 1988; 46: 144-151.

89. Lindner V, Majack RA, Reidy MA. Basic fibroblast growth factor stimulates endothelial regrowth and proliferation in denuded arteries. J Clin Inv 1990; 85: 2004-2008.

90. Lindner V, Lappi DA, Baird A, Majack RA, Reidy MA. Role of basic fibroblast growth factor in vascular lesion formation. Circ Res 1991; 68: 106-113.

91. McNeil PL, Muthukrishnan L, Warder E, D'Amore PA. Growth factors are released by mechanically wounded endothelial cells. J Cell Biol 1989; 811-822.

92. Gajdusek CM, Carbon S. Injury-induced release of basic fibroblast growth factor from bovine aortic endothelium. J Cell Physiol 1989; 139: 570-579.

93. Lindner V, Reidy MA. Proliferation of smooth muscle cells after vascular injury is inhibited by an antibody against basic fibroblast growth factor. Proc Nat Acad Sci USA 1991; 28: 3739-3743.

94. Olson NE, Chao S, Lindner V, Reidy MA. Intimal smooth muscle cell proliferation after balloon catheter injury. Am J Pathol 1992; 140: 1017-1023.

95. Levi-Montalcini R, Angeletti PU. Nerve growth factor. Physiol Rev 1968; 48: 534-569.

96. Thoenen H, Barde YA. Physiology of nerve growth factor. Physiol Rev 1980; 60: 1284-1335.

97. Korshing S, Thoenen H. Nerve growth factor in sympathetic ganglia and corresponding target organs of the rat: correlation with the density of sympathetic innervation. Proc Natl Acad Sci USA 1983; 80: 3513-3516.

98. Shelton DL, Reichardt LF. Expression of the ß-nerve growth factor gene correlated with the density of sympathetic innervation in effector organs. Proc Natl Acad Sci USA 1984; 81- 7951-7955.

99. Ichijima K. Morphological studies on the peripheral small arteries of spontaneously hypertensive rats. Jpn Circ J 1969, 33: 786-813.

100. Head RJ, Cassis LA, Robinson RL, Westfall DP, Stizel RE. Altered catecholamine contents in vascular and non-vascular tissues in genetically hypertensive rats. Bloods vessels 1985: 22: 196-204.

101. Cassis L, Stizel RE, Head RJ. Hyper-noradrenergic innervation of the caudal artery spontaneously hypertensive rats: an influence upon neuroeffector mechanisms. J Pharmacol exp ther 1985; 234: 792-803.

102. Donohue SL, Stizel RE, Head RJ. Time course of changes in the norepinephrine content of tissues from spontaneously hypertensive and wistar-kyoto rats. J Pharmacol Exp Ther 1988; 245: 24-31.

103. Donohue SJ, Head RJ, Stizel RE. Eleveted nerve growth factors levels in young spontaneously hypertensives rats. Hypertension 1989; 14:421-426.

104. Ueyama T, Hamada M, Hano T, Nishio I, Masuyama Y, Furukawa S. Increased nerve growth factor levels in spontaneously hypertensive rats. J Hypertens1992; 10: 215-219.

105. Lee RMKW, Triggle CR, Cheung DWT, Coughlin MD. Structural and functional consequence of neonatal sympathectomy on the blood vessels of spontaneously hypertensive rats. Hypertension 1987, 10:328-338.

106. Groopman JE, Mitsuyasu RT, DeLeo MJ, Oette DH, Golde DW. Effect of recombinant human granulocyte-macrophage colony-stimulation factor on myelopoiesis in the acquired immunodeficiency syndrome. N Engl J Med 1987; 317: 593-598.

107. Border WA, Noble NA, Yamamoto T, Harper JR, Yamaguchi Y, Pierschbacher MD, Ruoslahti E. Natural inhibitor of transforming growth factor-ß protects against scarring in experimental kidney disease. Nature 1992; 360:361-364.

108. Levy BI, Michel JB, Salzmann JB, Azizi M, Poitevin P, Safar M, Camilleri JP. Effects of chronic inhibition of converting enzyme on mechanical and structural properties of arteries in rat renovascular hypertension. Circ Res 1988; 63: 227-239.

109. Mulvany MJ. Resistance vessel structure; effects of treatment. J Cardiovasc Pharmacol 1991; 17 (supll 2): S58-S63.

110. Leenen FHH, Prowse S. Time course of changes in cardiac hyprtrophy and pressor mechanisms in two-kidney, one clip hypertensive rats during treatment with minoxidil, enalapril or after uninephrectomy. J Hypertens 1987; 5: 73-83.

111. Michel JB. Relationship between decrese in afterload and benefical effects of ACE inhibitors in experimental cardiac hypertrophy and congestive heart failure. Eur Heart J 1990; 11 (suppl D): 17-26.

112. Frohlich ED, Apstein C, Chobanian AV, Devereux RB, Dustan HP, Dzau V, Fauad-Tarazi F, Horan MJ, Marcus M, Massie B, Pfeffer MA, Re RN, Roccella EJ, Savage D, Shub C. The heart in hypertension. N Engl J Med 1992; 327: 998 - 1007.

113. Sen S, Tarazi RC, Bumpus FM. Cardiac hypertrophy and antihypertensive therapy. Cardiovasc Res 1977; 11: 427-433.

114. Tsoporis J, Leenen FHH. Effects of arterial vasodilators on cardiac hypertrophy and sympathetic activity in rats. Hypertension 1988; 11: 376-385.

115. Heagerty AM. Angiotensin II: vasoconstrictor or growth factor? J Cardiovasc Pharmacol 1991; 18 (supl 2): S14-S19.

116. Schneider MD, Parker TG. Cardiac myocytes as targets for the action of peptide growth growth factors. Circulation 1990; 81: 1443-1456.

117. Contard F, Koteliansky V, Marotte F, Dubus I, Rappaport L, Samuel JL. Specific alterations in the distribution of extracellular matrix components within rat myocardium during the development of pressure overload. Lab Invest 1991; 64: 65-75.

118. Samuel JL, Barrieux A, Dufour S, Dubus I, Contard F, Faradian F, Koteliansky V, Marotte F, Thiery JP, Rappaport L. Reexpression of a fetal pattern of fibronectin mRNAs during the development of rat cardiac hypertrophy induced by pressure overload. J Clin Invest 1991; 88: 1737-1746.

119. French JE, Jennings MP, Poole JCF, Robinson DS, Florey H. Intimal changes in the arteries of the aging swine. Proc R Soc Lond (Biol) 1963; 158: 24-42.

120. Gerrity RG, Cliff WJ. The aortic intima in young and aging rats. Exp Mol Patho 1972; 16: 382-402.

121. Haudenschild CC, Prescott MF, Chobanian AV. Aortic endothelial and subendothelial cells in experimental hypertension and aging. Hypertension 1981; 3 (supll I): I-148-I153.

122. Wolinsky H. Long term effects of hypertension on the rat aortic wall and their relation to concurrent aging changes: Morpholigic and chemical studies. Circ Res 1972; 30: 301-309.

123. Owens GK. Differential effects of antihypertensive drug therapy on vascular smooth muscle cell hypertrophy, hyperploidy, and hyperplasia in the spontaneously hypertensive rat. Circ Res 1985; 56: 525-536.

124. Barrett TB, Sampson P, Owens GK, Schwart SM, Benditt EP. Polyploid nuclei in human artery wall smooth muscle cells. Proc Natl Acad Sci USA 1983; 80: 882-885.

125. Arnal J-F, Warin L, Michel J-B. Determinants of aortic cyclic guanosine monophosphate in hypertension induced by chronic inhibition of nitric oxide synthase. J Clin Inv 1992; 90: 647-652.

18. Transforming growth factor-ß induction in carcinoid heart disease

JOHANNES WALTENBERGER

Carcinoid tumor disease

Carcinoid tumors are the most frequent neuroendocrine neoplasms and have an incidence of 2.1 per 100,000 per year in Sweden [1]. They are characterized by their ability to produce and secrete a variety of bioactive substances, e.g. serotonin, histamin, prostaglandins, kallikrein and tachykinins. These or related substances produce the clinical symptoms of flush, diarrhea and tachycardia as well as bronchospasm, cyanosis and edema.

The majority of the carcinoid tumors are located in the mid-gut (most often in the distal ileum or appendix) and are of benign nature. In patients with malignant carcinoid tumors, liver metastases can be found in 90% [2] and two thirds of these patients develop the classical "carcinoid syndrome", which includes flush, diarrhea and urinary excretion of 5-hydroxyindolacetic acid (5-HIAA). In about 50-66% of these patients, cardiac lesions can be found both by echocardiography [3-6] or during autopsy [7,8], described as carcinoid heart disease.

Within recent years mortality from carcinoid tumor disease decreased markedly and life expectancy increased secondary to new treatment regimens. The five year survival after diagnosis has increased during the last three decades from 21% (9) to 80% [10], namely due to the successful use of interferon [11] and the somatostatin analogue octreotide [10]. The increased survival of patients with malignant carcinoid tumors is accompanied by an increasing incidence of carcinoid heart disease.

312

Carcinoid heart disease

Carcinoid heart disease is a unique complication of a carcinoid tumor, and it represents the major cause of death in patients with carcinoid syndrome [2]. The carcinoid heart lesions appear as plaques, and are predominantly located in the right heart in the mural and valvular subendocardium. The plaques contain fibroblasts or phenotypically immature myofibroblasts expressing muscle actin in their cytoplasm [12]. The surrounding fibrous stroma is matrix-rich, composed of proteoglycans and mucopolysaccharides and devoid of elastic fibers [13,14].

The etiology of these lesions is still unknown and it has not been possible yet to induce them in an experimental animal model. However, positive correlations with the levels of circulating vasoactive substances such as serotonin and tachykinins have been demonstrated [5]. These findings would be compatible with the hypothesis, that substances produced and released by the carcinoid tumor, participate in a direct or indirect way in the development of these fibrotic lesions.

The clinical presentation of carcinoid heart disease is mostly right ventricular failure secondary to pulmonary stenosis, tricuspid regurgitation or both. Surgical repair appears to be the treatment of choice in progressed stages of carcinoid heart disease. This usually involves tricuspid valve replacement and the correction of pulmonary stenosis by valve replacement, valvulotomy or valvectomy [15].

The transforming growth factor-ß family of polypeptides

TGF-ß is a family of multifunctional growth factors (reviewed in [16]), which affects growth and differentiation of many cell types and which is produced by a variety of different cell types [17]. With regard to fibroblasts, TGF-ß stimulates them to produce extracellular matrix components [18]. Furthermore, TGF-ß has been demonstrated to be involved in fibroproliferative processes such as liver fibrosis [19,20], glomerulonephritis [21] and pulmonary fibrosis [22].

TGF-ß is a family of structurally related isoforms, TGF-ß1, -ß2 and -ß3, which are synthesized and secreted as large, latent complexes. Within these complexes the TGF-ß molecule is noncovalently associated with the N-terminal remnants of their precursors ("latency associated peptides", LAPs); TGF-ß1-complexes from certain sources, like e.g. platelets, have been shown to contain an additional component denoted latent TGF-ß1 binding protein (LTBP) [23]. LTBP associates with the

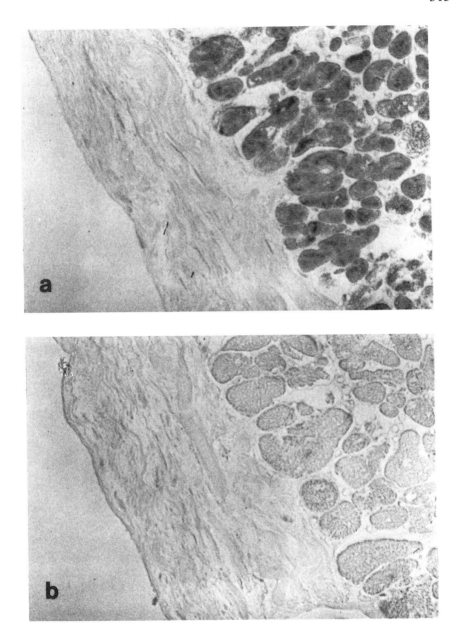

Figure 1. Normal papillary muscle from a patient of the control group stained for the latent TGF-ß1 (a) and LTBP (b). The immunoreactivity was visualized by the ABC-immunoperoxidase staining method. No immunoreactivity can be detected in the subendocardial space for both molecules, while the staining of the myocardium is the same as in the diseased material (Figure 2). The original magnification is 250x. Reproduced in part with permission from Amer J Pathol [29].

TGF-ß1 precursor in the large latent complex (24), and this association was shown to be important for an efficient secretion of TGF-ß1 [25, reviewed in [16,26]). LTBP may play a role in the extracellular matrix because of its structural homology to fibrillin [27], which represents an important component for the mechanical stability of the connective tissue, and which is impaired in the case of Marfan's syndrome [28].

TGF-ßs need to be activated in order to exert their biological effects via binding to specific cell surface receptors. The exact mechanisms for activation are unknown, but they may involve enzymatic degradation of the precursor molecules.

Expression of TGF-ß in carcinoid heart disease

In a recent study the TGF-ß isoforms were shown to be produced within the carcinoid plaques of nine patients undergoing valve replacement surgery [29]. Normal control tissue contained only few fibroblasts in the subendocardium, and these produced either no or only low levels of immunoreactive TGF-ß and latent TGF-ß1 binding protein LTBP, as demonstrated by the use of immuno-histochemistry (Figure 1). In contrast, the carcinoid heart lesions contained abundant fibroblasts or myofibroblasts, producing high levels of TGF-ß1 as well as TGF-ß3 and lower levels of TGF-ß2 (Table I; Figure 2a-c). Moreover, LTBP was found to be induced in the carcinoid plaques of three patients, being partly concordant with the presence of TGF-ß1, but located extracellularly (Figure 2d).

TGF-ß produced in these plaque fibroblasts might stimulate the production of extracellular matrix in an autocrine fashion, as it does in various other types of fibroproliferative disorders. The mechanism by which the TGF-ß precursors are induced in these fibroblasts is still unknown. It is possible that the vasoactive substances produced by the carcinoid tumor cells trigger the induction. In fact, it has been demonstrated that serotonin and tachykinins, which are frequently produced by carcinoid tumor cells in high amounts, contribute to the

Table 1. Immunostaining of fibroblasts in carcinoid plaques and in normal subendocardium for the various precursors of TGF-ß and LTBP.

Patient	Tissue	TGF-ß1	TGF-ß2	TGF-ß3	LTBP
# 1	Tricuspid Valve	(+)	++	++	-
	Right Atrial Wall	-	-	+	-
	Pulmonary Valve	(+)	+	++	-
# 2	Tricuspid Valve	+	(+)	++(+)	-
	Right Atrial Wall	+	-	+	-
# 3	Tricuspid Valve	-	(+)	+	-
	Right Atrial Wall	(+)	0	+	-
# 4	Papillary Muscle	+(+)	+	++	++
	Tricuspid Valve	+	(+)	++	+
	Right Atrial Wall	(+)	(+)	0	-
# 5	Papillary Muscle	++	(+)	++	-
	Tricuspid Valve	+++	-	++	-
# 6	Papillary Muscle	+	(+)	++	+
	Tricuspid Valve	++	-	+++	-
# 7	Papillary Muscle	-	-	+	-
	Right Atrial Wall	+	-	++	-
# 8	Papillary Muscle	+	(+)	+(+)	-
	Tricuspid Valve	+	(+)	++	-
# 9	Tricuspid Valve	+	-	++	(+)
	Right Atrial Wall	++	-	+(+)	+
Control	Papillary Muscle	(+)	-	-	-
	Tricuspid Valve	-	-	(+)	-
	Right Atrial Wall	(+)	(+)	(+)	-
	Pulmonary Valve	-	(+)	(+)	-

316

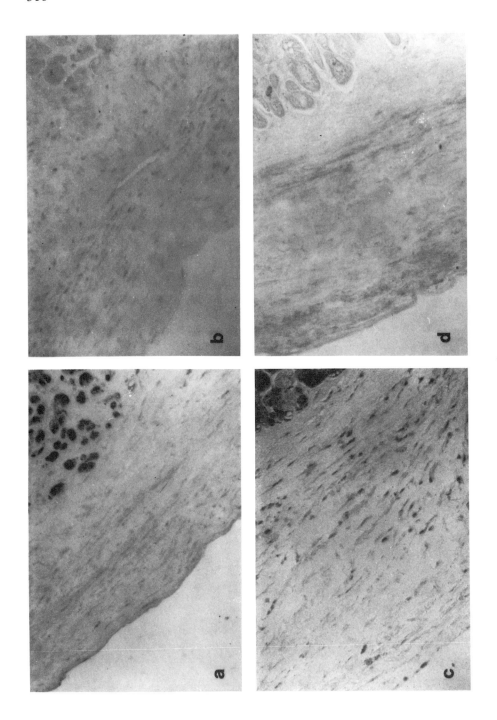

Table 1 (cont). Immunostaining is located intracellularly in the case of TGF-ß1, TGF-ß2 and TGF-ß3, extracellularly in the case of LTBP. Semiquantitative evaluation of immunostaining: - no iommunostaining; + few positive cells; ++ less than 50% of the cells positive; +++ more than 50%, but not all cells positive; ++++ all cells positive; ( ) weak staining; 0 plaque absent. Taken with permission from Amer J Pathol [29].

stimulation of DNA synthesis in cultured fibroblasts [30,31].

It is noteworthy that the mid-gut carcinoid tumors were found to produce all three TGF-ß isoforms themselves [32]. Whether these are involved in the pathogenesis of the cardiac lesions remains currently unknown.

Therapeutic implications

In carcinoid heart disease, the fibroproliferative process is associated with TGF-ß overproduction. Suppression of TGF-ß might prevent the development of the fibrotic lesions and may therefore contribute to decrease the disease related morbidity and mortality. The *in vivo* modulation of TGF-ß is feasible, as demonstrated in an animal model of glomerulonephritis (21), and it has been speculated, that this principle could be used to manipulate other TGF-ß related diseases (33). In the initial approach (21) an antiserum raised against TGF-ß1 was used for neutralizing the activity of TGF-ß1 *in vivo*. In a similar way one could think of antagonizing the different TGF-ß isoforms in carcinoid heart disease. This approach might suppress the excessive production of extracellular matrix and may therefore prevent or delay the onset of related signs and symptoms.

While the prolonged therapeutic application of antibodies might encounter serious side effects, alternative strategies for antagonizing TGF-ß *in vivo* have been suggested: These include the natural TGF-ß antagonist decorin (34) or TGF-ß antagonists, that may be developed, based on the recently discovered three-dimensional structure of TGF-ß (35).

Figure 2. Carcinoid plaque of a papillary muscle of the tricuspid valve containing the latent forms of TGF-ß1 (a), TGF-ß2 (b), TGF-ß3 (c) as well as LTBP (d) and treated in the same way as the samples shown in Figure 1. While the precursors are located inside the myofibroblasts of the plaque, LTBP is located extracellularly. Original magnification is 250x. Reproduced with permission from Amer J Pathol [29].

318

Acknowledgments

I'm indebted to Kohei Miyazono, Keiko Funa and Carl-Henrik Heldin for carefully reading the manuscript.

References

1.   Berge T, Linell F. Carcinoid tumors. Acta Pathol Microbiol Scand Sect A 1976; 84: 322-330.
2.   Norheim I, Öberg K, Theodorsson-Norheim E, Lindgren PG, Lundqvist G, Magnusson A, Wide L, Wilander E. Malignant carcinoid tumors: An analysis of 103 patients with regard to tumor localization, hormone production and survival. Ann Surg 1987; 206: 115-125.
3.   Callahan JA, Wroblewski EM, Reeder GS, Edwards WD, Seward JB, Tajik AJ. Echocardiographic features of carcinoid heart disease. Am J Cardiol 1982; 50: 762-768.
4.   Howard RJ, Drobac M, Rider WD, Keane TJ, Finlayson J, Silver MD, Wigle ED, Rakovski H: Carcinoid heart disease: Diagnosis by two-dimensional echocardiography. Circulation 1982, 66: 1059-1065
5.   Lundin L, Norheim I, Landelius J, Öberg K, Theodorsson-Norheim E. Carcinoid heart disease: relationship of circulating vasoactive substances to ultrasound-detectable cardiac abnormalities. Circulation 1988; 77: 264-269.
6.   Himelman RB, Schiller NB. Clinical and echocardiographic comparison of patients with the carcinoid syndrome with and without carcinoid heart disease. Am J Cardiol 1989; 63: 347-352.
7.   Spain M. Association of gastrointestinal carcinoid tumor with cardiovascular abnormalities. Am J Med 1955; 19: 366-369.
8.   Roberts WC, Sjoerdsma A. The cardiac disease associated with the carcinoid syndrome (carcinoid heart disease). Am J Med 1964; 36: 5-34.
9.   Moertel CG, Sauer WG, Dockerty MB, Baggenstoss AH. Life history of the carcinoid tumor of the small intestine. Cancer 1961; 14: 901-912.
10. Öberg K, Norheim I, Theodorsson E. Treatment of malignant midgut carcinoid tumours with a long-acting somatostatin analogue octreotide. Acta Oncologica 1991; 30: 503-507.
11. Öberg K, Eriksson B. The role of interferons in the management of carcinoid tumors. Acta Oncologica 1991; 30: 519-522.
12. Lundin L, Funa K, Hansson HE, Wilander E, Öberg K. Histochemical and immunohistochemical morphology of carcinoid heart disease. Path Res Pract 1991; 187: 73-77.

13. Ferrans VJ, Roberts WC. The carcinoid endocardial plaque. An ultrastructural study. Hum Pathol 1976; 7: 387-408.
14. Müller HG, Siebenmann RE. Ultrastruktur der Endokardveränderungen beim Carcinoidsyndrom. Virchows Archiv A. 1981; 391: 33-44.
15. Lundin L, Hansson HE, Landelius J, Öberg K. Surgical treatment of carcinoid heart disease. J Thorac Cardiovasc Surg 1990; 100: 553-561.
16. Roberts AB, Sporn MB. The transforming growth factor-ßs. In: Sporn MB, Roberts AB. editors. Peptide growth factors and thier receptors. Springer, Berlin 1990; 419-472.
17. Thompson NL, Flanders KC, Smith JM, Ellingsworth LR, Roberts AB, Sporn MB: Transforming growth factor-ß1 in specific cells and tissues of adult and neonatal mice. J Cell Biol 1989; 108: 661-669.
18. Ignotz RA, Massagué J: Transforming growth factor-ß stimulates the expression of fibronectin and collagen and their incorporation into the extracellular matrix. J Biol Chem 1986; 261: 4337-4345.
19. Nakatsukasa H, Nagy P, Everts RP, Hsia C-C, Marsden E, and Thorgeirsson SS: Cellular distribution of transforming growth factor-ß1 and procollagen types I, III and IV transcripts in carbon tetrachloride-induced rat liver fibrosis. J Clin Invest 1990; 85: 1833-1843.
20. Castilla A, Prieto J, Fausto N. Transforming growth factor ß1 and alpha in chronic liver disease - Effects of interferon alfa therapy. N Engl J Med 1991; 324: 933-940.
21. Border WA, Okuda S, Languino LR, Sporn MB, Ruoslahti E. Suppression of experimental glomerulonephritis by antiserum against transforming growth factor ß1. Nature 1990; 346: 371-374.
22. Broekelmann TJ, Limper AH, Colby TV, McDonald JA. Transforming growth factor-ß1 is present at sites of extracellular matrix gene expression in human pulmonary fibrosis. Proc Natl Acad Sci USA 1991; 88: 6642-6646.
23. Kanzaki T, Olofsson A, Morén A, Wernstedt C, Hellman U, Miyazono K, Claesson-Welsh L, Heldin C-H. TGF-ß1 binding protein: A component of the large latent complex of TGF-ß1 with multiple repeat sequences. Cell 1990; 61: 1051-1061.
24. Miyazono K, Hellman U, Wernstedt C, Heldin C-H: Latent high molecular weight complex of transforming growth factor ß1. Purification from human platelets and structural characterization. J Biol Chem 1988; 263: 6407-6415.
25. Miyazono K, Olofsson A, Colosetti P, Heldin C-H. A role of the latent TGF-ß1-binding protein in the assembly and secretion of TGF-ß1. EMBO J 1991; 10: 1091-1101.

320

26. Miyazono K, Heldin C-H: Latent forms of TGF-ß. In: Molecular structure and mechanisms of activation. Proceedings of Ciba Foundation Symposium No. 157 on Clinical Applications of TGF-ß, Wiley, Chichester 1991; 81-92.

27. Maslen CL, Corson GM, Maddox BK, Glanville RW, Sakai LY. Partial sequence of a candidate gene for marfan syndrome. Nature 1991; 352: 334-337.

28. Dietz HC, Cutting GR, Pyeritz RE, Maslen CL, Sakai LY, Corson GM, Puffenberger EG, Hamosh A, Nanthakumar EJ, Curristin SM, Stetten G, Meyers DA, Francomano CA. Marfan syndrome caused by a recurrent de novo missense mutation in the fibrillin gene. Nature 1991; 352: 337-340.

29. Waltenberger J, Lundin L, Öberg K, Wilander E, Miyazono K, Heldin C-H, Funa K. Involvement of transforming growth factor-ß in the formation of fibrotic lesions in carcinoid heart disease. Am J Pathol 1993; 142: in press.

30. Nilsson J, von Euler AM, Dalsgaard CJ. Stimulation of connective tissue cell growth by substance P and substance K. Nature 1985; 315: 61-63.

31. Seuwen K, Magnaldo I, Pouysségur J. Serotonin stimulates DNA synthesis in fibroblasts acting through $5\text{-}HT_{1B}$ receptors coupled to a G_i-protein. Nature 1988; 335: 254-256.

32. Beauchamp RD, Coffey RJ Jr, Lyons RM, Perkett EA, Townsend CM Jr, Moses HL. Human carcinoid cell production of paracrine growth factors that can stimulate fibroblast and endothelial cell growth. Cancer Res 1991; 51: 5253-5260.

33. Border WA, Ruoslahti E. Transforming growth factor-ß in disease: The dark side of tissue repair. J Clin Invest 1992; 90: 1-7.

34. Border WA, Noble NA, Yamamoto T, Harper JR, Yamaguchi Y, Pierschbacher MD, Ruoslahti E. Natural inhibitor of transforming growth factor-ß protects against scarring in experimental kidney disease. Nature 1992; 360: 361-364.

35. Daopin S, Piez KA, Ogawa Y, Davies DR. Crystal structure of transforming growth factor-ß2: An unusual fold for the superfamily. Science 1992; 257: 369-372.

19. Adrenergic stimulation and growth factor activity

CARLIN S. LONG and PAUL C. SIMPSON

Background

Myocardial hypertrophy is the common endpoint of many cardiovascular stimuli such as hypertension, myocardial infarction, valvular disease, and congestive failure. Although in some ways adaptive, this hypertrophic response is pathological in that it is associated with abnormalities in both diastolic and systolic myocardial function. Moreover, the Framingham study has identified myocardial hypertrophy as an independent risk factor for cardiovascular morbidity and mortality (reviewed in [1]). However, not all forms of myocardial hypertrophy are associated with either functional abnormalities or an increase in cardiovascular mortality. This type of hypertrophy, referred to as physiologic hypertrophy, occurs with normal development and exercise training. Because these two seemingly identical phenotypes have strikingly different causes and subsequently outcomes, there has been considerable interest in the pathogenesis of myocardial hypertrophy.

The catecholamine hypothesis of myocardial hypertrophy

While searching for potential causative agents, many investigators have implicated catecholamines in the pathogenesis of myocardial hypertrophy [2-11]. This theory was largely due to experiments showing that hypertrophy could be induced by catecholamine infusion in experimental animals [12-14] as well as observations that there is an increase in sympathetic activity in several types of experimental hypertrophy and in some hypertensive patients [6-10]. This "catecholamine hypothesis" was also bolstered by clinical studies showing that hypertrophy in hypertension was reversed by agents which block sympathetic activity and unaffected by those which produce unopposed reflex sympathetic stimulation [15-20]. Unfortunately, these types of in vivo studies are difficult to interpret since the subtle hemodynamic effects of catecholamine infusions which could secondarily induce hypertrophy might not be detected. Even if such effects are ignored, it is also very difficult to sort out catecholamine mechanisms in vivo. Norepinephrine (NE) and Epinephrine can activate at least four types of adrenergic receptors in the myocardium (α_1, α_2, β_1, and β_2), some present on myocytes, some on non-myocytes. For these reasons, it is very difficult to be sure about the extent to which cardiac myocyte adrenergic receptors are being activated when experiments are done in vivo with various agonists and antagonists. Furthermore, although catecholamine effects have always been assumed to result from a direct action on the myocytes themselves, recent work in our laboratory [21], and others [22], suggests a potentially important paracrine effect of catecholamine stimulation of the non-myocardial cells.

A cell culture model of myocardial hypertrophy

In an effort to study the effects of catecholamines on both cardiac myocytes and non-myocytes alike, we have developed a cell culture model which excludes hemodynamic effects and allows the assignment of receptor specificity to catecholamine effects [23-25]. Utilizing this system, we have shown that stimulation of myocyte adrenergic receptors leads to the development of myocyte hypertrophy [26]. This response is independent of contractile activity [27], although the development of beating does augment the hypertrophic process by 10-20 %. Supplementing this work, we have recently reported that medium conditioned by cardiac non-myocytes also has a myocyte growth-promoting effect in culture [25] and, as described below, stimulation of non-myocyte β adrenergic receptors appears to augment this growth effect [28].

In this culture system, myocytes are obtained from the hearts of neonatal rats by gentle trypsinization and plated at low density in serum-free medium. Under these conditions, the muscle cells are quiescent and there is no change in cell size, DNA synthesis or cell number over time [29]. "Contaminating" non-muscle cells (predominantly fibroblasts) are reduced by the process of differential attachment, and their proliferation is prevented by the use of a DNA synthesis inhibitor (bromodeoxyuridine). As such, over 90% of the cells in culture are cardiac myocytes. By taking advantage of this differential attachment property of the cardiac myocytes, the non-myocytes can also be cultured in relatively pure form (~ 2-3% "contaminating" muscle cells) and subjected to the same treatments as the myocytes. Under these stable culture conditions, catecholamines and other growth factors or their diluent are then added to the culture medium. Since the myocytes do not undergo cell division, the main variable examined is the induction of cell growth (hypertrophy). This can be assessed either by quantifying changes in cell size or ^{14}C-Phenylalanine incorporation into new protein. Cardiac fibroblasts, on the other hand, respond to stimuli predominantly through proliferation. This can be assessed by observing changes in ^{3}H-thymidine incorporation in response to the various growth stimulants. In this way, it is possible in vitro to reconstruct the complex environment of the cardiac myocyte in vivo in order to delineate the specific factor or factors which regulate myocardial growth and function. Since most of the work done up to the present time with catecholamines in culture has been directed at myocyte growth and gene expression, this will be addressed first. Subsequently, our preliminary work on catecholamine effects on the non-myocytes will be presented.

Myocyte effects of adrenergic stimulation

Stimulation of myocyte growth

Treatment of the myocyte cultures with the α_1 agonist NE causes a dose-dependent 1.5 to 2-fold increase in cell size and protein content which occurs within 12 hours after stimulation and becomes maximal with 24 to 48 hours of treatment [24, 26, 27]. This response has an EC_{50} of approximately 200 nM, a level which is physiologic for an active sympathetic nerve terminal [30]. Pharmacologic studies carried out with other selective adrenergic agonists and antagonists indicate that this hypertrophic response is directly related to the α_1 adrenergic receptor, a specificity which has been confirmed by others [31, 32].

Similar to in vivo hypertrophy, this α_1 stimulated growth in culture does not involve myocyte proliferation and relates to a specific increase in per cell size and protein content [25]. This is in contrast to the recent observation that cultured fetal cardiac myocytes proliferate in response to NE [33], but similar to the observations of some in an adult rat cardiac myocyte culture system [34]. As such, these differences in growth responses of fetal, neonatal, and adult cardiac myocytes may indicate important fundamental changes in the differentiation program of the cardiac myocyte.

Additionally, the cell culture model has allowed us to investigate the role of contractility in the development of the hypertrophic phenotype. Although α_1 stimulated hypertrophy does not require myocyte contractile activity [27, 35], the stimulation of contractility is an important α_1 effect [27] which requires stimulation of both α_1 and β_1 adrenergic receptors. As such, treatment with NE and a β receptor antagonist results in hypertrophic cells which do not beat. Isolated stimulation with a β receptor agonist such as Isoproteronol does result in a modest increase in myocyte size and contractility; however, the mechanism of this increase is not entirely clear at this time and may involve, at least in part, the non-myocytes (see below). Of note, blockade of calcium channels does prevent NE induced contractility (but not hypertrophy), suggesting the importance of ion fluxes in this phenomenon [35].

Contractile-protein isoform switching and gene transcription in alpha1-stimulated hypertrophy.

Similar to the induction of clinical hypertrophy by a heterogeneous group of stimuli, different types of hypertrophy in the in vivo rat heart are also accompanied by different patterns of contractile protein isogene expression. For example, in hypertrophy induced by exercise or thyroid hormone, there is an increased expression of the a-myosin heavy chain (MHC) isogene, the normally occurring isoform [36]. In contrast, pressure overload hypertrophy results in the selective up-regulation of isogenes whose expression is normally limited to the fetal/neonatal heart. Specifically, aortic banding increases the mRNAs for skeletal α-actin and β-MHC [37, 38] as well as those encoding the nuclear protooncogenes c-fos and c-myc (for review see [39]) Although the functional significance of these isoform switches is unclear, there are differences in ATPase activity for the individual MHC isoforms [40-42] suggesting a potential attempt at a conservation of energy with hypertrophy. This heterogeneous response of the hypertrophic cardiac myocytes suggests that there may be multiple signals for hypertrophy. Therefore, we were interested in examining the changes in gene expression in our cell culture model of induced hypertrophy.

Quantitation of the myocyte content of specific mRNAs and proteins in our system of α_1 stimulated myocyte hypertrophy indicates that the α_1-adrenergic receptor is coupled to both general and specific changes in gene expression during hypertrophy. In addition to the 1.5 to 2-fold increase in the per cell total protein and RNA, stimulation of the α_1 receptor also results in the selective up-regulation of mRNAs encoding c-myc, skeletal α-actin and ß-MHC [43-45], a pattern similar to that descibed above with in vivo hypertrophy, and possibly indicating similar mechanisms. Similar changes in contractile protein gene expression are also seen with non-myocyte conditioned medium (Long, C.S., unpublished data) and, as described by Dr Schneider in this text, with the administration of members of the fibroblast growth factor and transforming growth factor ß families to the cultured myocytes. However, not all hypertrophic stimuli induce such changes in gene expression. For example, in culture, thyroid hormone (T_3) also produces hypertrophy, however T_3 stimulation increases α-MHC and decreases ß-MHC while other stimuli, such as serum, up-regulates both MHC isoforms [45]. Thus, the cell culture system mimics the varied changes in gene expression seen with the different types of experimentally-induced hypertrophy in vivo.

Since the changes in mRNA levels reported above could result from action either at the level of mRNA production (transcriptional) or from changes in mRNA stability (post-transcriptional), we performed nuclear run-on experiments with α_1 stimulated myocardial cells in culture [29]. These studies indicated that α_1 stimulation led to a specific temporal sequence of gene activation. This was characterized by a rapid but transient increase in cardiac α-actin transcription which occured within 3 hours of agonist administration, followed by a more sustained increase in skeletal α-actin transcription over the next 6-12 hours. This stimulation of transcription was not prevented by cyclohexamide, indicating that it did not require new protein synthesis. This latter observation is consistent with the postulate that α_1 receptor stimulation leads to modification of a pre-existing factor(s) that activates transcription. These studies also indicated that while the α_1-stimulated increase in total messenger RNA synthesis (α-amanitin-sensitive transcription) was transient, the increase in ribosomal and transfer synthesis (α-amanitin-insensitive transcription) was sustained, leading to an overall increase in the translational potential of the cardiac myocyte.

In summary, these experiments indicated that stimulation of a cell surface receptor resulted in an alteration in the transcriptional program of the nucleus. In order to effect this change, however, the signal must be transmitted from the cell surface to the nucleus. Unlike the case with steroid hormone receptors, the α_1 receptor has not been shown to be able to act as "second messenger" itself, suggesting that there must be some other substance responsible. As has been shown for other second messenger systems, the phosphorylation of a transcription factor was an attractive hypothesis.

The role of protein kinase C in alpha1 stimulated gene transcription

As noted above, evidence from many systems suggests a common theme in the regulation of gene expression by hormones and growth factors: post-translational modification of pre-existing protein transcription factors that interact with promoter elements of a particular gene (reviewed in [39]). The independence of gene transcription from new protein synthesis in our culture system is consistent with this theme.

As shown by others, stimulation of the α_1 receptor in our system activates phospholipase C (PLC) [46], and the activation of PLC implies production of diacylglycerol (DAG), the endogenous activator of protein kinase C (PKC). Although DAG has not been assayed directly, we have documented that α_1 receptor stimulation does activate myocyte PKC. This α_1 stimulated increase in PKC is similar to the PKC activation which occurs with phorbol ester in the cardiac myocytes, however, there are also important differences between these two agents both of whom increase myocyte size. Whereas both phorbol myristate acetate (PMA) and the α_1-adrenergic agonist NE stimulate acute translocation of PKC activity to the particulate fraction [47], acute activation of PKC by PMA differs from that by NE in several respects: (1) PMA-induced activation is more pronounced and is accompanied by loss of PKC activity and generation of calcium/lipid-independent kinase activity and (2) Chronic treatment with NE up-regulates PKC, measured as total PKC activity per cell and ^{3}H-phorbol dibutyrate binding sites per cell, whereas chronic treatment with PMA down-regulates PKC. These differing effects of PMA and NE on PKC activation suggest caution in extrapolating from PMA effects to those of natural PKC-activating agonists, such as NE.

As shown previously by our collaborators, of the various PKC isoforms known, the cultured cardiac myocytes express at least three, namely α-PKC, ß-PKC, and a PKC isoform recognized by the monoclonal antibody CK 1.4 which is not α, ß, or γ [48]. We have used immunofluorescence with monoclonal antibody CK 1.4, and a monoclonal specific for ß-PKC, to determine the intracellular site of translocation of these PKC isoforms after stimulation of the myocytes with both PMA and NE [48]. Within seconds of stimulation, the PKC isoform recognized by CK 1.4 is translocated to myofibrils. In contrast, ß-PKC is translocated to the surface membrane and the perinuclear area, suggesting that different PKC isoforms might phosphorylate different substrates, and thus subserve different functions in the cardiac myocytes.

Because of this translocation to the perinuclear area, we felt that ß-PKC was ideally suited to be the second messenger for the α_1 stimulated changes in contractile protein gene transcription described above. Utilizing a co-transfection protocol, we have recently obtained data that provide direct support for a role of this PKC isoform in activation of the ß-MHC gene [49]. In these experiments, expression plasmids encoding normal α- or ß-PKC, or constitutively-activated mutants of α- or ß-PKC, were introduced into the cultured cardiac myocytes, along with a plasmid containing 3300 bp of the ß-MHC promoter fused to the chloramphenicol acetyltransferase (CAT) reporter gene. Assay of the CAT protein product thus served as an index of activation of the ß-MHC promoter by one of the expressed PKCs. Results of these studies indicated that the activated mutant of the ß-PKC isoform increased expression from the ß-MHC promoter, and was more than twice as potent as activated a-PKC, providing the first direct evidence that the ß-PKC isozyme is in a pathway regulating transcription of the ß-MHC isogene. The specific DNA sequences in the ß-MHC promoter that mediate the ß-PKC response are presently under study in our laboratory and have been localized to an 20 base pair element which can transfer both PKC and adrenergic responsiveness to a heterologous promoter [50]. This element also shows specific protein binding to cardiac myocyte nuclear extracts in a gel retardation assay

[50]. It is interesting to note that, in contrast with the ß-PKC stimulation of ß-MHC transcription, no increase in skeletal α-actin transcription occurs using the co-transfection system (Karns, L. and Simpson, P. C., unpublished data), suggesting the involvement of a different second messenger system, or at least a different PKC isoform, in the α_1 stimulation of this contractile protein isoform.

The Beta-Adrenergic Receptor in Cardiac Myocyte Hypertrophy

As recorded above, our work has supported the notion that catecholamines can be important non-hemodynamic factors in myocardial hypertrophy. However, for the most part, it has focused attention on the α_1-adrenergic receptor as a mediator of these effects.

We have previously suggested that isoproterenol-stimulated hypertrophy may be mediated by ß-adrenergic stimulated increases in NE release from sympathetic nerve terminals and by the increased sympathetic activity seen with isoproterenol infusions [27].

Recent studies may require revision of this postulate, since we have recently been able to show a growth-promoting effect of ß-adrenergic stimulation in the cultured cardiac myocytes (Simpson, P. C. unpublished data). This ß-adrenergic growth effect differs from that mediated through the a_1 receptor in several respects. To our surprise, cardiac myocyte hypertrophy induced by ß stimulation in the culture system appears to be dependent on the particular culture medium used, being seen in MEM but absent in M199. Further, it has a lower EC_{50} (200 nM for NE vs 2 nM for isoproterenol) and shows desensitization. Additionally, some experiments carried out in high (50 mM) KCl suggests that ß stimulated hypertrophy may be, at least in part, dependent upon myocyte contractile activity (Rocha-Singh, K. and Simpson, P. C. , unpublished data). One of the most intriguing aspects of the ß stimulated myocyte growth, however, relates to the potential role played by the non-muscle cells present in the culture system.

Non-myocyte effects and adrenergic stimulation

As mentioned previously, we have only recently begun to appreciate the role of the cardiac non-myocytes in the process of myocyte growth. Furthermore, our work using medium conditioned by cardiac non-myocytes in culture suggests that this may be, in fact, a profound effect. Since it is assumed that such indirect non-myocyte-induced growth effects result from the production of growth factors by the cardiac non-myocytes, it is interesting to note that many of these factors have been found in myocardium. These include PDGF ß chain [51], FGF (both acidic and basic) [52-57], TGFß [58-60], IGF-1 and IGF-2 [61, 62], TNFα [63], NGF [64, 65], and the factor identified in our laboratory which we have tentatively called the "non-myocyte derived growth factor" or NMDGF [25]. All of these factors have been found to induce cardiac myocyte hypertrophy in culture [25].

Our initial interest in the possibility that the ß-adrenergic system might have an effect on the non-myocyte fraction of the heart related to observations by others suggesting that adrenergic stimulation of cardiac myocyte gene transcription appeared to differ with respect to receptor subtype purely as a function of plated cell density [66]. In brief, when plated at low density, the myocyte growth effect and induction of contractile protein isoform switching was predominantly α_1 in origin.

In apparent contrast, when cultured at higher densities, both α and ß adrenergic stimulation seemed to result in these same changes in myocyte growth and transcriptional program. Given our previous work on the effects of increasing cell density on myocyte growth [25], we wondered whether this apparent discrepancy might in fact relate to an indirect ß adrenergic response. In other words, was it possible that the ß adrenergic effects seen at high density were the result of a paracrine effect of ß stimulation of the cardiac non-myocytes? In support of this theory, we have found that, in addition to the production of a growth-promoting conditioned medium under "baseline" conditions, these cells respond to ß-adrenergic stimulation by producing a more potent conditioned medium [28].

In an attempt to explain the efects of isoproterenol on the non-myocyte conditioned medium, we asked whether there was anything peculier to ß stimulation which might result in an increase in the production of growth factor(s) by the non-myocytes. The obvious answer was that ß stimulation leads to an increase in adenyl cyclase acivity and cAMP production by these cells. Since it had been recently reported that the TGFß$_3$ isoform of the TGFß family contained a functional cAMP response element, this was an attractive candidate. In subsequent experiments, we found that within 24-48 hours of isoproterenol treatment, the steady state level of non-myocyte TGFß$_3$ mRNA did indeed increase in response to the increase in cAMP in contrast to that of the TGFß$_1$ isoform which does not contain a functional CRE and did not change with isoproterenol treatment [21]. In addition to this paracrine myocyte growth effect, isoproterenol stimulation also resulted in the autocrine stimulation of non-myocyte DNA synthesis (Long, C S, unpublished observations). Since these non-myocytes are also involved with the elaboration of the extracellular matrix (reviewed by Drs Rappaport and Samuel in this text), such a ß stimulated increase in cell numbers may have an important impact on the composition of the cardiac interstitium.

In summary, the prevalence of myocardial hypertrophy and its prognostic significance for the development of cardiovascular morbidity and mortality has stimulated interest in the factors responsible for the development of the hypertrophic phenotype. We have developed a cell culture model of myocardial hypertrophy in which stimulation of the α_1 adrenergic receptor results in a hypertrophic phenotype which is quite similar to that seen with other forms of experimentally-induced myocardial hypertrophy in vivo. In this model, growth is largely independent of contractility and results in a change in the transcriptional program of the cardiac myocytes. As a result of our co-transfection studies, we postulate that protein kinase C plays a role as second messenger in this system, although it does not appear to account for the α_1 stimulated increase in skeletal actin gene transcription. In response to the new data regarding the production of growth factors by both muscle and non-muscle cells in myocardium, our culture system has also allowed us to study the interaction between the cardiac myocytes and the surrounding non-myocytes. Using this system we have shown a dramatic effect of medium conditioned by the non-myocytes on both myocyte growth and gene expression. Furthermore, studies with adrenergic stimulation of these non-myocytes indicates that their expression of at least one growth factor, namely TGFß, is not fixed and may be responsive to changes in the hormonal environment. Further work is presently underway in our laboratory to define with certainty how all of these factors act, both individually and together, to produce the different forms of myocardial hypertrophy seen clinically.

References

1. Levy D, Clinical significance of left ventricular hypertrophy: insights from the framingham study. J Cardiovasc Pharm 1991: 17(Suppl 2); S1-S6.

2. Laks MM, Morady F. Norepinephrine - the myocardial hypertrophy hormone? Am Heart J 1976; 91: 674-675.
3. Rossi MA, Carillo SV. Does norepinephrine play a central causative role in the process of cardiac hypertrophy ? Am Heart J 1985; 109: 622-624.
4. Tarazi RC et al. The multifactorial role of catecholamines in hypertensive cardiac hypertrophy. Eur Heart J 1982; 3 (Suppl A): 103-110.
5. Genovese A et al. Adrenergic activity as a modulating factor in the genesis of myocardial hypertrophy in the rat. Exp Mol Pathol 1984; 41: 390-396.
6. de Champlain J et al. Circulating catecholamine levels in human and experimental hypertension. Circ Res 1976; 38: 109-114.
7. Ostman-Smith I. Cardiac sympathetic nerves as the final common pathway in the induction of adaptive cardiac hypertrophy. Clin Sci 1981 61; 265-272.
8. Lake CR. Essential hypertension: are catecholamines involved? Fed Proc 1984; 43: 45-46.
9. Corea L et al. Plasma norepinephrine and left ventricular hypertrophy in systemic hypertension. Am J Cardiol 1984; 53: 1299-1303.
10. Trimarco B et al. Participation of endogenous catecholamines in the regulation of left ventricular mass in progeny of hypertensive parents. Circulation 1985; 72: 38-46.
11. Zierhut W, Zimmer H-G. Significance of myocardial α- and ß-adrenoceptors in catecholamine-induced cardiac hypertrophy. Circ Res 1989; 65: 1417-1425.
12. Stanton G, Brenner G, Mayfield EDJr. Studies on isoproterenol-induced cardiomegaly in rats. Am Heart J 1969; 77: 72-80.
13. Laks M, Morady F, Swan H. Myocardial hypertrophy produced by chronic infusion of subhypertensive doses of norepinephrine in the dog. Chest 1969; 64: 75-78.
14. King BD et al. Absence of hypertension despite chronic marked elevations in plasma norepinephrine in conscious dogs. Hypertension 1987; 9: 582-590.
15. Pfeffer JM et al. Regression of left ventricular hypertrophy and prevention of left ventricular dysfunction by captopril in the spontaneously hypertensive rat. Proc Natl Acad Sci USA 1982; 79: 3310-3314.
16. Pfeffer MA, Pfeffer JM. Reversing cardiac hypertrophy in hypertension. N Engl J Med 1990; 322: 1388-1390.
17. Leenen FHH et al. Vasodilators and regression of left ventricular hypertrophy: hydralazine versus prazosin in hypertensive human. Am J Med 1987; 82: 969-978.
18. Sugishita Y et al. Cardiac determinants of regression of left ventricular hypertrophy in essential hypertension with antihypertensive treatment. J Am Coll Cardiol 1990; 15: 665-671.

19. Schulman SP et al. The effects of antihypertensive therapy on left ventricular mass in elderly patients. N Engl J Med 1990; 322: 1350-1356.

20. Strauer BE et al. The influence of sympathetic nervous activity on regression of cardiac hypertrophy. J Hypertension 1985; 3 (Suppl 4): S39-S44.

21. Long CS et al. ß-adrenergic stimulation of cardiac non-myocytes increases non-myocyte growth factor production. J Mol Cell Cardiol 1992; 24(Suppl I): S245.

22. Bhambi B, Eghbali M. Effect of norepinephrine on myocardial collagen gene expressionm and response of cardiac fibrblasts after norepinephrine treatment. Am J Pathol 1991; 139: 1131-1142.

23. Simpson P, Savion S. Differentiation of rat myocytes in single cell cultures with and without proliferating nonmyocardial cells: cross-striations, ultrastructure, and chronotropic response to isoproterenol. Circ Res 1982; 50: 101-116.

24. Simpson P, McGrath A, Savion S, Myocyte hypertrophy in neonatal rat heart cultures and its regulation by serum and by catecholamines. Circ Res 1982; 51: 787-801.

25. Long CS, Henrich CJ, Simpson PC. A growth factor for cardiac myocytes is produced by cardiac nonmyocytes. Cell Reg 1991; 2: 1081-1095.

26. Simpson P. Norepinephrine-stimulated hypertrophy of cultured rat myocardial cells is an alpha1-adrenergic response. J Clin Invest 1983; 72: 732-738.

27. Simpson P. Stimulation of hypertrophy of cultured neonatal rat heart cells through an a1-adrenergic receptor and induction of beating through an α1-and β1-adrenergic receptor interaction: evidence for independent regulation of growth and beating. Circ Res 1985; 56: 884-894.

28. Long CS, Paningbatan M, Simpson PC. A ß-adrenergic receptor stimulates paracrine growth factor activity. J Cell Biochem 1991; Suppl 15C: H213.

29. Long CS, Ordahl CP, Simpson PC. α1-Adrenergic receptor stimulation of sarcomeric actin isogene transcription in hypertrophy of cultured rat heart muscle cells. J Clin Invest 1989; 83: 1078-1082.

30. Bevan JA. Norepinephrine and the presynaptic control of adrenergic transmitter release. Fed Proc 1978; 39: 187-190.

31. Meidell RS et al. α1-adrenergic stimulation of rat myocardial cells increases protein synthesis. Am J Physiol 1986; 251: H1076-H1084.

32. Lee HR et al. α1-adrenergic stimulation of cardiac gene transcription in neonatal rat myocardial cells: effects on myosin light chain-2 gene expression. J Biol Chem 1988; 263: 7352-7358.

33. Marino TA et al. Effects of catecholamines on fetal rat cardiocytes in vitro. Am J Anat 1989; 186: 127-132.

34. Fuller SJ, Gaitanaki CJ, Sugden PH. Effects of catecholamines on protein synthesis in cardiac myocytes and perfused hearts isolated from adult rats: stimulation of translation is mediated through the a1-adrenoceptor. Biochem J 1990; 266: 727-736.

35. Simpson P. Calcium entry blockers inhibit catecholamine-induced beating but not catecholamine-stimulated hypertrophy of cultured rat heart cells (abstract). Clin Res 1984; 33: 90A.

36. Gustafson TA, Markham BE, Morkin E. Effects of thyroid hormone on α-actin and myosin heavy chain gene expression in cardiac and skeletal muscles of the rat: measurement of mRNA content using synthetic oligonucleotide probes. Circ Res 1986; 59: 194-201.

37. Schwartz K et al. α-skeletal muscle actin mRNAs accumulate in hypertrophied adult rat hearts. Circ Res 1986; 59: 551-555.

38. Izumo S et al. Myosin heavy chain messenger RNA and protein isoform transitions during cardiac hypertrophy: Interaction between hemodynamic and thyroid hormone-induced signals. J Clin Invest 1987; 79: 970-977.

39. Simpson PC. Proto-oncogenes and cardiac hypertrophy. Ann Rev Physiol 1989; 51: 189-202.

40. Scheuer J. Bahn AK. Cardiac contractile proteins: adenosine triphosphatase activity and physiological function. Circ Res 1979; 45: 1-12.

41. Schwartz K et al. Myosin isoenzyme distribution correlates with speed of myocardial contraction. J Mol Cell Cardiol 1981; 13: 1071-1075.

42. Pagani ED, FJ Julian. Rabbit papillary muscle myosin isoenzymes and the velocity of muscle shortening. Circ Res 1984; 54: 586-594.

43. Starksen NF et al. Cardiac myocyte hypertrophy is associated with c-myc proto-oncogene expression. Proc Natl Acad Sci USA 1986; 83: 8348-8350.

44. Bishopric NH, Simpson PC, Ordahl CP. Induction of the skeletal α-actin gene in α1-adrenoceptor-mediated hypertrophy of rat cardiac myocytes. J Clin Invest 1987; 80: 1194-1199.

45. Waspe LE, Ordahl CP, Simpson PC. The cardiac ß-myosin heavy chain isogene is induced selectively in α1-adrenergic receptor-stimulated hypertrophy of cultured rat heart myocytes. J Clin Invest 1990; 85: 1206-1214.

46. Karliner JS, Kagiya T, Simpson PC. Effects of pertussis toxin on α1-agonist-mediated phosphatidylinositide turnover and cell hypertrophy in neonatal rat ventricular myocytes. Experientia 1990; 46: 81-84.

47. Henrich CJ, Simpson PC. Differential acute and chronic response of protein kinase C in cultured neonatal rat heart myocytes to α1-adrenergic and phorbol ester stimulation. J Mol Cell Cardiol 1988; 20: 1081-1085.

48. Mochly-Rosen D et al. A protein kinase C isozyme is translocated to cytoskeletal elements on activation. Cell Regul 1990; 1: 693-706.

49. Kariya K, Karns LR, Simpson PC. Expression of a constitutively activated mutant of the ß-isozyme of protein kinase C in cardiac myocytes stimulates the promoter of the promoter of the ß-myosin heavy chain isogene. J Biol Chem 1991; 266: 10023-10026.

50. Kariya K-I, Karns LR, Simpson PC. Myocyte-specific and α1-adrenergic and protein kinase c (PKC)-stimulated transcription of the ß-myosin heavy chain (MHC) gene are mediated through interaction of a 20-base pair (bp) promoter element with cardiac myocyte nuclear factors. Circ (abstract) 1992 : in press.

51. Sarzani R, Arnoldi G, Chobanian AV. Hypertension-induced changes of platelet-derived growth factor receptor expression in rat aorta and heart. Hypertension 1991; 17: 888-895.

52. Speir E et al. Fibroblast growth factors are present in adult cardiac myocytes, in vivo. Biochem Biophys Res Commun 1988; 157: 1336-1340.

53. Kardami E, Fandrich RR. Basic fibroblast growth factor in atria and ventricles of the vertebrate heart. J Cell Biol 1989; 109: 1865-1875.

54. Sasaki H et al. Purification of acidic fibroblast growth factor from bovine heart and its localization in the cardiac myocytes. J Biol Chem 1989; 264: 17606-17612.

55. Weiner HL, Swain JL. Acidic fibroblast growth factor mRNA is expressed by cardiac myocytes in culture and the protein is localized to the extracellular matrix. Proc Natl Acad Sci USA 1989; 86: 2683-2687.

56. Quinckler W, Pfeffer J. Isolation of Heparin Binding Growth Factors from Bovine, Porcine, and Canine Hearts. Eur J Biochem 1989; 181: 67-73.

57. Casscells W et al. Isolation, characterization, and localization of heparin-binding growth factors in the heart. J Clin Invest 1990; 85: 433-441.

58. Eghbali M. Cellular origin and distribution of transforming growth factor-ß1 in the normal rat myocardium. Cell Tissue Res 1989; 256: 553-558.

59. Casscells W et al. Transforming growth factor beta-1 in normal heart and myocardial infarction (abstract). Circulation 1989; 80: II-452.

60. Wunsch M et al. Expression of transforming growth factor ß1 (TGFß1) in collateralized swine heart (abstract). Circulation 1989; 80: II-453.

61. Cercek B et al. Induction of vascular insulin-like growth factor-1 mRNA after balloon denudation precedes neointimal proliferation (abstract). Circulation 1989; 80: II-453.

62. Engelmann GL et al. Insulin-like growth factors and neonatal cardiomyocyte development: ventricular gene expression and membrane receptor variations in normotensive and hypertensive rats. Mol Cell Endocrinol 1989; 63: 1-14.

63. Friedman G et al. Lipoprotein lipase in heart cell cultures is suppressed by bacterial lipopolysaccharide: an effect mediated by production of tumor necrosis factor. Biochem Biophys Acta 1988; 960: 220-228.

64. Furukawa Y, Furukawa S, Satoyoshi E. Nerve growth factor secreted by mouse heart cells in culture. J Biol Chem 1984; 259: 1259-1264.

65. Norrgren G, Ebendal T. Nerve growth factor in medium conditioned by embryonic chicken heart cells. Int J Develop Neuroscience 1986; 4: 41-49.

66. Bishopric NH, L. Kedes L. Adrenergic regulation of the skeletal α-actin gene promoter during myocardial cell hypertrophy. Proc Natl Acad Sci (USA) 1991; 88: 2131-2136.

20. Effects of transforming growth factor-beta on cardiac fibroblasts

MAHBOUBEH EGHBALI

Introduction

Cardiac cells consist of cardiac myocytes and non-myocyte cells. The non-myocyte population includes cardiac fibroblasts that are present in the interstitium, endothelial cells that form the lining of blood vessels and myocardial cavities, smooth muscle cells, and nerve cells. By the use of monospecific antibodies to each cell type and immunofluorescent staining of freshly isolated non-myocyte heart cells, we have established that greater than 90% of the heart cells in the non-myocyte population are cardiac fibroblasts [1]. In the ventricular myocardium, cardiac fibroblasts are responsible for biosynthesis of extracellular matrix proteins [1,2]. In the heart, extracellular matrix provides structural and functional support for cardiac myocytes and the vasculature. Major protein of this matrix is collagen. Collagens are a family of related molecules with distinct genes and variable tissue distribution. Major collagens of the adult heart are classical fiber-forming collagen types I and III, and basement membrane-specific collagen type IV. Collagen type I accounts for greater than 80% of total collagens in the heart [3]. A normal collagen matrix that is the result of a balanced collagen synthesis and degradation process is critical for maintaining the integrity of myocardial function. In the interstitium, cardiac fibroblasts are exposed to the regulatory effects of various hormones, neurotransmitters and growth factors that are present in the myocardium or gain access to the ventricular tissue by blood vessels. Regulation of gene expression in cardiac fibroblasts and modulation of their phenotype by those regulatory factors may occur under various pathophysiological conditions. Transforming growth factor-beta (TGF-ß$_1$) is a multi-functional growth factor peptide that is present in the myocardium in areas surrounding the blood vessels [4]. It has been shown that TGF-ß$_1$ regulates biosynthesis of collagen type I both at transcriptional and post-transcriptional levels [5]. In this chapter, I review the results of our studies that indicate cardiac fibroblasts are cellular targets for the regulatory effects of TGF-ß$_1$ in the heart and that the interstitial compartment of the heart may be altered both structurally and functionally as the result of the effects of TGF-ß$_1$, both on collagen gene expression and on cardiac fibroblast phenotype.

Functional importance of cardiac fibroblasts and their properties in culture

While the importance of cardiac muscle cells in the myocyte compartment of the heart is based on their contractile ability, functional significance of cardiac fibroblasts lies in the fact that they are the cellular origin of extracellular matrix proteins. The major protein of the cardiac extracellular matrix is collagen. Studies by scanning electron microscopy have shown that collagen matrix of the heart is an intricate and highly organized structure that serves to interconnect cardiac myocytes to one another and to their neighboring capillaries [1]. This arrangement provides support for cardiac myocytes and prevents cardiac myocyte slippage and maintains their alignment during a cardiac cycle. Collagen fibers of the heart are composed of fibrillar collagen types I and III. In addition, collagen type IV, a basement membrane-specific protein is synthesized by both cardiac fibroblasts and cardiac myocytes. Collagen type I accounts for greater than 80% of total collagen of the ventricular myocardium. Due to differences in physical and mechanical properties of collagen type I and III, alterations in the proportion of these collagen types may result in altered cardiac performance. Immunofluorescent studies with monospecific antibodies to attachment molecules have demonstrated that the interaction of collagen fibers, in the heart, with cardiac myocytes occurs at regions near the Z band and the attachment is mediated by specific molecules that belong to the family of integrins [6]. It is, therefore, reasonable to speculate that in addition to its important role in providing structural support for cardiac myocytes, collagen matrix may also act as a link between the contractile element of adjacent cardiac myocytes and as a conduit of information that are necessary for cell function. Remodeling of collagen matrix under pathophysiological conditions such as increased blood pressure has been shown to occur in conjunction with alterations in the myocyte compartment of the heart [7,8]. Therefore, alterations in mechanical and physical properties of the heart, as seen in conditions such as myocardial hypertrophy, could be due, to a large extent, to an altered collagen matrix. Study of collagen synthesis and degradation in cardiac fibroblasts is critical to better understanding of molecular basis of the regulatory mechanisms that are involved in the remodeling of myocardial matrix. Although understanding of in vivo regulatory mechanisms is best achieved by investigating the intact tissue, cultured cells provide a valuable system that allows study of cell function and behavior under defined and controlled conditions. It also allows studies of individual factors or in vivo conditions that may regulate cell behavior and gene expression. We have established cultured cardiac fibroblasts from rat and rabbit ventricular tissue and identified their phenotypic properties in culture. Cells from both rat and rabbit heart share many characteristics with fibroblasts obtained from other tissues, such as typical cell morphology and synthesis of extracellular collagen fibrils [9]. Using monospecific antibodies and immunofluorescent light microscopy, we showed that cardiac fibroblasts synthesize types I, III and IV collagen, laminine and fibronectin [9]. Cardiac fibroblasts synthesize collagen type I even in the absence of ascorbate. However, the presence of ascorbate in the culture medium is essential for deposition of crosslinked collagen fibrils [9]. Cultured cardiac fibroblasts express mRNAs for cytoskeletal actin, TGF-ß$_1$ [8] and the gap junction-specific protein, connexin-43 [10]. Expression of gap junction-specific protein by cardiac fibroblasts is an additional evidence in support of their active participation in the myocardial function and cell communication.

Expression and regulation of TGF-ß1 in the myocardium and in cardiac fibroblasts.

Previously, we have shown that TGF-ß$_1$ is present in the myocardium [4] In those studies, by immunofluorescent light microscopy and specific antibody to TGF-ß$_1$, we showed that this growth factor is located in areas surrounding the blood vessels. By the use of freshly isolated heart cells and Northern analysis of total RNA extracted from those cells, we also showed that the mRNA for TGF-ß$_1$ was detected in the non-myocyte fraction of freshly isolated heart cells in the adult rat heart [4]. Our studies on several models of cardiac hypertrophy have demonstrated that TGF-β_1 gene expression in the ventricular myocardium is subject to regulation by various pathophysiological stimuli such as increased blood pressure, induced by hormones and neurotransmitters. In a rat model of cardiac hypertrophy, induced by intravenous perfusion of hypertensive doses of norepinephrine [8], we have demonstrated that abundance of mRNA for TGF-β_1 was increased in the heart of norepinephrine-treated rats compared with that in the heart of normal untreated animals. This enhancement of mRNA for TGF-β_1 was parallel to increased mRNA for proα_2 (I) collagen. In the same model, as shown by immunofluorescent light microscopy, ventricular hypertrophy was accompanied by myocardial fibrosis and remodeling of collagen matrix [8]. Although in vivo administration of norepinephrine led to increased collagen gene expression, norepinephrine-treatment of cardiac fibroblasts did not seem to induce any significant changes in the abundance of mRNA for collagen type I [8]. Considering the proven effects of TGF-β_1 on collagen type I gene transcription [5], it is likely that TGF-β_1 is the regulatory factor for myocardial collagen gene expression that comes into play as the result of norepinephrine-induced hormonal or hemodynamic changes and is indirectly responsible for in vivo alterations in collagen type I mRNA in the heart of norepinephrine-treated rats. In a different model of ventricular hypertrophy, induced by intraperitoneal injections of thyroid hormone (L-thyroxine), it was shown that while mRNA for collagen type I was decreased drastically, the abundance of mRNA for TGF-β_1 in the heart of thyroxine-treated rats was increased compared with that in the heart of untreated rats [11]. Interestingly, in this model of hypertrophy, and unlike models induced by pressure overload and hypertensive dosage norepinephrine, cardiac fibrosis did not occur even after prolonged treatment with thyroxine [11]. Our in vitro studies with cardiac fibroblasts in culture showed that treatment of cells with thyroxine led to increased abundance of mRNA for TGF-β_1 in treated cells compared with that in untreated control cells [11]. However, thyroxine, unlike norepinephrine, had a direct impact on collagen gene expression in cardiac fibroblasts, in that thyroxine-treatment of cardiac fibroblasts led to decreased levels of mRNA for collagen type I. Therefore, although thyroid hormone is an enhancer of TGF-β_1 gene expression in ventricular myocardium, it seems unlikely that TGF-β_1 would be the mediator of in vivo inhibitory effects of thyroid hormone on collagen gene expression.

Regulation of collagen gene expression in cardiac fibroblasts by TGF-ß1

Studies of regulatory mechanisms that alter cardiac fibroblast behavior are critical to the understanding of underlying mechanisms that are involved in maintaining a balanced collagen matrix in the myocardium. TGF-ß$_1$ is a known enhancer of collagen gene expression [5] and its own expression is regulated by various pathophysiological conditions such as cardiac hypertrophy [8,11]. To understand the cellular basis of its regulatory role, we examined the effects of TGF-ß$_1$ on cardiac fibroblasts in culture with respect to collagen gene expression [12]. In those studies, we used Northern analysis of total RNA and immunofluorescent light microscopy to determine alterations in collagen synthesis. Our findings indicated that TGF-ß$_1$-treatment of cardiac fibroblasts leads to increased abundance of mRNA for pro α_2 (I) and pro α_1 (III) collagens. Stimulatory effect of TGF-ß$_1$ on collagen mRNA was shown to cause increased collagen synthesis as it was evident by enhanced immunofluorescent staining of intracellular collagen type I in TGF-ß$_1$-treated cardiac fibroblasts compared with normal untreated cells [12]. Studies with the inhibitor of protein synthesis, cycloheximide, revealed that the increased mRNA for collagen type I in cardiac fibroblasts, following treatment with TGF-ß$_1$, required de novo protein synthesis. We had previously shown that in a norepinephrine-induced model of cardiac hypertrophy, increased abundance of TGF-ß$_1$ mRNA was accompanied, at early stages of treatment, with the induction of mRNAs for transcription factors, c-fos, and c-jun proto-oncogenes and early growth response gene, Egr-1. These early response genes are known to encode transcription factors that are widely implicated as nuclear signal transducers which initiate diverse responses such as cell proliferation and differentiation [13]. Interestingly, TGF-ß$_1$ treatment of cardiac fibroblasts did not cause induction of mRNA for proto-oncogenes or Egr-1. It is important to note that during cardiac myocyte growth [14] and in the course of myocardial hypertrophy [15], these transcription factors have been shown to be induced at the level of mRNA. Therefore, although TGF-ß$_1$ gene expression is enhanced in the myocardium in several models of cardiac hypertrophy, it seems that effects of this growth factor on collagen gene expression is independent of those mechanisms that are involved in the process of cell hypertrophy. However, TGF-ß$_1$-treatment caused stimulation of cardiac fibroblast proliferation, and led to a modest increase in DNA synthesis as it was shown by increased ^{3}H-thymidine incorporation into the cell nuclei of TGF-ß$_1$-treated cells compared with that in control untreated cardiac fibroblasts [12]. This effect of TGF-ß$_1$ on cell proliferation, when compared with the effect of mitogen and tumor promoter, 12-0-tetradecanoyl phorbol myristate 13-acetate (PMA), was proved to be relatively low. It was also shown that unlike TGF-ß$_1$-treatment, PMA-treatment of cardiac fibroblasts led to the induction of mRNAs for early transcription factors c-fos, c-jun and Egr-1, within 45 minutes of treatment [12]. More importantly, in contrast to the effect of TGF-ß$_1$ on pro α_2 (I) collagen gene expression, PMA treatment of cardiac fibroblasts resulted in a diminished abundance of mRNA for pro α_2 (I) collagen.

Modulation of cardiac fibroblast phenotype by TGF-ß1

TGF-ß$_1$ is a multifunctional growth factor with proven effects as mitogen, transforming agent and growth enhancing factor in a variety of cell types. In cardiac fibroblasts, in addition to its regulatory effect on collagen gene expression, TGF-ß$_1$ exerts a transforming effect on cardiac fibroblasts phenotype [15]. It was shown that rabbit cardiac fibroblasts when exposed to TGF-ß$_1$, display several characteristics of cardiac myocytes [16] and undergo phenotypic modulation. Modulation of cardiac fibroblast phenotype was based on several evidence: 1) appearance of morphological features, characteristic to cardiac myocytes, in TGF-ß$_1$-treated cells; 2) induction of sarcomeric actin mRNA in cardiac fibroblasts following treatment with TGF-ß$_1$; 3) appearance of sarcomeric actin filaments in TGF-ß$_1$-treated cells; and 4) disappearance of intermediate filament vimentin, following treatment with TGF-ß$_1$ as evidenced by immunofluorescent light microscopy. While expression of sarcomeric actin mRNA and appearance of sarcomeric actin filaments in cardiac fibroblasts could be the result of the effects of TGF-ß$_1$ on actin gene expression, loss of vimentin filaments in TGF-ß$_1$-treated cells is an indication of phenotypic modulation of cardiac fibroblasts by TGF-ß$_1$, since terminal differentiation of myoblasts is associated with reduced expression of vimentin in differentiated cells. Transforming effect of TGF-ß$_1$ on cardiac fibroblasts phenotype seems to be specific for cardiac fibroblasts. This view is supported by the observation that skin fibroblasts and NIH 3T3 cells were not affected by TGF-ß$_1$ with respect to modulation of their phenotype. On the other hand, induction of sarcomeric actin mRNA in cardiac fibroblasts did not occur following treatment of those cells with other regulatory factors such as PMA, angiotensin II, interleukin-1, or norepinephrine. Together, these data suggest that modulation of cardiac fibroblasts phenotype by TGF-ß$_1$ is a specific effect of this growth factor that cannot be mimicked by other factors to which cardiac fibroblasts are naturally exposed. Modulation of cardiac fibroblasts phenotype by TGF-ß$_1$ was proved to be a permanent effect. We showed that second generation of cells, stemmed from TGF-ß$_1$-treated cardiac fibroblasts, expressed sarcomeric actin filaments as shown by immunofluorescent light microscopy. In addition, those cells had a diminished rate of proliferation compared with that in untreated cardiac fibroblasts. Together, these findings suggest that cardiac fibroblasts are predisposed to convert into a phenotype with characteristics common to cardiac myocytes and TGF-ß$_1$ is the specific inducer of such phenotypic modulation. In view of the fact that TGF-ß$_1$ is an in vitro stimulus of cardiac fibroblasts gene expression and that it is present in the ventricular tissue, the phenotypic modulation of cardiac fibroblasts by this growth factor could be of significant biological relevance. Mechanisms of myogenesis in the heart are not elucidated. Stem cells or cell lines that could convert into cardiac myocytes in the cardiac muscle, have not been identified. Our finding are highlighted by the observation that phenotypic modulation occurred in cardiac fibroblasts obtained from the adult rat heart. Therefore, these findings suggest that TGF-ß$_1$ alone or in combination with other factors that are present in the myocardium, may be exploited to induce terminal phenotypic modulation of cardiac fibroblasts. They also raise the possibility of compensation for the lack of regenerative capacity of adult cardiac myocytes by the newly converted cardiac fibroblasts in the adult heart.

Summary and concluding remarks.

TGF-ß$_1$ is an endogenous myocardial growth factor peptide. Freshly isolated cardiac fibroblasts and cardiac fibroblasts in culture express mRNA for TGF-ß$_1$. Our studies with animal models of cardiac hypertrophy indicated up-regulation of TGF-ß$_1$ gene expression in hypertrophied myocardium irrespective of the presence of cardiac fibrosis. Our studies with cultured cardiac fibroblasts and related studies by other investigators on other cell types, however, demonstrated that TGF-ß$_1$ enhances collagen type I gene expression. Cardiac fibroblasts also are targets for other regulatory effects of TGF-ß$_1$. TGF-ß$_1$ has a modest stimulatory effect on DNA synthesis in cardiac fibroblasts. Most importantly, TGF-ß$_1$ was shown to have modulatory effects on cardiac fibroblasts phenotype. This effect of TGF-ß$_1$ was evidenced by induction of muscle-specific morphology, sarcomeric actin gene expression and loss of intermediate filament, vimentin in cardiac fibroblasts. Together, these results point to a dual effect of TGF-ß$_1$ on cardiac fibroblasts, in that, on the one hand it induces myocyte-specific characteristics, and on the other, it potentiates some residual properties of cardiac fibroblasts such as collagen gene expression and proliferation. As the result of such effects, TGF-ß$_1$ may alter structural and functional aspects of myocardial interstitium, hence physical and mechanical properties of the heart under various pathophysiological conditions.

Acknowledgements

This work was supported by NHLBI grants R01-HL-42666 and R01-HL43557.

References

1. Eghbali M, Weber KT. Collagen and the myocardium: Fibrillar structure, biosynthesis and degradation in relation to hypertrophy and its regression. Mol Cell Biochem 1990; 96: 1-14.
2. Eghbali M, Czaja MJ, Zeydel M, Weiner FR, Zern MA, Seifter S, Blumenfeld 00. Collagen mRNAs in isolated adult heart cell. J Mole Cell Cardiol 1988; 20: 267-276.
3. Eghbali M, Blumenfeld 00, Seifter S, Buttrick PM, Leinwand LA, Robinson TF, Zern MA, Giambrone MA. Localization of types I, III and IV collagen mRNAs in rat heart cells by in situ hybridization. J Mole Cell Cardiol 1989; 21: 103-113.
4. Eghbali M. Cellular origin and distribution of transforming growth factor-ß1 in the normal rat myocardium. Cell Tiss Res 1989; 256: 553-558.

5. Rossi P, Karsenty G, Roberts AB, Roche NS, Sporn MB, deCrumbrugghe B. A nuclear factor 1 binding site mediates the transcriptional activation of type I collagen promoter by transforming growth factor-ß. Cell 1988; 52: 405-414.

6. Terracio L, Rubin T, Gullberg D, Balog ED, Carver W, Jyring R, Borg TK. Expression of collagen binding integrins during cardiac development and hypertrophy. Circ Res 1991; 68: 734-744.

7. Chapman D, Weber KT, Eghbali M. Regulation of fibrillar collagen types I and III and basement membrane type IV collagen gene expression in hypertrophied rat myocardium. Circ Res 1990; 67: 787-794.

8. Bhambi B, Eghbali M. Effect of norepinephrine on myocardial collagen gene expression and response of cardiac fibroblasts following norepinephrine treatment. Am J Pathol 1991; 139: 1131-1142.

9. Zeydel M, Puglia K, Eghbali M, Fant J, Seifter S, Blumenfeld OO. Heart fibroblasts of adult rats: Properties and relation to deposition of collagen. Cell Tiss Res 1991; 265: 353-359.

10. Eghbali M. Cardiac fibroblasts: Function, regulation of gene expression and phenotype modulation. Basic Res Cardiol 1992; (in press).

11. Yao J, Eghbali M. Decreased collagen gene expression and absence of fibrosis in thyroid hormone-induced myocardial hypertrophy: Response of cardiac fibroblasts to thyroid hormone in vitro. Circ Res 1992; 71: 831-839.

12. Eghbali M, Tomek R, Sukhatme V, Woods C, Bhambi B. Differential effects of transforming growth factor-ß1 and phorbol mirystate acetate on cardiac fibroblasts: Regulation of fibrillar collagen mRNAs and expression of early transcription factors. Circ Res 1991; 69: 483-490.

13. Curran T. FOS. In: Reddy EP, Skalka AM, Curran T editors. The Oncogene Handbook. Amsterdam, Elsevier Science Publishing Co Inc. 1988; 307-325.

14. Starksen NF, Simpson PC, Bishopric N, Coughlin SR, Lee WMF, Escobeno JA, Williams LT. Cardiac myocyte hypertrophy is associated with c-myc proto-oncogene expression. Proc Natl Acad Sci USA 1986; 83: 8348-8350.

15. Izumo S, Nadal-Ginard B, Mahdavi V. Proto-oncogene induction and reprogramming of cardiac gene expression produced by pressure overload. Proc Natl Acad Sci USA 1988; 85: 339-343.

16. Eghbali M, Tomek R, Woods C, Bhambi, B. Cardiac fibroblasts are predisposed to convert into myocyte phenotype: Specific effects of transforming growth factor-beta. Proc Natl Acad Sciences USA 1991; 88: 795-799.

21. Transforming growth factor ßs and cardiac development

ROSEMARY J. AKHURST, MARION DICKSON, FERGUS A. MILLAN

Introduction

Most studies of the action of growth factors on the cardiovascular system, and of the endogenous growth factor synthetic profiles of cardiac myocytes, endothelial cells and fibroblasts, have focused on tissues or cells derived from adult or, at most, neonatal material. Investigation of how these molecules might regulate early cardiogenesis is, however, fundamental to our understanding of congenital malformation of the heart, as well as being of relevance to studies of adult cardiovascular disease.

Our approach has been to undertake an analysis of those cells of the early mouse embryo which synthesise each of the three TGFß isoform RNAs. This has been compared with the distribution patterns of the encoded polypeptides. In this chapter, we will review the evidence that TGFßs are important in early murine cardiogenesis, placing our descriptive data in context with what is known about the biological activities of TGFßs on cardiac cells *in vitro*.

A summary of cardiac development

The heart primordium appears very early in development. Lateral plate mesoderm migrates anteriorly from the primitive streak, to form a crescent of cardiogenic mesoderm, anterior and ventral to the head folds of the 7.5 day post-coitum (p.c.) mouse embryo (Figure1). The

348

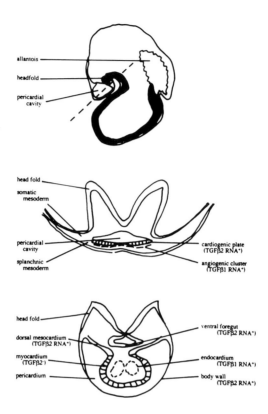

Figure 1. Early development of the mouse heart, indicating the first sites of TGFß gene expression. Top cartoon depicts sagittal section through a 8.0 day p.c.embryo; lower cartoons represent transverse sections of 7.5 and 8.0 day p.c. embryos, respectively. Dashed line in the upper cartoon denotes the plane of the transverse section shown in the lower cartoons. Blocked-in area is the definitive body of the embryo. Striped area is the future myocardium. N.B. No protein staining for TGFß1 or TGFß2 is seen at these stages.

intra-embryonic coelom appears, splitting the lateral plate mesoderm into dorsal somatic and ventral splanchnic mesoderm. Within the latter cell layer, a distinct cuboidal "epithelium" develops, known as the cardiogenic plate or pro-myocardium. Endothelial cells, the progenitors of the endocardium, appear ventral to the cardiogenic plate (Figure1)[1-3]. In urodeles, it has been shown that cardiac mesoderm is induced to form by the underlying pharyngeal endoderm, since removal of the endoderm results in a cardiac embryos [4]. Experimental evidence for cardiac mesoderm induction by foregut does not exist in mammals, though Jacobson and Sater [4] noted that some human fetuses with pharyngeal endoderm defects also have cardiac abnormalities.

Between 7.5 and 8.0 days p.c., the anterior heart-forming region undergoes a rotation through 180^0, as it is pulled in a caudo-dorsal direction along with the invaginating foregut. The myocardium thus becomes suspended from the dorsal wall of the pericardium by the splanchnopleuric mesoderm, with which it is continuous, and from which it continues to differentiate. The myocardium now engulfs the endocardium, to produce the primitive bilayered cardiac tube, the two layers being separated by a large expanse of acellular cardiac jelly (Figure 1).

Over the next 24-36 hours, the heart tube grows at an astonishing rate and, due to differential growth rates along thet ube, and the constraints of the pericardium, the tube bends and dilates. The dorsal mesocardium disintegrates along the length of the heart, such that the tube is now only continuous with the splanchnic mesoderm at its aortic and venous ends. The splanchnic mesoderm continues to differentiate into cardiomyocytes, mainly at the venous end, but also within the outflow region. Additionally, the newly formed septum transversum, caudal to the heart, contributes to the myocardium of the sinus venosus [1,5].

A major contribution to septation of the heart is made by mesenchymal cushion tissue, which also contributes to formation of heart valves. The cushion tissue arises by transformation of endothelial cells into mesenchymal cells, which occurs in the atrio-ventricular (AV) and proximal outflow regions of the heart [6], commencing at around 9.0 days p.c. in the mouse. In the chick, the process of this endothelial-mesenchymal transformation has been extensively studied by the groups of Markwald and Runyan [7,8]. Tissue recombination experiments, using a collagen gel culture system, suggest that a regional induction signal emanating from the myocardium, acts on the endocardium to initiate this event. There is both regional specificity in the ability of the myocardium to produce the inducer(s) and in the ability of the endothelium to respond.

By 10.5 days p.c. in the mouse, the AV cushions are begining to fuse, contributing to septation, and the heart already has the four-chambered appearance characteristic of the adult heart. Between 10.5 and 13.5 days p.c. septation reaches completion and, although morphogenesis continues up until birth and beyond, the second half of gestation is characterised mainly by cardiac growth, rather than morphogenesis.

Functional studies indicative of a role for TGFßs in cardiogenesis

TGFßs in cardiac mesoderm induction

The formation of mesoderm is a prerequiste for cardiac development. In Xenopus, TGF-like proteins are one of three families of molecule capable of inducing mesoderm in animal cap explants [9]. The earliest reports showed that TGF2 was a more potent inducer than TGF1,but the most potent mesoderm-inducers in the TGF superfamily are, however, the activins [9]. In the Axolotl, TGF enhances differentiation of cardiac mesoderm, suggestive of a role in cardiac mesoderm induction [10].

TGFs in induction of mesenchymal cushion tissue formation.

In a series of experiments, Runyan et al [8] have demonstratedt hat, in the chick, TGFß3 might be a component of the regional myocardial induction signal which initiates transformation of AV endocardial cells into mesenchyme. They showed that AV endothelial cells could be induced to undergo mesenchymal cell transformation, if TGFß was added to a co-culture of these cells with ventricular myocardium, but not if TGFß was omitted. Neither TGFß alone, nor ventricular myocardium alone, was capable of eliciting this response, suggesting synergy with some other soluble factor(s). They also demonstrated that blocking antibody against "generic" TGFß inhibited this transformation of endothelial cells [11].

More recently, the same group have further investigated this phenomenon using modified anti-sense oligonucleotides designed to block translation of each of four chick TGFß isoforms specifically [12]. When added to explant cultures of AV canal tissue, they demonstrated that modified anti-sense TGFß3 oligonucleotides, but not anti-sense oligonucleotides against the other three chick TGFß isoforms, blocked the transformation of endothelial cells. Interestingly, anti-sense TGFß3 did not inhibit the characteristic loss of endothelial cell-cell contactobserved prior to invasion of cardiac jelly, whereas theanti-TGFß antibody did.

TGFß isoform expression during murine embryogenesis

We have used in situ hybridisation, either to 7μm tissue sections with radioactive gene probes, or to whole mount embryo preparations with non-radioactive gene probes, to investigate which cells of the early- and mid-postimplantation embryo synthesise each of the three mammalian TGFß isoforms. Additionally, we have used two antibodies, one which recognises extracellular forms of TGFß1, and one which recognises intracellular TGFß2, to compare immunohistochemical localisation of the proteins with these sites of synthesis [13-15]. The early embryonic distributions of RNA and protein for TGFß1 and TGFß2 are highly indicative that these molecules play a role in cardiogenesis, as discussed in detail below. In contrast, TGFß3 RNA expression was not seen at high levels until relatively late in cardiac development [14,15], mainly in well established mesenchymal tissues of the heart valves. Thus, we did not examine TGFß3 protein distributions in the embryo. This has, however, been performed by Mahmood et al. [16], who saw very little immunostaining with an anti-TGBß3 antibody up to 10.5 days p.c..

TGFβ1 RNA and protein localisations during cardiac development

The only cells transcribing detectable quantities of TGFß1RNA in the heart are endothelial cells or their precursors [13]. In the presomite embryo, at 7.25-7.5 days p.c., a number of mesodermal cells, anterior and ventral to the head fold, expressed this mRNA species (Fig.2). At this stage, the TGFß1-expressing cells are indistinguishable from surrounding mesoderm cells, but by their position, and from the knowledge that 12 hours later the only TGFß1-expressing cells are endothelial, we concluded that these are probably angioblast progenitors derived from cardiac mesoderm. At this early stage, cells of the blood islands within the yolk sac also express TGFß1 RNA. Again, it is difficult to distinguish endothelial progenitors from haematopoietic progenitors. However, later in development, both cell types express TGFß1 RNA [13,17].

By 8.0 days p.c. (Figure 1), it is very clear that most endothelial cells within the primitive heart tube express TGFß1 RNA, as do endothelial cells forming the capillary networks within the head mesenchyme, and the plexus of blood vessels forming around the neural tube at 9.0 days p.c.. Endothelial cells of the major blood vessels all

352

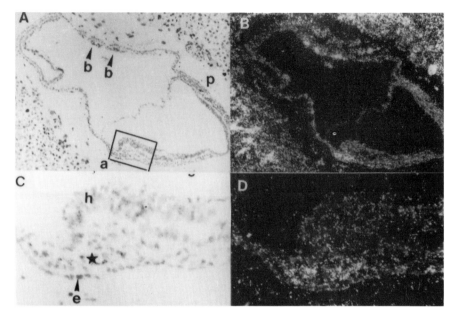

Figure 2 In situ hybridisation to sagittal section of 7.5 day p.c. embryo, showing expression of TGFß1 RNA in region of the cardiac mesoderm, and in yolk sac blood islands. A and B are bright and dark field images at low power. Boxed-in area in A, is shown at high magnification in C and D as light and dark field images, respectively. b, blood islands; a, anterior and p, posterior ends of embryo; h, headfold; e, endoderm. Star denotes the presumptive region of cardiac mesoderm. Reproduced from [13].

showed hybridisation to the TGFß1 probe at early stages of embryogenesis, but by 11.5 days p.c., this RNA is down-regulated except for regions of the vessels most proximal to the heart.

Later in development, as regionalisation of the tube is apparent, and endothelial cells start to invade the underlying cardiac jelly and transform into mesenchymal cells, endocardial TGFß1 RNA expression also become regionalised. Between 9.0 and 12.5 days p.c., most intense expression is seen in cells overlying mesenchymal cushion tissue [13]. Ventricular endothelial expression is still apparent, as determined by whole mount in situ hybridisation [15], albeit at lower levels, whereas, in the atrium expression is undetectable. Indeed, there appears to be a correlation between levels of TGFß1 RNA expression, and the quantity of underlying cardiac jelly. This endocardial TGFß1

RNA expression progressively becomes more restricted, eventually only to cells overlying heart valve leaflets. This pattern persists to one week post-partum. In the adult heart, TGFß1 RNA is no longer detectable.

The immunolocalisation of extracellular TGFß1 protein is entirely consistent with that of the RNA. The first detectable protein stain is seen at 9.0 days p.c., 36 hours after the appearance of RNA, within the cardiac jelly of the AV canal and outflow tract [13]. The delay in appearance of the protein is presumably due to the time taken for translation of sufficient quantities of protein to be detected immunohistochemically. This temporal delay between appearance of RNA and protein has been seen in another biological system examined by us [18].

The differential spatial localisation of RNA and protein is significant, suggesting a paracrine mode of action [17]. The TGFß1 protein staining of mesenchymal cushion tissue persists thoughout the remainder of development, and is seen in the valve leaflets beyond birth. Persistence of TGFß1 protein staining within the valve leaflets of the adult heart, suggests that there is residual localised endocardial transcription of this gene, but at levels undetectable by in situ hybridisation.

Interestingly, in our studies on TGFß1 expression during cardiogenesis, we noted a correlation between endothelial sites of TGFß1 RNA synthesis, and mesenchymal localisation of the extracellular matrix molecule, tenascin [13]. This correlation, in fact, also extends to many sites of TGFß1-expressing epithelia, and is pertinent, since tenascin is known to bet ranscriptionally activated by TGFß [19].

TGF1 in vasculogenesis and angiogenesis

Vascular development in vertebrates occurs by two processes "vasculogenesis", the laying down of new blood vessels in situ, and "angiogenesis", the outgrowth of new vessels from existing ones [20]. From the localisation of TGFß1 RNA to the cardiac meosderm and blood islands of the 7.5 day p.c. embryo, it would appear that TGFß1 might be involved in the neovascularisation of the embryo. The expression of TGFß1 in the major blood vessels would also suggest an involvement in angiogenesis. It should be noted that one of the first reported biological activities of exogenously applied TGFß in vivo, was induction of angiogenesis[21].

TGFß has a number of biological effects on endothelial cells in culture, all of which are relevant to the growth and morphogenesis of vascular structures. It induces the elaboration of extracellular matrix (ECM), which in turn affects endothelial cell growth [22,23]. It is also a potent inhibitor of endothelial cell growth [24,25], though its mitogenic effects depend on the exact endothelial cell type, and can be modulated by the culture conditions [23,26]. Indeed, when microvascular endothelial cells (possibly most akin to early endocardial cells) are grown in a three dimensional collagen gel culture system, TGFß has no effect on proliferative rate, but induces the formation of tube-like structures [22]. This type of response to endogenously synthesised TGFß would contribute to the neovascularisation of the embryo.

It is significant that the TGFß isoform expressed in embryonic endothelia is TGFß1 rather than TGFß2, since the former is one to two orders of magnitude more potent in eliciting both mitogenic and non-mitogenic biological effects on endothelial cells in culture [27,28]. This is due to differential expression of receptor sub-sets on endothelial cells [29].

TGFβ1 in cardiac morphogenesis

We have previously noted the differential localisation of TGFß1 RNA and protein between several morphogenetically-active epithelia and their underlying mesenchymal tissues. We attributed this to a possible paracrine function for epithelially-synthesised TGFß1, acting to modulate tissue remodelling in the underlying mesenchyme [17]. The differential localisation of TGFß1 RNA and protein in the forming endocardial cushions and, at later stages of morphogenesis, in the heart valves, suggests a similar function for TGFß1 in cardiac morphogenesis.

TGFß is well known to have major effects in modulating ECM deposition from many cell types. In general, TGF increases deposition of ECM molecules, by increasing the synthesis of ECM molecules and inhibitors of extracellular proteases, and by decreasing production of extracellular proteases [reviewed in 13]. It alters expression of cell adhesion molecules and substrate adhesion molecules [13], and can modulate the effects of other growth factors on ECM [30], thus having profound effects on cell adhesion and migration. TGFß1 may act in an autocrine fashion, modulating these parameters of the endothelial cell, especially at very early stages of cardiogenesis. Additionally, it could act on the mesenchymal cells of the cushion tissue, in a paracrine fashion.

We have previously proposed that tenascin may help mediate some of these morphogenetic effects [13], though obviously therei s a large spectrum of extracellular molecules induced by TGFß1, each of which probably has a mediating role. However, tenascin is particularly interesting as an example, since its localisation within the early embryo is tightly correlated with sites of TGFß1 synthesis. Tenascin is known to disrupt cell-substratum and cell-cell interactions, promoting cell mobility and invasive behaviour [31]. This type of cellular behaviour is essential to the transformation of endothelial cells into mesenchymal cells that occurs during cushion tissue formation, and it also important in subsequent morphogenesis of the cardiac septae and valves.

Endothelially-synthesised TGFß1 may also contribute to growth of cardiac cushion tissue in a paracrine manner, by increasing cell proliferation. Choy et al. [32] have shown that cardiac mesenchyme has a mitogenic response to TGFß1.

TGFβ2 RNA and protein localisations during early cardiac development

The first expression of TGFß2 RNA in the developing mouse embryo, seen by in situ hybridisation, is in the cuboidal cells of the crescent-shaped cardiogenic plate at 7.25-7.5 days p.c., i.e the progenitor cells of the myocardium which overly TGFß1-expressing endothelial cells (Figure 1). As the heart undergoes its very rapid and quite amazing genesis, over the next 24-48 hours, there is a gradual shift in the expression domains of TGFß2 RNA [15].

At all stages from 7.5 up to 9.5 days p.c., the splanchnic mesoderm, feeding into the myocardium, expresses high levels of TGFß2 RNA, as does the endoderm of the invaginating foregut. At 8.0 days p.c. there is obvious continuity between the splanchnic mesoderm and the differentiating myocardium, and there is a clear demarcation between the TGFß2-expressing mesoderm, and the cardiomyocytes, which have down-regulated this mRNA. There is also a caudo-rostral gradient of TGFß2 RNA from high levels within the relatively immature cells of the venous region (sinus venous and vitelline veins) to barely detectable levels in the ventricular myocardium. This gradient reflects the gradient ofmyocardial differentiation, the cells of the sinus region being relatively undifferentiated [1,5]. The outflow myocardium also expresses higher levels of TGFß2 RNA [15].

As the heart becomes regionalised, between 8.5 and 9.5 days p.c., the basic TGF ß2 expression pattern, described above, persists.

356

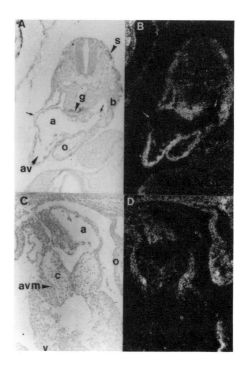

Figure 3. In situ hybridisation showing expression of TGFß2 RNA in: A,B, a transverse section through the heart of a 9.0 day p.c. heart; C, D, a sagittal section through a 10.5 day p.c. heart. A,C, are bright field images; B, D, are dark field images. g, gut endothelium; a, atrium; o, outflow tract; av, cardiac jelly of atrio-ventricular canal; c, mesenchymal cushion tissue; avm, specialised atrio-ventricular region of myocardium; v, ventricular myocardium; s, somite; b, mesoderm of body wall. Arrows denote atrial myocardium, which does not express TGF ß2 RNA. Reproduced from [14].

Superimposed on this, there is an increase in TGF ß2 RNA levels within the myocardia of the outflow tract and AV canal (Figure 3). The septum transversum, which appears between 8.5 and 9.0 days p.c. and contributes to the myocardium of the sinus venosus, is a rich source of TGFß2 RNA.

TGFß2 protein staining is first apparent at around 8.75 days p.c., at least 24 hours after the RNA is first detectable. It is striking that the protein localisation is virtually mutually exclusive with that of the RNA. TGF ß2 protein is seen only in myocardial cells, and there is a slight gradient in intensity of expression along the myocardial tube, opposite

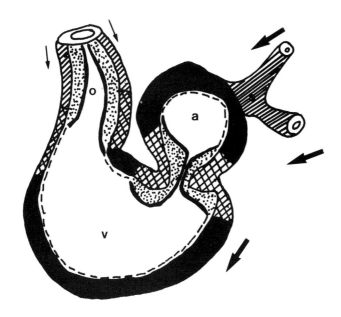

Figure 4 Expression of TGF isoforms in a 8.5-9.0 day p.c.heart. Cartoon shows schematically the localisation of TGFß1 and TGFß2 RNA and protein in the rapidly developing heart. Bold line indicates TGFß1 RNA-expressing endothelia; stippled regions indicate TGFß1 protein in cardiac jelly / mesenchyme; striped regions show areas expressing TGFß2 RNA only; cross-hatched areas show regions expressing both TGFß2 RNA and protein; blocked-in areas contain TGFß2 protein but little RNA. Arrows denote the direction of cell movement, as splanchnic mesoderm feeds into the heart. Note that at this stage, and earlier, the surrounding splanchnic mesoderm expresses large amount of TGFß2 RNA but not protein. Note also the opposing "gradients" of TGFß2 RNA and protein expression, as the splanchnic mesoderm migrates into the heart and differentiates into myocardium.

to that seen for the RNA. Ventricular myocardium, which is most highly differentiated, stains most intensely, with diminished levels towards the venous and aortic ends. Non-myocardial mesenchymal tissues, which express the highest levels of TGF ß2 RNA, do not stain for TGFß2 protein, though the septum transversum shows weak staining. Thus, the only two areas of the embryo where cells contain considerable levels of both TGFß RNA and protein, are the outflow and AV canal myocardia (summarised in Figure 4).

At 10.5 days p.c., by which time the AV cushions are large and begining to fuse, myocardial TGFß2 RNA expression is limited to the outflow tract and, at a reduced level, to a very narrow band of cells underlying the cushions in the AV canal (Figure 3). Myocardial TGFß2 RNA expression continues to diminish, until it is no longer detectable by 12.5 days p.c. Over the next four days, TGFß2 RNA appears within the cardiac mesenchyme, as does TGFß3 RNA. The function of these molecules is possibly related to morphogensis of the valves [14,32].

TGFß2 protein staining is seen ubiquitously in cardiomyocytes, increasing in intensity to 12.5 days p.c., and persisting even in the adult heart. It is noticable that, even at later stages, RNA and protein distributions are mutually exclusive. Thus, at 14.5 days p.c., mesenchymal cushion tissue contains large quantities of TGFß2 RNA, but does not stain for protein, whereas the myocardium does not have detectable levels of the RNA, but stains heavily with the antibody [15].

A role for TGFβ2 in cardiomyogenesis

The disparate distributions of TGFß2 RNA and protein in the early embryo might, at first, appear incongruous. However, this observation may be explained by either autocrine and/or paracrine action of TGFß2 protein in cardiomyocytes. Classical studies on cardiogenesis in the chick and mouse [1,5,33,34] have demonstrated the inward movement and incorporation of splanchnic mesoderm, including the derivative septum transversum, into the myocardium. It has been suggested that this continues to occur even as late as 10 days p.c. [1,5]. It is quite clear, from our studies, that all cells which have the potential to differentiate into cardiomyocytes, express TGFß2 RNA. In contrast, cardiomyocytes per se, contain TGFß2 protein, but only very low levels of the RNA, if any. Bearing in mind the temporal delay between appearance of RNA and protein which has been seen for TGFß1 (discussed above [18]), andt he very rapid nature of cell movement that occurs over this period [34], the appearance of TGFß2 protein in early cardiomyocytes could be explained as autocrine production by rapidly moving cells. This effect could also be amplified if one postulates a change in degree of translational control, as the progenitor cell moves inward and differentiates into a cardiomyocyte. TGFßs, in particular TGFß2, are known to be under translational control in other systems [35]. This type of regulation of growth factor synthesis would explain the opposing gradients of TGFß2 RNA and protein observed in the myocardial tube at around 9.0 days p.c.

An equally plausible explanation is that TGFß2 protein appears in the cardiomyocyte as a consequence of paracrine uptake of the protein, produced from cells around the pericardial cavity. Taking this consideration into account, it is notable that the ventral foregut endoderm, which is closely apposed to the forming heart tube, synthesises high levels of TGFß2 RNA.This growth factor is known to have mesoderm inducing capacity and, in urodeles, it has been shown that foregut endoderm specifically induces formation of cardiac mesoderm [4]. More recently, it has been demonstrated that cultures of presumptive cardiac mesoderm of the Axolotl, are enhanced in their ability to differentiate into cardiac muscle tissue, by exogenously-added TGFß [10]. Thus endodermally-derived TGFß2 might be involved in early induction of cardiac mesoderm tissue and, more likely, in supporting cardiomyogenesis at later stages. Indeed, synthesis of TGFß2 by the entire pericardial region of 8.0 to 9.5 day p.c.embryos, may be important in such "formative influences" [4,10].

It has generally been accepted that TGFß is an inhibitor of myogenesis, since early studies on skeletal myoblasts grown in culture showed that this growth factor prevents differentiation to skeletal myotubes [37-39]. This, of course, could not be reconciled with our data, unless one proposed that TGFß2 had a negative effect, to prevent terminal cardiomyocyte differentiation too soon in development. However, over the past two years there has been mounting evidence that this growth factor is in fact an inducer of myogenesis. In addition to the observations made with Axolotl pre-cardiac mesoderm cultures [10], Eghbali et al. [40], demonstrated that adult cardiac mesenchyme cells are converted into cardiomyocyte-like cells by TGFß1. Parker et al. [41] showed that TGFß1, added to cultures of neonatal cardiomyocytes, shifted the profile of contractile protein gene expression towards a fetal phenotype, rather than preventing their differentiation. Finally, and more recently, Zentrella and Massague [42] have shown that skeletal myoblasts can be induced to differentiate by TGFß1. They demonstrated that the exact response of myoblasts, whether differentiation-inhibitory or -stimulatory, depends on culture conditions, particularly prescence of mitogens and extent of cell contact. Only actively proliferating myoblasts are induced to differentiate by TGFß1, and this is a consequence of resultant withdrawal from the cell cycle, in combination with down-regulation of the inhibitor of differentiation, Id. Thus, it appears from the localisations of TGFß2 RNA and protein in early embryo, that this growth factor might be an inducer of cardiomyocyte differentiation in this rapidly proliferating embryonic tissue, whether acting via autocrine and/or paracrine mechanisms.

The role of TGFßs in mesenchymal transformation of endocardial cells

As discussed in the Introduction, experiments on chick heart explants, have suggested that TGFßs (specifically TGFß3) are important in the induction of transformation of endothelial cells to mesenchymal cells within the AV canal. There are a number of observations which need to be reconciled between our own data on the mouse [13-15] and that on the chick [11,12].

Potts and Runyan [11] showed that TGFß added to AV endothelium, would synergise with ventricular myocardium to induce the transformation of the AV cells. However, we have demonstrated that mouse AV canal endothelium is already a rich source of TGFß1. This could be reconciled if a function of the AV myocardium is to maintain high levels of TGFß1 expression within the overlying endocardium, and that this expression is essential to some aspect of the transformation event. Alternatively, there may be threshold effects, such that the quantity of TGFß1,produced endogenously by the endothelium, is not sufficient to initiate transformation. Additional, myocardially-derived TGFß may be needed [11].

An excellent candidate for this putative myocardial TGFß, in the mouse, is TGFß2. Very high levels of this RNA are seen in the myocardium of both the outflow tract and the AV canal. Maximal expression is seen just prior to the initiation of mesenchymal transformation and subsequently falls to barely detectable levels by 11.5 days p.c., when transformation is complete. TGFß2 protein was not, however, localised to cushion tissue or AV endothelium until 11.5 days p.c., by which time transformation is virtually complete. Even then, protein expression is at barely detectable levels, despite localisation of the RNA in this tissue. One might have expected to have seen early cardiac jelly/endothelial localisation of the protein, if TGFß2 did have an inductive role. However, TGFß2 exists in several conformational states, and we do not know precisely which one was recognised by the antibody used in our studies (possibly latent TGFß2?).

A major difference between the data of Runyan's group and our own, is the conclusion that different TGFß isoforms must be implicated in chick heart development as compared to that of the mouse. We have suggested that TGFß2 and 1 could be involved in induction and morphogenesis of cushion tissue. In contrast, Runyan implicates TGFß3 as directly involved in this process. Furthermore, preliminary data would suggest that the TGFß expression pattern in the mouse heart differs from that in the chick [8].

Although it is tempting to speculate that TGFß2 is part of the regional induction signal required for endothelial transformation, an alternative explanation for the AV localisation of TGFß2 RNA, would be that this is related to control of cardiomyocyte differentiation. The AV myocardium, in particular, has very distinct differentiative properties from the rest of the myocardium, related to its specialised function in the primitive conduction system of the heart [43]. The cells in this region have been described as immature in character [44]. It should be borne in mind, however, that the alternate possibilities of TGFß2 being involved in regulation of differentiation of the specialised AV cardiomyocytes, or in inductive interactions on the overlying AV endocardium, are not mutually exclusive.

The AV canal is an interesting region of the embryo. Several key developmental genes are expressed in this critical region of the heart at the time of cushion tissue formation. These include sother TGFß-related molecules, such as BMP2 [45] and BMP4 [46], other growth factors, such as bFGF [47], HOX genes [48], the retinoid binding protein genes, RAR, CRBP and CRABP [49], to name a few. These classes of molecules have been functionally implicated as being of central importance in early inductive and morphogenetic interactions which result in mesoderm formation and the establishment of body plan [9]. It would therefore be wrong to dismiss the possibilty that TGFß2 plays a role in inductive interactions in the AV canal.

Conclusions

By examining the temporal and spatial patterns of expression of the TGFß genes and their encoded polypeptides, during murine cardiogenesis, and comparing these with the documented bio-activities of these growth factors on cells in culture, we have drawn several conclusions as to their putative endogenous functions in this developing system. TGFß1 is probably involved in the initial neo-vascularisation of the embryo, acting in an autocrine fashion on early endothelial cells. Later, the primary function of this molecule probably shifts to that of

362

modulation of morphogenesis of the valves and septae, acting in both paracrine and autocrine modes. TGFß2 might play an important role in induction and maintainance of cardiomyogenesis, and/or be involved in inductive interactions between myocardium and endocardium, which result in mesenchymal cushion tissue formation. These postulates now need to be tested by functional assay in the mouse.

Acknowledgements

Work in the authors' laboratory has been supported by the MRC, Wellcome Trust and CRC.

References

1. Viragh S, Challice CE. Origin and differentiation of cardiac muscle cells in the mouse. J Ultrasructure Research 1973; 42: 1-24.
2. Kaufman MH, Navaratnam V. Early differentiation of the heart in mouse embryos. J Anat 1981; 2: 235-24.
3. DeRiuter, MC, Poelmann RE, VanderPlas-de Vries I, Mentink MMT, Gittenberger-de Groot AC. The development of the myocardium and endocardium in mouse embryos: Fusion of two heart tubes ? Anat Embryol 1992; 185: 461-473.
4. Jacobson AG, Sater A.K. Features of embryonic induction. Development 1988; 104: 341-359.
5. Challice CE, Viragh S. The architectural development of the early mammalian heart. Tissue Cell Res 1973; 3: 447-462.
6. Bernanke DH, Markwald RR. Migratory behaviour of cardiac cushion tissue cells in a collagen lattice system. Dev Biol 1982; 91: 235-245.
7. Mjaatvedt CH, Markwald RR. Induction of an epithelial-mesenchymal transition by an in vivo adheron-like complex. Dev Biol 1989; 136: 118-128.
8. Runyan RB, Potts JD, Weeks DL. TGFß-3-mediated tissue interaction during embryonic heart development. 1992; Mol Reprod Devel 1992; 32: 152-159.
9. Melton DA. Pattern formation during animal development.Science 1991; 252: 234-241.

10. Muslin AJ, Williams LT. Well-defined growth factors promote cardiac development in axolotl mesodermal explants. Development 1991; 112: 1095-110.

11. Potts JD, Runyan RB. Epithelial-mesenchymal cell transformation in the embryonic heart can be mediated, in part,by transforming growth factor beta. Dev Biol 1989; 134: 392-401.

12. Potts JD, Dagle JM, Walder JA, Weeks DL, Runyan RB. Epithelial-mesenchymal transformation of embryonic cardiac endothelial cells is inhibited by a modified antisense to transforming growth factor ß3. Proc Natl Acad Sci. USA 1991; 88: 1516.

13. TGF beta in murine morphogenetic processes: the early embryo and cardiogenesis. Development 108:645-656, 1990.

14. Millan FA, Kondaiah P, Denhez F, Akhurst RJ. Embryonic gene expression patterns of TGF betas 1, 2 and 3 suggest different developmental functions in vivo. Development 1991; 111: 131-144.

15. Dickson M, Slager HG, Duffie E, Akhurst RJ. TGFß2 RNA and protein localisations in the early embryo suggest a role in cardiac development and myogenesis. 1992, submitted.

16. Mahmood R, Flanders KC, Morriss-Kay, G. Interactions between retinoids and TGFßs in mouse morphogenesis. Development115: 67-74, 1992.

17. Lehnert SA, Akhurst RJ. Embryonic expression pattern of TGF beta type-1 RNA suggests both paracrine and autocrine mechanisms of action. Development 1988; 104: 263-273.

18. Fowlis DJ, Flanders K, Duffie E, Balmain A, Akhurst RJ. Discordant TGFß1 RNA and protein localisations during chemical carcinogenesis of the skin. Cell Growth Diff 1992; 3: 81-91.

19. Pearson CA, Pearson D, Shibahara S, Hofsteenge J. Tenascin: cDNA cloning and induction by TGF-beta. EMBO J 1988; 7: 2977-2982.

20. Poole TJ, Coffin JD. Vasculogenesis and angiogenesis: Two distinct morphogenetic mechanisms establish embryonic vascular pattern. J Exp Zool 1989; 251: 224-231.

21. Roberts AB, Sporn MB, Assoian RK et al. Transforming growth factor type beta: rapid induction of fibrosis and angiogenesis in vivo and stimulation of collagen formation in vitro. Proc Natl Acad Sci USA 1986; 83: 4167-4171.

22. Madri, J.A., Pratt BM, Tucker AM. Phenotypic modulation of endothelial cells by transforming growth factor-beta depends upon the composition and organization of the extracellular matrix. J Cell Biol 1988; 106: 1375-1384.

23. Madri JA, Bell L, Merwin JR. Modulation of vascular cell behaviour by transforming growth factors . Mol Reprod Devel 1992; 32: 121-126.

24. Takehara K, LeRoy EC, Grotendorst GR. TGF-beta inhibition of endothelial cell proliferation: alteration of EGF binding and EGF-induced growth-regulatory (competence) gene expression. Cell 1987; 49: 415-422.

25. Heimark RL, Twardzik DR, Schwartz SM. Inhibition of endothelial regeneration by type-beta transforming growth factor from platelets. Science 1986; 233: 1078-1080.

26. Baird A, Durkin T. Inhibition of endothelial cell proliferation by beta-type transforming growth factor: interactions with acidic and basic fibroblast growth factors. Biochem Biophys Res Comm 1986; 138: 476-482.

27. Jennings JC, Mohan S, Linkhart TA, Widstrom R, Baylink DJ. Comparison of the biological actions of TGF beta-1 and TGF beta-2: differential activity in endothelial cells. J Cell Physiol 1988; 137: 167-172.

28. Merwin JR, Newman W, Beal D, Tucker A, Madri JA. Vascular cells respond differentially to transforming growth factors-beta 1 and beta 2. Am J Pathol 1991; 138: 37-51.

29. Cheifetz S, Hernandez H, Laiho M, ten Dijke P, Iwata KK, Massague J. Distinct transforming growth factor-ß (TGF-ß) receptor subsets as determinants of cellular responsiveness to three TGF-ß isoforms. J Biol Chem 1990; 265: 20533-20538.

30. Pepper MS, Belin D, Montesano R, Orci L, Vassalli J-D. Transforming growth factor-beta 1 modulates basic fibroblast growth factor-induced proteolytic and angiogenic properties of endothelial cells. J Cell Biol 1990; 111: 743-755.

31. Chiquet-Ehrismann R, Kalla P, Pearsor CA. Participation of tenascin and transforming growth factor beta in reciprocal epithelial-mesenchymal interactions of MCF7 cells and fibroblasts. Cancer Res 1989; 49: 4322-4325.

32. Choy M, Armstrong MT, Armstrong PB. Regulation of proliferation of embryonic heart mesenchyme: Role of transforming growth factor beta 1 and the interstitial matrix. Developmental Biology 1990; 141:421-425.

33. DeHaan RL. Morphogenesis of the vertebrate heart. In: Organogenesis, edited by DeHaan RL. USA: Holt, Rinehart and Wilson 1965, p. 377-419.

34. Rosenquist GC, DeHaan RL. Migration of precardiac cells in the chick: A radioautographic study. Carnegie Inst Contr EmbryoL 1966; 38: 111-121.

35. Glick AB, Flanders KC, Danielpour D, Yuspa SH, Sporn MB. Retinoic acid induces transforming growth factor-beta 2 in cultured keratinocytes and mouse epidermis. Cell Regulation 1989; 1: 87-97.

37. Olson EN, Sternberg E, Hu JS, Spizz G, Wilcox C. Regulation of myogenic differentiation by type beta transforming growth factor. J Cell Biol 1986; 103: 1799-1805.

38. Massague J, Cheifetz S, Endo T, Nadal-Ginard B. Type beta transforming growth factor is an inhibitor of myogenic differentiation. Proc Natl Acad Sci USA 1986; 83: 8206-8210.

39. Florini JR, Roberts AB, Ewton DZ, Falen SL, Flanders KC, Sporn MB. Transforming growth factor-beta. A very potent inhibitor of myoblast differentiation, identical to the differentiation inhibitor secreted by Buffalo rat liver cells. J. Biol. Chem. 261: 16509-16513.

40. Eghbali M, Tomek ?, Woods C, Bhambi B. Cardiac fibroblasts are predisposed to convert into myocyte phenotype: Specific effects of transforming growth factor ß. Proc Natl Acad Sci USA 1991; 88: 795-799.

41. Parker TG, Chow K-L, Schwartz RJ, Schneider MD. Differential regulation of skeletal α-actin transcription in cardiac muscle by two fibroblast growth factors. Proc Natl Acad Sci USA 1991; 87: 7066-7070.

42. Zentrella A, Massague J. Transforming growth factor ß induces myoblast differentiation in the presence of mitogens. Proc Natl Acad Sci USA 1992; 89: 5176-5180.

43. Viragh S, Challice CE. The development of the conduction system of the heart. I. The first embryonic A-V conduction pathway. Dev Biol 1977; 56: 382-396.

44. Viragh S, Challice CE. The development of the conduction system of the mouse embryo heart. II. Histogenesis of the atrioventricular node and bundle. Dev Biol 56: 397-411.

45. Lyons KM, Pelton RW, Hogan BL. Organogenesis and pattern formation in the mouse: RNA distribution patterns suggest a role for Bone Morphogenetic Protein-2A (BMP2A). Development 1990; 109: 833-844.

46. Jones CM, Lyons KM, Hogan BLM. Involvement of Bone Morphogenesis Factor-4 (BMP-4) and Vgr1 in morphogenesis and neurogenesis in the mouse. Development 1991; 111: 531-542.

47. Parlow MH, Bolender DL, Kokan-Moore NP, Lough J. Localisation of bFGF-like proteins as punctate inclusions in the preseptation myocardium of the chicken embryo. Dev Biol 1991; 146:139-147.

48. Robert B, Sassoon D, Jacq B, Gehring W, Buckingham M. Hox-7, a mouse homeobox gene with a novel pattern of expression during embryogenesis. EMBO J 1989; 8: 91-100.

49. Dolle P, Ruberte E, Leroy P, Morriss-Kay G, Chambon P. Retinoic acid receptors and cellular retinoid binding proteins I: A systematic study of their differential pattern of transcription during mouse organogenesis. Development 1990; 110: 1133-1152.

Index

Acidic fibroblast growth factor 19; 20
    angiogenesis 120
    cardiac myocytes 23-24
    content in heart 23
    immunocytochemistry 22
    skeletal myogenesis 20
Acromegaly 108
Actin 79-88; 106
    cytoskeletal 83
    fibroblasts 342
    response element 81
    skeletal promoter 80-86
Alpha adrenergic stimulation 290
    contractile protein switching 324
    growth factor activity 321
Angiogenesis 10; 121; 149-160
    coronary collaterals 119
    embryonic 150
    epithelial growth factor 156
    fibroblast growth factors 149;
        153-155
    growth factors 140
    restenosis 262-263
    transforming growth factor 155-
        156; 353-354
    tumor angiogenesis factor 151
Angiogenin 158
Angioplasty 175; 227
    platelet derived growth factor 261
Angiotensin II
    as growth promoter 290
Angiotensin converting enzyme
inhibitor 240
Angiotropin 158
Arteriosclerosis 170
Atherectomy 227
Atherogenesis 169
    growth factors 177
    platelet derived growth factor 180

Atherosclerosis 108
    angioplasty 175
    hypercholesterolemia 175
    lipoproteins 174
    macrophage colony stimulating
        factor 173
    oxygen free radicals 174
    platelet derived growth factor 169;
        277
    thrombocytopaenia 181
    transforming growth factor beta
        197
    transplantation 176
Atrial natriuretic factor 80
Autoimmune diseases 12
Basic fibroblast growth factor 19-20;
    55
    actin promoter 82
    bioassay 65-66
    cardiac injury 70
    cardiac myocytes 23-24
    content in heart 23
    human myocytes 111
    immunocytochemistry 22
    isoforms 66
    localisation 63; 66-69
    nucleus 69
    receptors 232
    regenerative potential 63
    skeletal myogenesis 20
    smooth muscle cell proliferation
        227
    thyroid hormone 58
    vascular injury 228
Beta adrenergic stimulation
    myocyte hypertrophy 328
Calmodulin 216
Carcinoid heart disease 311
    fibroblasts in plaques 315
Cardiac hypertrophy 36-37; 108

Cardiac injury 70
Cardiac morphogenesis
    transforming growth factor beta
        354
Cardiac myocytes 17
    adrenergic stimulation 322-324
    atrial myocytes 18
    basic fibroblast rowth factor 55-
        56; 67-69
    collagen synthesis 33
    human 105-114
    hypertrophy and hyperplasia 18
    injury and basic fibroblast growth
        factor 70
    laminin synthesis 33
    mitosis 17
Cardiogenesis
    transforming growth factor beta
        350
Cardiomyopathy 109
Cardioprotection 47; 249
    transforming growth factor
        beta.250-258
Catecholamine 321
Cell adhesion 59
Chicken chorioallantoic membrane
    152
Chronic inflammatory conditions 11
Collagen 25
    cardiac localisation 31-32
    fibroblasts 33; 337-338
Coronary artery by-pass grafting 176
Coronary collaterals 119-140
    fibroblast growth factors 126-130
    interleukin-1 134; 136
    porcine model 122
    transforming growth factor 130
    tumor necrosis factor 134
Coronary heart disease 170
    plaque formation 171
Creatine kinase 82
Cuff injury 279
Development
    atrio ventricular canal 356
    cardiac primordium 347
    cardiogenic plate 349

transforming growth factor beta
    347-362
Diabetes 108
    diabetic retinopathy 120
Dystrophin 82
Embryogenesis 130
    cardiac jelly 352
    transforming growth factor beta
        351
Endothelial cells 119
Epidermal growth factor 112
    atherosclerosis 173
Epithelial growth factor 156
    signal transduction 213
Extra-cellular matrix 31-43
    angiogenesis 35-36
    cardiac hypertrophy 36-37
    fibroblasts 337
    myocardial infarction 35
    ontogenic development 33
Fetal cardiac genes 91
Fibroblast growth factors
    vascular remodelling 296
Fibroblasts 323
    transforming growth factor beta
        337-343
Fibronectin 25
    cardiac localisation 31-32
    isoforms during development 34
Fibrosis 39
Gap junctions 63
    basic fibroblast growth factor 71
Growth hormone 108
Hepatocyte growth factor 11
Homeodomain protein 91
Hydrogen peroxide 59
Hyperlipidemia 172
Hypertension 108
    smooth muscle cell proliferation
        240
    transforming growth factor beta
        196
    vascular remodelling 287
Hypertrophy 71; 79
    alpha adrenergic stimulation 321
    beta adrenergic stimulation 328

Insulin 107; 110
Insulin-like growth factor 56; 107-108
    coronary collaterals 131
    mRNA's 108
    vascular remodelling 295
Interleukin 47-48
    atherosclerosis 173
    coronary collaterals 134; 136
    macrophages 136
    monocytes 136
    signal tramnsduction 208
Laminin 31
Lipoproteins
    atherosclerosis 174
Mesenchymal cells 107
Myocardial infarction 46; 71
Myocardial ischemia 50; 59; 123
    mitotic cell activity 123
    plasminogen activator 139
    reperfusion injury 59; 253-258
    transforming growth factor beta
        120; 130; 249
Myocyte specific enhancer factor
(MEF2) 88-89
Myo D 83; 87
Myogenin 82; 87
Myosin heavy chain 79; 106
    alpha adrenergic stimulation 325
Myosin light chain 82
Nerve growth factor
    vascular remodelling 298
Neuroectodermal cells 107
Nitric oxide 48
    endothelial preservation 253
Oxidative stress 59
Phosphoinositol pathway
    signal transduction 212; 290
    turnover 214
Plasminogen activator 139
    inhibitor 139
Platelet derived growth factor 112
    angiogenesis 157
    angioplasty 261; 264-267
    antagonists of hyperplasia 181
    atherosclerosis 178-179
    endothelial cell growth factor 158

receptor 179; 275
receptor and vascular injury 275-
    282
receptor tyrosine kinase 276
restenosis 269
transforming growth factor 191
vascular remodelling 294
vascular smooth muscle cells 194

Polymorphonuclear neutrophil 251-
    252
    endothelial cell adherence 256
Prostacyclin 172
Proto-oncogenes 38; 83-85; 89
    fibroblasts 341
    signal transduction 290
    vascular smoooth muscle 211;
        217; 219
Receptors 4
    autophosphorylation 6
    interleukin 4
    serine / threonine kinase 4
    tyrosine kinase 4
Rous sarcoma virus 66
Saporin
    basic fibroblast growth factor 231-
        239
Sarcoplasmic reticulum 79
Serum response element 77
Signal transduction pathways 4; 77-
        79; 207-208
    angiotensin II 208
    downstream signalling 9
    endothelin 208
    platelet-derived growth factor 8;
        276
    protein kinase C 326-327
    serotonin 208
    vascular smooth muscle cells 207
Skeletal myoblasts 65; 108
    epidermal growth factor 113
Smooth muscle cells
    fibroblast growth factor receptors
        232-236
    pulmonary vascular 237
Ternary complex factor 89

Thrombospondin 194
Thyroid hormone 58; 71
    fibroblasts 340
    hypertrophy 325
Transcriptional control 87
Transforming growth factor beta 19;
    45
    actin 78
    atherosclerosis 197
    binding protein 46
    carcinoid heart disease 311-317
    cardiac hypertrophy 38
    cardiac myocytes 24-25
    cardioprotection 25
    collagen 341
    contractile proteins 22
    extracellular matrix 34-35
    fibroblasts 337-344
    hemodynamic overload 22; 25; 79
    hypertension 196; 292
    immunocytochemistry 20-21; 45
    interleukins 48
    isoforms 45; 155
    latent 46; 155
    latent binding protein 314
    mRNA in heart 21
    myocardial infarction 46
    myocardial ischemia 120; 249
    nitric oxide 49
    receptors 155
    serum response element and actin
        85
Transgenic animals 92
Troponin T 82
Tumor necrosis factor 47; 121
    angiogenesis 159
    carcinoid 311-317
    cardioprotection 250
    coronary collaterals 134
Tumors 11
    vascularization 120
Vascular endothelial growth factor
    120; 125-126; 157-158
Vascular injury 228
    baloon injury 235; 279-280
    endothelial loss 236

platelet derived growth factor
    receptor 275
    restenosis 241
Vascular remodelling 287-301
    extracellular matrix 287
    hypertension 287
    platelet derived growth factor 294
    transforming growth factor beta
        292
Vascular smooth muscle cells
    cell cycle efects 192
    extra cellular matrix 193
    growth promoters 290
    hypertension 288
    phosphoinositol pathways 214
    proliferation 191
    response element 218
    signal transduction 207
    transforming growth factor beta
        190
Vasculogenesis 353
Wound healing 56; 130
Xenopus 10